T5-CVF-713

Nurse's Clinical Guide

MATERNITY CARE

Second Edition

Nurse's Clinical Guide

MATERNITY CARE

Second Edition

Pennie Sessler Branden, RN, MSN, CNM
Associate Editor
Journal of Nurse-Midwifery
Cheshire, Conn.

Springhouse Corporation
Springhouse, Pennsylvania

STAFF

Senior Publisher
Matthew Cahill

Editorial Director
Donna O. Carpenter

Clinical Director
Judith Schilling McCann, RN, MSN

Art Director
John Hubbard

Managing Editor
David Moreau

Acquisitions Editor
Patricia A. Fischer, RN, BSN

Associate Acquisitions Editor
Louise Quinn

Clinical Editors
Collette Bishop Hendler, RN, CCRN
Lori Musolf Neri, RN, MSN

Senior Editor
Karen Diamond

Copy Editors
Cynthia C. Breuninger (manager),
Karen C. Comerford, Brenna H.
Mayer, Pamela Wingrod

Designers
Arlene Putterman (associate art director), Stephanie Peters, Jeff Sklarow,
STELLARViSIONs

Manufacturing
Deborah Meiris (director), Patricia K.
Dorshaw (manager), Otto Mezei

Production Coordinator
Stephen Hungerford, Jr.

Editorial Assistants
Beverly Lane, Mary Madden

Printed in the United States of America.

NCGMC2-010298

Ⓡ A member of the Reed Elsevier plc group

Library of Congress Cataloging-in-Publication Data

Branden, Pennie Sessler.
  Maternity care / Pennie Sessler Branden.—2nd ed.
      p. cm.—(Nurse's clinical guide)
  Rev. ed. of: Maternity care / [edited by] Aileen MacLaren. © 1992. Includes bibliographical references and index.
      1. Maternity nursing—Handbooks, manuals, etc. I. Title. II. Series
  [DNLM: 1. Obstetrical Nursing—handbooks. WY 39 B817m 1998]
RG951.N867   1998
610.73'67—DC21
DNLM/DLC   97-42636
ISBN 0-87434-883-8 (alk. paper)   CIP

CONTENTS

APPENDICES

CONTRIBUTORS AND REVIEWERS

CLINICAL CONSULTANT

Barbara Decker, RN, EdD, CNM, FaCNM
Clinical Associate Professor; Institute of Midwifery, Women, and
Health; Philadelphia College of Textiles and Science
Former Director, Nurse Mid-Wifery Program, Yale School of Nursing,
New Haven, Conn.

CONTRIBUTORS

Bernadine Adams, RN, BSN, MN
Assistant Professor, School of Nursing, Northeast Louisiana University,
Monroe

Cynthia Armstrong, RN,C, MSN
Perinatal Clinical Nurse Specialist, School of Nursing, University of
Pennsylvania, Philadelphia

Constance A. Bobik, RN, MSN
Assistant Professor, Brevard Community College, Cocoa, Fla.

Pennie Sessler Branden, RN, MSN, CNM
Associate Editor, Journal of Nurse-Midwifery, Cheshire, Conn.

Ann Brodsky, MS, RD
Nutritionist, Women's Health Practice, Champaign, Ill.

Susan M. Cohen, RN, DSN
Associate Professor, School of Nursing, University of Texas Health
Science Center at Houston

Leonard V. Crowley, MD
Professor, Century College, St. Paul, MN; Clinical Assistant Professor,
University of Minnesota Medical School, Minneapolis

Debra C. Davis, RN, DSN
Associate Dean and Director of Graduate Studies, University of South
Alabama, Mobile

Deborah S. Davison, MSN, CRNP
Assistant Professor, La Roche College, Pittsburgh

viii

Catherine Dearman, RN, PhD
Associate Professor, School of Nursing, Troy State University, Montgomery, Ala.

Peggy J. Drapo, RN, PhD
Professor, College of Nursing, Texas Woman's University, Denton

JoNell Efantis, RN, MSN, ARNP
Adjunct Instructor, School of Medicine, University of Miami, Fla.

Joan Engebretson, RN, MS, DrPH
Associate Professor, University of Texas Health Science Center at Houston

Harriett W. Ferguson, RN,C, EdD
Associate Professor, Department of Nursing, Temple University, Philadelphia

Florencetta Gibson, RN, MSN, MEd
Clinical Nurse Specialist, Associate Professor, School of Nursing, Northeast Louisiana University, Monroe

Bonnie Mauger Graff, RN, MSN, CRNP
Clinical Faculty-Clinical Research, School of Nursing, University of Pennsylvania, Philadelphia

Annette Gupton, RN, MN, PhD
Associate Professor, School of Nursing, University of Manitoba, Winnipeg, Canada

Kathleen Convery Hanold, RN, MS
Director, Women and Infant Services, Barnes Hospital, Washington University Medical Center, St. Louis

Andrea O. Hollingsworth, RN, PhD
Director, Undergraduate Program, College of Nursing, Villanova (Pa.) University

Lynne Hutnik, RN,C, MSN, MHA
Nursing Program Director— Maternal-Child Health, Allegheny University Hospital, Elkins Park, Pa.

Christabel A. Kaitell, RN, BN, MPH, SCM
Assistant Professor, School of Nursing, Faculty of Health Sciences,
University of Ottawa, Ontario, Canada

Virginia H. Kemp, RN, PhD
Professor and Associate Dean, Graduate Programs and Research,
School of Nursing, Medical College of Georgia, Augusta

Carole Kenner, RN,C, DNS, FAAN
Professor and Department Head, College of Nursing and Health,
University of Cincinnati

Harriett Linenberger, RN,C, ACCE-R, MSN
Clinical Instructor, School of Nursing, University of Texas Health
Science Center at Houston

Aileen MacLaren, CNM, MSN, PhD(c)
Acting Assistant Professor, Director of Nurse-Midwifery Educational
Program, University of Washington, Seattle

Paula C. Maisano, RN, MS
Nursing Education Coordinator, Saint Francis Hospital, Tulsa, Okla.

Connie Marshall, RN, MSN
Perinatal Clinical Specialist, Vice President, Conmar Publishing, Inc.,
Citrus Heights, Calif.

Sylvia A. McSkimming, RN, PhD
Director of Nursing—Quality and Research, St. Vincent Hospital and
Medical Center, Portland, Ore.

Patricia Anne Mynaugh, RN, PhD
Assistant Professor, College of Nursing, Villanova (Pa.) University

Tommie P. Nelms, RN, PhD
Assistant Professor, School of Nursing, Georgia State University,
Atlanta

Charlotte R. Patrick, RN, MS, MEd
Associate Clinical Professor Emerita, College of Nursing, Texas
Woman's University, Denton

Constance Sinclair, RN, MSN, CNM
Faculty, Valley Medical Center, University of California Medical
School at San Francisco

Gale Robinson Smith, RN, PhD, CS
Assistant Professor, College of Nursing, Villanova (Pa.) University

Jan Weingrad Smith, CNM, MS, MPH
Clinical Nurse Specialist, Maternal-Child Health, Lawrence Hospital,
Bronxville, N.Y.

Donna J. van Lier, CNM, PhD
Nurse-Midwife, Private Practice, Atlanta OB/GYN Associates

Sarah Elizabeth Whitaker, RN,C, MSN, DNSc(c)
Lecturer, College of Nursing and Health Sciences, University of Texas
at El Paso

Janet K. Williams, RN, PhD, CPNP, CGC
Associate Professor, College of Nursing, University of Iowa, Iowa City

REVIEWERS

Lynne Hutnik, RN,C, MSN, MHA
Nursing Program Director— Maternal-Child Health
Allegheny University Hospital
Elkins Park, Pa.

Rita Tobler, RN, MSN
Professor Emeritus
Northern Kentucky University
Highland Heights

As the 20th century draws to a close, nursing once again finds its role changing. Clinical practice is adapting rapidly to keep up with new treatments, new technologies, and newly identified diseases. Major changes in health care delivery systems are also occurring with the increase of health maintenance organizations and other managed care organizations. This constant flux greatly affects health care access and practice patterns. The health care team is increasingly challenged to continue to provide high quality patient care and education.

Maternity nurses have a unique role in today's health care system: They are among the few health care professionals who provide holistic care for the mother and her family. They serve as caregivers, educators, and advocates for their maternity patients and families.

The first edition of this guide was developed to give practicing and student maternity nurses a concise pocket guide to use in clinical practice. The *Nurse's Clinical Guide to Maternity Care*, Second Edition, is updated to provide comprehensive information reflecting the current changes in maternity care. The nursing process is used to organize the entire text, with an eye to the ever-increasing role nurses are assuming in home care. This increased focus on home care is in direct response to shorter hospital stays and the efforts of the health care team to try to meet more of the maternity patient's needs.

This pocket reference guide is organized into four units that provide the clinical maternity nurse with in-depth information as well as easy-to-use charts. Unit I is an overview of maternity and obstetric care, including components of comprehensive maternity care as well as reproductive anatomy and physiology. Units II, III, and IV map out care for the patient's pregnancy and postpartal periods. Each unit is structured with a comprehensive overview of physiologic and psychological changes; fetal or neonatal development and assessments; the normal antepartal, intrapartal, and postpartal periods; the high-risk patient in each period; and possible complications during each period. Maternal home care is discussed in Unit IV as it applies to the postpartal and long-term health of the mother and her family.

This book provides a current, accurate, and quick reference for nurses who strive to give optimal, comprehensive health care to patients and their families throughout the maternity cycle. In a nurse's journey to update her knowledge, this guide will serve as a clinical reference guide as well as an adjunct to books dedicated solely to obstetric care. Armed with this information, maternity nurses will be able to enter the 21st century as indispensable members of the health care team.

Pennie Sessler Branden, RN, MSN, CNM

OVERVIEW OF MATERNITY CARE

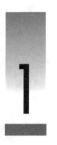

COMPONENTS OF COMPREHENSIVE MATERNITY CARE

Maternity nursing involves many of the concerns for which today's family seeks care, including women's health care, maternity care, birth options, contraception, and neonatal care. For the childbearing family, nursing care and health care delivery have changed significantly in the past few decades.

Before obstetric nursing was a specialty, nurses working in obstetrics usually took care of mothers during delivery as labor room nurses or after delivery as postpartal nurses. They were supported by nurses who cared for neonates in the nursery. Each of these nurses had a specific role.

Today's maternity nurse is more of a generalist, taking care of the pregnant woman from labor to delivery and then caring for the woman and neonate until discharge. The maternity nurse typically works in a labor-delivery-recovery-postpartal (LDRP) unit which has replaced the separate labor, delivery, and postpartal units.

In order to give the best possible care, the maternity nurse must understand and teach the woman and her family about reproductive anatomy and physiology, preconception issues, conception, and fetal development in a comprehensive way. The nurse must also answer questions and evaluate how these interventions affect the outcome of pregnancy and delivery. The nursing process is an excellent tool with which to accomplish these goals.

The nursing process is a simple, highly versatile tool that helps map out the nurse's caring relationship with the woman. A system for making nursing decisions, it includes assessment, nursing diagnosis, planning, implementation, and evaluation. Regardless of the setting, the nursing process guides the nurse in providing quality care to the childbearing family. By following this process and supporting it with thorough documentation, the nurse can develop effective strategies to respond to current and potential needs and problems while promoting family health.

Family health, or a family's ability to function constructively, depends on several factors. Cultural patterns, religious influences, socioeconomic status, and stage of family development shape each member's roles and functions within the family. These factors also influence how the family perceives and copes with everyday problems and crisis situations.

The nurse promotes the health of the childbearing family by providing family-centered nursing care. This approach includes assessing each family member's health needs, identifying health deficiencies and strengths, and intervening with education and counseling to improve family health. The nurse also involves the woman and her partner in health care decision making during preconception and throughout pregnancy and childbirth.

NURSE-PATIENT COMMUNICATION

Effective communication must occur at the appropriate stages of the nursing process for maternity nursing care to benefit the patient. Communication, teaching, and motivation are critical components of an effective nurse-patient relationship. (See *Components of an effective nurse-patient relationship*, page 4.)

By using effective communication, teaching, and motivation, the nurse—with the patient's input—can establish appropriate patient goals for each situation. The typical pregnant woman requires goals that address the following issues:

- acquiring knowledge about and planning for pregnancy, childbirth, and parenthood
- adapting sexual patterns to pregnancy
- adapting community activities to pregnancy
- developing new patterns for earning and spending money
- evaluating family roles, responsibilities, and authority
- reorienting relationships with relatives, friends, and associates
- expanding communication systems for present and anticipated emotional needs
- arranging for physical care of the neonate
- maintaining morale and an acceptable lifestyle during pregnancy and as a parent.

ASSESSMENT

Assessment, the first step in the nursing process, involves the orderly collection and careful interpretation of a woman's health status information. This information includes subjective data and objective data. Information gleaned from interviews with the patient or family members is classified as subjective data. Information collected from physical examination, medical records, diagnostic test results,

Components of an effective nurse-patient relationship

The following chart provides examples of the three critical components in establishing a nurse-patient relationship.

Communication
The nurse and woman can exchange information more easily and effectively if the nurse uses the following methods:
• establishing a trusting relationship
• listening actively
• respecting the patient's rights
• asking open-ended questions
• looking and acting professionally
• encouraging questions
• respecting cultural and language differences
• using touch appropriately.

Teaching
To teach effectively, the nurse must determine what the woman already knows, her readiness to learn, any obstacles to learning, and her preferred learning style. Important teaching principles include:
• knowing the subject matter
• being flexible in the nurse-patient relationship and adopting the type of instruction that most benefits the woman
• evaluating learning readiness and capability
• encouraging mutual respect and bonding
• using varied presentations of information
• considering needs of significant others, as appropriate
• evaluating effectiveness of teaching.

Motivation
Motivating the woman to assimilate and act on new information, thus taking charge of her own health care, is integral to each phase of the nurse-patient relationship. Methods to assist the nurse in patient motivation include:
• showing concern and caring for the woman
• determining self-care ability and adjusting the plan accordingly
• encouraging questions at all times.

and other medical or nursing sources is classified as objective data. Together, subjective and objective data give the nurse information that is essential for developing an effective plan of care.

Assessment begins during the first meeting with a patient and her family and continues throughout the nurse-patient relationship.

Any change in the family—such as its composition, socioeconomic status, health status, or relationships among members—requires reassessment and possible alteration in the nursing plan of care. For a childbearing woman, the nurse will find frequent reassessment necessary to identify the woman's changing needs during pregnancy, childbirth, and the postpartal period.

Assessment consists of two parts: health history (the major subjective data source) and physical assessment (the objective portion of the complete health assessment).

Health history

The health history gives insights into actual or potential problems and provides the nurse with pertinent physiologic, psychological, cultural, and socioeconomic information in light of such factors as family lifestyle and relationships. The health history interview enables the nurse to identify questions, concerns, or misconceptions the woman and her family may have. (See *Performing a health history*, page 54.)

Throughout the interview, the nurse must remain aware of verbal and nonverbal cues communicated by the woman and family members. To interpret these cues accurately, the nurse must consider them in the context of psychosocial, ethnic, and cultural influences on the woman's life. These influences may affect the way a woman or family member responds to pregnancy, labor and delivery, neonatal care, and other aspects of childbearing.

Physical assessment

After gathering the appropriate subjective information and establishing a rapport with the patient during the health history, the nurse performs a physical assessment to collect objective data, which may substantiate or refute the nurse's or patient's health concerns.

Complete physical assessment involves evaluating all physiologic systems in an organized manner, typically from head to toe or from least invasive procedure (general observation) to most invasive (such as pelvic examination). Diagnostic studies such as bloodwork or ultrasound studies provide additional, important assessment information.

NURSING DIAGNOSIS

After completing the assessment step, the nurse analyzes the subjective and objective data obtained. Such analysis allows the nurse to formulate nursing diagnoses, the next step in the nursing process.

A nursing diagnosis is a statement of an actual or potential health problem that nurses are capable of treating and licensed to treat.

Determining one or more applicable nursing diagnoses for a patient provides the basis for formulating an individualized, effective nursing plan of care. Each diagnosis must be supported by clinical information obtained during assessment.

Nursing diagnoses provide a common language to convey the nursing management necessary for each patient among the many nurses involved in that patient's care. To help ensure standardized nursing diagnosis terminology and usage, the North American Nursing Diagnosis Association (NANDA) has formulated and classified a series of nursing diagnosis categories based on nine human response patterns. These patterns include:

- Exchanging (mutual giving and receiving)
- Communicating (sending messages)
- Relating (establishing bonds)
- Valuing (assigning worth)
- Choosing (selection of alterations)
- Moving (activity)
- Perceiving (reception of information)
- Knowing (meaning associated with information)
- Feeling (subjective awareness of information).

Within each pattern are NANDA-approved nursing diagnosis categories specific to that topic. For example, the human response pattern devoted to relating includes such diagnostic categories as "sexual dysfunction" and "parental role conflict." The complete list of NANDA diagnostic categories, arranged by human response pattern, is called the nursing diagnosis taxonomy. (For the complete list, see Appendix 1: NANDA taxonomy of nursing diagnoses.)

Assigning specific nursing diagnoses to a patient involves several steps, including clustering assessment data, choosing the appropriate category, and adding specific patient information.

Clustering assessment data

Clustering is designed to identify broad areas of a person's need; it begins with the nurse's review of assessment data for completeness and accuracy. When possible, the nurse collects assessment data from all involved family members before making a diagnosis. Next, the nurse analyzes assessment data from different perspectives using standards of care, established physiologic norms, and information from other disciplines (such as psychology or social work to assess family relationships, or sociology to assess cultural influences). Finally, the nurse determines how various data groups relate to one another, clustering them in appropriate groups. This step requires broad-based health care knowledge; thus, the nurse should consult current literature or other health care professionals for help with unfamiliar subject areas.

Choosing nursing diagnosis categories

Using clustered assessment data to identify broad areas of the patient's needs, the nurse chooses one or more appropriate nursing diagnosis categories from the NANDA taxonomy. Each category may address an actual or potential problem.

PLANNING

After completing the assessment and formulating appropriate nursing diagnoses, the nurse develops a plan of care appropriate for the patient and her family. Effective planning focuses on the woman's specific needs, considers her strengths and weaknesses, incorporates her participation, sets achievable goals, includes feasible interventions, and occurs within the scope of the nursing practice setting.

Planning involves three basic steps: setting and prioritizing goals, formulating nursing interventions, and developing a plan of care. The plan of care acts as a written guide for and documentation of a patient's care and can be revised and updated as needed. It also helps ensure continuity of care, collaboration by all involved health care providers, and compliance with treatment.

IMPLEMENTATION

Implementation, the next step in the nursing process, involves working with the woman and her family to accomplish the designated interventions and move toward the desired outcomes. Effective implementation requires a sound understanding of the plan of care and collaboration among the patient, her family, and other members of the health care team, as needed. The implementation phase begins as soon as the plan of care is completed and ends when the established goals are achieved. Before and during implementation of any interventions, the nurse reassesses the patient as needed to ensure that planned interventions continue to be appropriate. Periodic reassessment helps ensure a flexible, individualized, and effective plan of care.

EVALUATION

Through evaluation, the nurse obtains additional subjective and objective assessment data relating to the goals identified in the nursing diagnoses. The nurse then uses these data to determine whether the goals have been met. Although evaluation is the final step in the nursing process, it actually occurs throughout the process, particularly during implementation, where the nurse continually reassesses the effects of interventions. Evaluation is directly linked to and must be based on the goals developed for each nursing diagnosis.

DOCUMENTATION

Although documentation of nursing care is not usually identified as a nursing process step, it is essential to effective care. Documentation serves several functions: It provides communication among members of the health care team, it functions as a discharge planning and quality-assurance tool, and it establishes a legal record of care provided. The nurse can be instrumental not only in establishing a plan of care and implementing it but also in facilitating patient record accessibility in any setting. The complete patient record must be readily accessible to all health care team members at all times. Each institution also must develop mechanisms for ensuring confidentiality of records.

Regulations regarding the minimal frequency of documentation relative to the patient's status may differ among states and institutions. Some institutions have standard documentation forms to use during all phases of nursing care. In all cases, the nurse must use sound professional judgment and document all care provided to help ensure appropriate communication of information and provision of quality care. This should include all assessments, interventions, patient teaching, and standard and emergency medications and treatments.

2

REPRODUCTIVE ANATOMY AND PHYSIOLOGY

Whatever the practice setting, every nurse will encounter women concerned about reproduction and other sexuality issues such as family planning, contraception, fertility, and infertility. To provide effective nusing care for these women, the nurse will need in-depth knowledge of reproductive system anatomy and physiology.

FEMALE REPRODUCTIVE SYSTEM

The female reproductive system includes the external and internal genitalia and the accessory organs, the breasts. The genitalia and their related structures respond to sexual stimulation, facilitate reproduction, and produce several hormones that regulate the development of female secondary sex characteristics, the reproductive cycle, and the physiologic changes associated with pregnancy and childbirth.

External genitalia

The vulva consists of the female external genitalia, most of which are visible upon inspection: the mons pubis, labia majora, labia minora, clitoris, ducts from Skene's (paraurethral) glands and Bartholin's (vulvovaginal) glands, vaginal orifice, hymen, fossa navicularis, and fourchette.

Internal genitalia

The female internal genitalia are highly specialized organs with one primary function: reproduction. (See *Internal female genitalia*, page 10.) They include the vagina, uterus, fallopian tubes, ovaries, and related structures. Hormones, especially estrogen and progesterone, regulate their development and function. Their blood supply passes through a network of arteries and veins, and innervation is provided through the autonomic nervous system.

Internal female genitalia

This illustration shows the internal genitalia of the mature female.

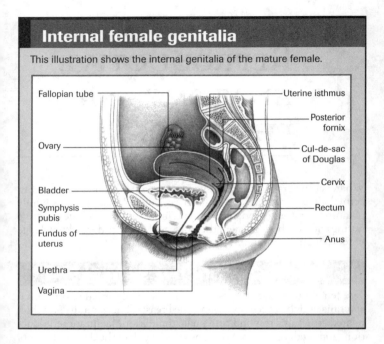

Fallopian tube

Ovary

Bladder

Symphysis pubis

Fundus of uterus

Urethra

Vagina

Uterine isthmus

Posterior fornix

Cul-de-sac of Douglas

Cervix

Rectum

Anus

Bony pelvis

The female bony pelvis, which resembles a basin, supports the upper torso, protects pelvic structures, and forms the fixed axis of the birth canal. Age, sex, race, and heredity affect pelvic size and shape. The most significant differences between the female and male pelvis are the contours and thickness of the bones. The female pelvic bones are lighter and thinner, and the female pelvis is wider, shallower, and rounder. (For more information about pelvic diameters and planes, see Chapter 8, Physiology of labor and childbirth.)

Pelvic floor

Muscle pairs and deep fascia in the pelvic floor are accessory structures to the bony pelvis. The pelvic floor contains the upper and lower (urogenital) pelvic diaphragms and muscles of the external genitalia and anus. Pelvic diaphragm ligaments, fascia, and muscles are anchored to the perineal body. Perineal muscles protect pelvic viscera; perform the sphincter action of the urethra, vagina, and rectum; and contract during orgasm.

Related pelvic structures

The pelvis contains urinary and intestinal structures as well as reproductive structures. Urinary structures include the ureters, bladder, urethra, and urethral meatus. The pelvis contains four intestinal segments: the rectum, colon, cecum, and ileum. These structures can be affected by changes in the reproductive tract.

Breasts

The breasts are highly specialized, cutaneous glands situated on either side of the anterior chest wall over the greater pectoral and the anterior serratus muscles. Vertically, they lie between the third and seventh ribs; horizontally, between the sternal border and the midaxillary line. A nipple is centrally located on each breast. A triangular-shaped portion of breast tissue known as the tail of Spence, or axillary tail, extends into the axilla. (See *Female breast*, page 12, for illustrations of breast structure and lymph drainage.)

Female reproductive cycle

The female reproductive cycle, or menstrual cycle, actually involves two simultaneous cycles: the ovarian cycle and the endometrial cycle. (See *Female reproductive cycle*, page 13.) The menstrual cycle begins at menarche, continues throughout a woman's reproductive life, and ceases at menopause. The average cycle is 26 to 28 days long.

Ovarian cycle

This cycle begins as the corpus luteum of the previous phase degenerates and hypothalamic stimulation occurs. There are two phases in this cycle. The follicular phase, during which a graafian follicle develops and ruptures, begins on the first day of menstruation and usually lasts 14 days, culminating in ovulation. The luteal phase begins on the 15th day and lasts through the end of the cycle. During the first 24 to 48 hours of this phase, the ovum is susceptible to fertilization. Variations in the length of the follicular phase account for variations in menstrual cycle length.

Follicular phase. On the first day of menses, primary follicles in the ovary begin to mature under the influence of pituitary gland hormones. Between the 5th and 7th days, a single graafian follicle dominates and continues to mature while other follicles undergo involution. On the 12th and 13th days, hormonal influence triggers swelling of the graafian follicle. Around the 14th day, it ruptures and ovulation occurs, as the mature ovum emerges and enters the fimbriated (fringed) end of the fallopian tube.

Ovulation can produce several clinical signs. Mittelschmerz, abdominal pain in the ovarian region, signals ovulation in many women.

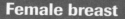

Female breast

The illustrations below show the structure and lymph drainage of the mature female breast.

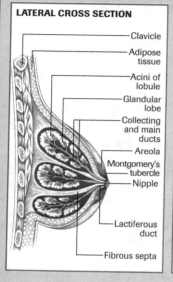

LATERAL CROSS SECTION

- Clavicle
- Adipose tissue
- Acini of lobule
- Glandular lobe
- Collecting and main ducts
- Areola
- Montgomery's tubercle
- Nipple
- Lactiferous duct
- Fibrous septa

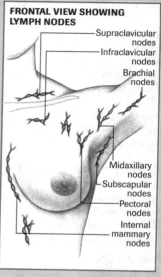

FRONTAL VIEW SHOWING LYMPH NODES

- Supraclavicular nodes
- Infraclavicular nodes
- Brachial nodes
- Midaxillary nodes
- Subscapular nodes
- Pectoral nodes
- Internal mammary nodes

Body temperature changes—typically a drop of 0.5° to 1.1° F (0.3° to 0.6° C) and then an increase above basal temperature—may signal ovulation. Evaluation of spinnbarkheit, the elasticity of cervical mucus discharge, can help pinpoint ovulation in many women. On the day of ovulation, estrogen stimulation enables stretching of the cervical mucus into long threads.

Luteal phase. After ovulation, the ruptured graafian follicle becomes a compact mass of tissue known as the corpus luteum. The corpus luteum produces small amounts of estrogen and progesterone that stimulate changes in the uterine endometrium, preparing it to receive a fertilized ovum. The corpus luteum continues to secrete hormones for about 8 days. If the ovum is not fertilized, the output of estrogen and progesterone decreases as the corpus luteum degenerates. The decreased hormone levels cannot support the endometrium; menstruation then occurs in about 6 days, initiating the next cycle. If fertilization occurs, the gonadotropins produced by the trophoblast (outside layer of the em-

Female reproductive cycle

The female reproductive cycle or menstrual cycle typically lasts 28 days, although cycles from 22 to 34 days are normal. During the cycle, hormones influence the release of a mature ovum from a graafian follicle in the ovary. Hormones also stimulate changes in the endometrial layer of the uterus that prepare the uterus for ovum implantation. The hormones involved in this cycle are estrogen, progesterone, follicle-stimulating hormone (FSH), and luteinizing hormone (LH). The diagrams illustrate all aspects of the cycle.

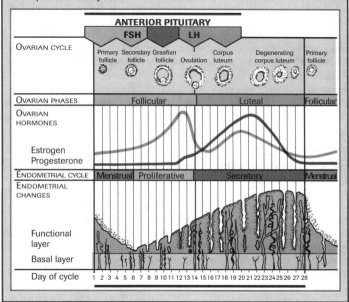

bryonic cell) prevent the decline of the corpus luteum, stimulating it to produce large amounts of estrogen and progesterone.

Endometrial cycle

During this cycle, changes occur in the uterine endometrium that prepare it for implantation of a fertilized ovum. The endometrial cycle has three phases: menstrual, proliferative, and secretory.

Menstrual phase. During this phase, which begins on the first day of menses and lasts approximately 5 days, the compact, spongy layers of the endometrium that developed during the previous cycle are sloughed off and expelled. Menstrual flow is typically dark red from the daily loss of 50 to 60 ml of blood. Approximately 0.5 mg of iron is lost with each ml of blood. While endometrial tissue, cells, and mucus are being discharged, the endometrial basal layer regenerates.

Proliferative phase. This phase begins on the 5th day and lasts until ovulation, typically on the 14th day. Early in this phase, the endometrium is 1 to 2 mm thick and undergoes few changes; cervical mucus is sparse and viscous. As estrogen secretion increases, the endometrium proliferates and the thickness of the uterine lining increases eight to ten times before ovulation.

Secretory phase. After ovulation, progesterone released by the corpus luteum increases endometrial vascularity and stimulates elongation of the glycogen-producing endometrial glands. The secretory phase lasts from the 14th day to the 25th day. At the end of this phase, the endometrium is soft, velvety, edematous, and about 4 to 6 mm thick. Rich with blood and glycogen, it is ready to nourish an implanted fertilized ovum. When fertilization and implantation do not occur, endometrial circulation decreases as blood vessels constrict in an ischemic process. Tissue necrosis follows ischemia. The subsequent sloughing of the compact and spongy endometrial layers marks the beginning of the next menstrual phase.

Hormonal regulation

Three endocrine structures—the hypothalamus, the pituitary gland, and the ovaries—produce the hormones that regulate the female reproductive cycle. These structures comprise a regulatory loop known as the hypothalamic-pituitary-gonadal axis, which generates physiologic changes through positive and negative feedback mechanisms. Prostaglandins, the fatty acid derivatives present in many tissues, also affect the reproductive cycle through smooth-muscle contraction and subsequent vasoconstriction and uterine contraction.

Hypothalamus. The nervous system provides the hypothalamus with sensory data. The hypothalamus then stimulates the pituitary gland to release or suppress appropriate gonadotropic hormones (hormones that regulate gonadal function). Stimulation takes one of two forms. The hypothalamus stimulates or suppresses the release of follicle-stimulating hormone (FSH) or luteinizing hormone (LH) from the anterior pituitary by releasing gonadotropin-releasing hormone (GnRH) or gonadotropin-inhibiting hormone (GnIH). Nerve impulses from the hypothalamus stimulate the release of oxytocin by the posterior pituitary.

Pituitary gland. The anterior pituitary gland (adenohypophysis) produces the gonadotropic hormones FSH, LH, and prolactin. FSH and LH regulate ovarian hormone secretion, and prolactin stimulates milk secretion. The posterior pituitary gland (neurohypophysis) stores oxytocin, a hormone that regulates uterine muscle contractility and the release of milk into the mammary glands during lactation.

Ovaries. The ovaries produce estrogen, progesterone, and a small amount of testosterone. Estrogen and progesterone help regulate the reproductive cycle, testosterone increases the sex drive, and estrogen stimulates pubic and axillary hair growth and sebaceous gland secretion during puberty.

Prostaglandins. All cells in the body produce prostaglandins, but they are especially plentiful in the endometrium of females and the prostate gland of males. In females, prostaglandins affect ovulation, fertility, and uterine motility and contractility. During ovulation, prostaglandins and LH stimulate ovum release and corpus luteum regression. During labor and delivery, they help stimulate uterine motility and cervical dilation.

Hypothalamic-pituitary-gonadal axis function. On the first day of the reproductive cycle, low levels of estrogen and progesterone in the bloodstream stimulate the release of GnRH by the hypothalamus. GnRH stimulates the release of FSH and LH by the pituitary gland. During the first five or six days of the reproductive cycle, these hormones stimulate follicle development in the ovaries. The maturing graafian follicle releases a potent form of estrogen into the bloodstream, which stimulates the proliferation of uterine endometrium.

As the cycle approaches ovulation on day 14, the level of estrogen in the blood is maintained in a pulsatile manner, and the hypothalamus signals the pituitary to slow FSH secretion and increase LH secretion. A day or so before ovulation, LH production peaks and the follicle reduces estrogen secretion and begins secreting progesterone. LH and progesterone cause follicle swelling and rupture during ovulation.

After ovulation, LH and prostaglandins stimulate corpus luteum regression. However, the corpus luteum continues to produce progesterone for several days. The high level of progesterone in the blood signals the hypothalamus to stimulate a reduction in FSH and LH secretion by the pituitary gland. Progesterone also stimulates secretory changes in the uterine endometrium that reduce contractility and prepare the uterus for ovum implantation, stimulates changes that prepare the fallopian tube mucosal lining to nourish the ovum, and stimulates lobule and acini development in the breasts and initiates their secretory phase.

After day 21 of the cycle, the corpus luteum begins to regress if fertilization has not occurred. Blood levels of progesterone decrease as the corpus luteum regresses, the uterine endometrium becomes ischemic and menstruation occurs.

NURSING CARE DURING THE ANTEPARTAL PERIOD

3

CONCEPTION AND FETAL DEVELOPMENT

A precise timetable governs the development of a functioning human being. Each developmental step occurs concurrently with other related phases. During this time, the fetus and mother form a relationship via the placenta that provides an environment conducive to fetal growth and well-being.

The gestation period spans the time from fertilization to birth. Its length can be calculated using two methods. One method calculates from the last ovulation (called ovulation age): gestation length from last ovulation approximates 38 weeks. Because few women know when ovulation occurs, however, the method using menstrual flow (called menstrual age) is more commonly used. In this method, gestation is calculated from the beginning of the last normal menstrual period: gestation length approximates 40 weeks. (See *Estimated date of confinement [EDC]*, page 18.)

PRE-EMBRYONIC PERIOD

Beginning with fertilization, the pre-embryonic period lasts for three weeks. During this crucial developmental stage, implantation occurs, cells divide rapidly and begin to differentiate, and the placenta and embryo begin to form.

Fertilization and implantation

Penetration of a female gamete (ovum) by a male gamete (spermatozoon) marks the beginning of conception. Called fertilization, this event requires coordination of a complex array of physical and chemical factors, some of which begin long before the spermatozoon and ovum join to form a zygote.

The first step needed for fertilization is gametogenesis, in which gonadotropic hormones stimulate testicular and ovarian precursor cells to develop into mature gametes.

Estimated date of confinement (EDC)

To calculate the EDC use the following formula (Nägele's Rule):

Last menstrual period date + 7 days – 3 months = EDC.
*(first day of the
last normal
menstrual period)*

The second step in fertilization is the introduction of spermatozoa into the vagina, either through ejaculation or artificial means. In normal ejaculate, spermatozoa are suspended in seminal fluid, which is composed of viscous secretions from the seminal vesicles, prostate, and bulbourethral (Cowper) glands. Ejaculate volume may vary from less than 2 ml to more than 5 ml, depending primarily on the interval between ejaculations. It typically contains about 3 ml of seminal fluid and up to 100 million spermatozoa per ml. Many of the spermatozoa aggregate in the portion of fluid ejaculated first rather than in a uniform distribution throughout the fluid.

Only spermatozoa (not seminal fluid) migrate through the cervix and into the uterus. Spermatozoa pass through the cervix primarily by active transport. The middle section of each spermatozoon's tail contains enzymes that catalyze energy needed for propulsion, resulting in a lashing motion, propelling the spermatozoon forward. Rhythmic uterine contractions move spermatozoa passively through the uterus and toward the fallopian tubes. The spermatozoa spread diffusely over the endometrium and enter both fallopian tubes, where they retain their fertilizing capability for at least 48 hours after intercourse.

Meanwhile, under the influence of follicle-stimulating hormone and luteinizing hormone, several ovarian follicles begin to mature during the female reproductive cycle. Granulosa cells surrounding the follicles proliferate, and a layer of acellular material called the zona pellucida forms on the surface of the developing follicle. Fluid accumulates within the layer of granulosa cells, eventually forming a central, fluid-filled cavity within the follicle known as a graafian follicle. At ovulation, the graafian follicle discharges its ovum, which is surrounded by the zona pellucida and several layers of adherent granulosa cells called the corona radiata. The ovum is swept into the adjacent fallopian tube by beating cilia that cover the tubal epithelium; peristaltic contractions of smooth muscles in the fallopian tube wall propel the ovum toward the uterus.

Fertilization is possible only when a descending ovum meets an ascending spermatozoon that has spent several hours in the female reproductive tract. Several conditions must be met before fertilization may occur, including:

- Seminal fluid must protect spermatozoa from destructively acid vaginal secretions.
- Cervical mucus must be thin and conducive to spermatozoa passage.
- Spermatozoa count typically must exceed 20 million per milliliter of seminal fluid.
- Contact must occur between a spermatozoon and an ovum.

When a spermatozoon penetrates an ovum, its tail degenerates and its head enlarges and fuses with the nucleus of the ovum. This restores the cell's genetic component to 46 chromosomes: 23 from the spermatozoon and 23 from the ovum. The fertilized ovum, known as a zygote at the one-cell stage, undergoes a series of mitotic divisions as it continues to travel down the fallopian tube toward the uterus. By the end of the first week after fertilization, the morula (small mass of cells) has begun to implant in the uterine wall.

EMBRYONIC PERIOD

Early in the fourth week, the flat, pre-embryonic structure becomes a cylindrical embryo that nearly triples in size over the next 4 weeks. Embryonic cells undergo complex differentiation and develop into primitive organ systems. (See *System development: Weeks 2 to 40*, pages 20 to 22 and *External appearance: Weeks 4 to 40*, page 23 for further information about pre-embryonic, embryonic, and fetal development.)

During this period, two major events begin: cell differentiation and cell organization. Specialized structures that protect and nurture the embryo—including the maternal decidua and fetal membranes—also become fully functional.

At this time, it is especially important for the mother to avoid teratogenic agents that can cause fetal malformations. Examples of these agents include drugs ingested by the mother, various viral infections, radiation, and some environmental factors. (See *Effects of teratogens on development*, page 24.)

Each of the germ layers derived from the inner cell mass will form specific tissues and organs within the embryo. In general, the ectoderm forms the embryo's external covering and the organs that come into contact with the environment. The endoderm forms the embryo's internal lining: the epithelium of the pharynx, the respiratory and gastrointestinal tracts, related organs, and parts of the urogenital tract.

(Text continues on page 22.)

System development: Weeks 2 to 40

Significant events occur during pre-embryonic, embryonic, and fetal developmental stages. The chart below lists these events along with the weeks during which they occur.

Nervous system

4 weeks
- Midbrain flexure is well-marked.
- Neural groove is closed.
- Spinal cord extends entire length of spine.

8 weeks
- Differentiation of cerebral cortex, meninges, ventricular foramina, and cerebrospinal fluid circulation occurs.

12 to 16 weeks
- Structural configuration of brain is roughly completed.
- Cerebral lobes are delineated.
- Cerebellum assumes prominence.

20 to 24 weeks
- Brain is grossly formed.
- Myelination of spinal cord begins.
- Spinal cords ends at S-1.

28 to 36 weeks
- Cerebral fissures appear.
- Convolutions appear.
- Spinal cord ends at L-3.

40 weeks
- Myelination of brain begins.

Musculoskeletal system

4 to 5 weeks
- Limb buds appear and are most vulnerable to teratogenic injury.

8 weeks
- Ossification (mandible, humerus, occiput) can be identified.

12 weeks
- Some bones are well-outlined.
- Ossification continues.

16 weeks
- Joint cavities are present.
- Muscular movements are detectable.

20 weeks
- Sternum ossifies.
- Mother can detect fetal movements (quickening).

28 to 32 weeks
- Ossification continues.
- Fetus can turn head to side.

36 weeks
- Muscle tone is developed; fetus can turn and elevate head.

System development: Weeks 2 to 40 (continued)

Cardiovascular system

2 to 4 weeks
- Heart begins to form.
- Blood circulation begins.
- Primitive red blood cells circulate.
- Tubular heartbeat can be detected by 24 days.

5 to 7 weeks
- Atrial division begins.
- Heart chambers are present.
- Fetal heartbeat is present.
- Groups of blood cells are identifiable.

8 weeks
- Development of heart is complete.
- Circulation through umbilical cord is well established.

16 to 20 weeks
- Fetal heart tone is audible with fetoscope.

Gastrointestinal system

4 weeks
- Oral cavity and primitive jaw are present.
- Stomach, ducts of pancreas, and liver form.

8 to 11 weeks
- Intestinal villi form.
- Small intestine coils in umbilical cord.

12 to 16 weeks
- Bile is secreted.
- Intestine withdraws from umbilical cord to normal position.
- Meconium is present in bowel.
- Anus is open.

20 weeks
- Enamel and dentin are deposited.
- Ascending colon appears.
- Fetus can suck and swallow.
- Peristaltic movements begin.

Hepatic system

4 weeks
- Liver function begins.

6 weeks
- Hematopoiesis by liver begins.

Genitourinary system

4 to 7 weeks
- Rudimentary ureteral buds present.

8 to 12 weeks
- Bladder and urethra separate from rectum; bladder expands as a sac.
- Kidneys secrete urine.

13 to 20 weeks
- Kidneys are in proper position with definitive shape.

36 weeks
- Formation of new nephrons ceases.

(continued)

System development: Weeks 2 to 40 *(continued)*

Respiratory system

4 to 7 weeks
- Primary lung, tracheal, and bronchial buds appear.
- Nasal pits form.
- Abdominal and thoracic cavities separated by the diaphragm.

8 to 12 weeks
- Bronchioles branch.
- Pleural and pericardial cavities appear.
- Lungs assume definitive shape.

13 to 20 weeks
- Terminal and respiratory bronchioles appear.

21 to 28 weeks
- Nostrils open.
- Surfactant production begins.
- Respiratory movements possible.
- Alveolar ducts and sacs appear.

38 to 40 weeks
- Pulmonary branching is two-thirds complete.
- Lecithin-sphingomyelin ratio is 2:1.

Reproductive system

6 to 8 weeks
- Sex glands appear.
- Differentiation of sex glands into ovaries or testes begins.
- External genitalia appear similar.

12 to 24 weeks
- Testes descend into the inguinal canal.
- External genitalia are distinguishable.

Endocrine system

4 weeks
- Thyroid can synthesize thyroxine.

10 weeks
- Islets of Langerhans are differentiated.

12 weeks
- Thyroid secretes hormones.
- Insulin is present in pancreas.

The mesoderm, which is sandwiched between the other two cell layers, forms various supporting tissues, muscles, the circulatory system, and major portions of the urogenital system.

Cell differentiation in each germ layer depends more on location than on inherent characteristics. For example, ectoderm cells transplanted during early development into locations normally oc-

External appearance: Weeks 4 to 40

The fetus' external appearance changes at various points throughout the gestation period, as indicated below.

4 weeks
- Body is C-shaped, pigment is present in eyes, and auditory pit is enclosed.

8 weeks
- Fetus has flat nose, eyes are far apart, digits are well-formed. Eyes, ears, nose, and mouth are recognizable.

12 weeks
- Nails appear.
- Skin is pink and delicate.
- Lacrimal ducts develop.

16 weeks
- Head is dominant.
- Scalp hair is present.
- Sweat glands develop.

20 weeks
- Vernix, lanugo, and sebaceous glands appear.
- Legs are considerably longer.

24 weeks
- Skin is red and wrinkled.
- Eyes are structurally complete.

28 weeks
- Eyelids are open.

32 weeks
- Fetus has an increasing amount of subcutaneous fat.
- Skin is pink and smooth.

36 weeks
- Lanugo is disappearing.
- Earlobes are soft with little cartilage.

40 weeks
- Copious vernix present.
- Hair is moderate to profuse.
- Lanugo on shoulders and upper body.
- Earlobes are stiffer with cartilage.

cupied by endoderm will differentiate as endoderm cells. The converse is also true. These transplantations suggest that embryonic cells, which may develop in various ways, are induced into specific development.

FETAL PERIOD

The fetal period, weeks 8 to 40, involves further growth and development of organ systems established in the embryonic period. When fully developed, fetal organs begin to function and supply part of the fetus's metabolic needs. In addition, the placenta continues to develop.

Effects of teratogens on development

During the first two weeks of embryonic development, exposure to a teratogen can result in spontaneous abortion or have no effect on the embryo at all. Later, depending upon the developmental stage in which it occurs, teratogen exposure can result in the formation of major congenital anomalies or functional defects (during highly sensitive stages), or minor congenital anomalies (during less sensitive stages). The following chart shows the approximate developmental stages during which nine body regions are highly sensitive and less sensitive to the effects of teratogens.

BODY REGION	HIGHLY SENSITIVE STAGES	LESS SENSITIVE STAGES
Central nervous system	3 to 16 weeks	20 to 38 weeks
Heart	3 to 6 weeks	6 to 8 weeks
Upper limbs	4 to 5 weeks	5 to 8 weeks
Eyes	4 to 8 weeks	8 to 38 weeks
Lower limbs	4 to 6 weeks	6 to 8 weeks
Teeth	6 to 8 weeks	9 to 38 weeks
Palate	6 to 9 weeks	9 weeks
External genitalia	7 to 9 weeks	9 to 38 weeks
Ears	4 to 9 weeks	9 to 16 weeks

PLACENTA

The placenta is a flattened, disk-shaped structure that weighs about 500 g and is derived from the trophoblast and from maternal tissues. The chorion and the villi are formed from the trophoblast, and the decidua basalis, in which the villi are anchored, is derived from the endometrium. The fused amnion and chorion extend from the margins of the placenta to form the fluid-filled sac enclosing the fetus; the sac ruptures at birth.

Placental circulation

The placenta circulates blood between the mother and fetus so that oxygen and nutrients may be exchanged. This is accomplished through a specialized circulation system in which fetal and maternal blood do not mix.

The fetus is connected to the placenta by the umbilical cord, which contains two arteries and a single vein. The arteries follow a spiral course in the cord, divide on the surface of the placenta, and branch to the chorionic villi. Maternal blood travels through a single large umbilical vein to the intervillous spaces. Fetal blood vessels within the villi are thus bathed in maternal blood. Nutrients and oxygen are transferred across capillary walls to the fetus while waste products from the fetus enter the maternal circulation via the umbilical arteries and the placenta. (See *Fetal circulation*, page 26.)

Placental transfer

The fetal-placental unit (umbilical cord, placental layers, and chorionic villi) must have developed properly and be functioning for placental transfer to occur. Substances from the mother (such as oxygen, water, antibodies, and many drugs) and substances from the fetus (such as carbon dioxide, urea, and waste products) are transferred across the placenta via four mechanisms: simple diffusion, facilitated diffusion, active transport, and pinocytosis.

Maternal protein hormones are not transferred through the placenta, with the exception of small amounts of thyroxin and triiodothyronine. Steroid hormones (the major ones are estrogen and progesterone) traverse the placenta freely. Viruses as well as some bacteria and protozoa may cross the placenta and infect and affect the fetus.

Endocrine functions

In addition to providing nourishment from the mother to the developing fetus, the placenta also functions as an endocrine organ, producing various peptide, neuropeptide, and steroid hormones. The two major peptide hormones are human chorionic gonadotropin (hCG) and human placental lactogen (hPL). The neuropeptides include gonadotropin-releasing hormone, thyrotropin-releasing factor, and adrenocorticotropic hormone. Synthesized by the cytotrophoblast, they may regulate the synthesis and release of peptide hormones from the syncytiotrophoblast.

Human chorionic gonadotropin (hCG)

The hCG hormone is a glycoprotein. Produced by the syncytiotrophoblast, it can be detected in the mother's serum as early as 8 days

Fetal circulation

The illustration below depicts the flow of oxygenated and deoxygenated blood in fetal circulation.

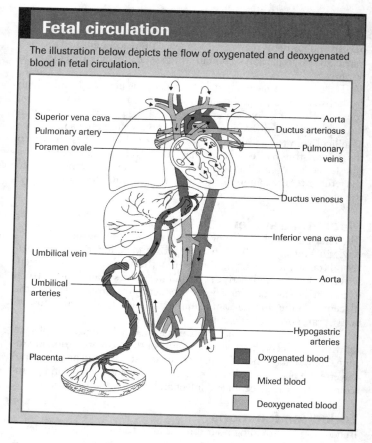

after conception, which corresponds to the time the blastocyst is burrowing into the endometrium.

Levels of hCG rise rapidly to about 100 IU/ml at about the 10th week of gestation, and then gradually decline, reaching a low of about 10 IU/ml by the 20th week and remaining at low levels for the remainder of gestation. For the first eight weeks of pregnancy, hCG maintains the corpus luteum, which provides the progesterone essential to the pregnancy until the placenta takes over hormone production. This hormone also may regulate maternal and fetal synthesis of steroid hormones, and it stimulates testosterone production by the testes of a male fetus.

The detection of hCG in the blood and urine by immunologic tests specific for the beta subunit of hCG is the basis of widely used pregnancy tests. Highly sensitive and specific pregnancy tests can detect hCG in blood and urine even before the first missed menstrual period, and sensitive tests almost invariably are positive if pregnancy causes a missed menstrual period.

Human placental lactogen (hPL)

Also known as human chorionic somatomammotropin, hPL is a single-chain polypeptide hormone that is produced by the syncytiotrophoblast and has properties similar to pituitary growth hormone. Human placental lactogen stimulates the maternal metabolism of protein and fat to ensure adequate amino and fatty acids for the mother and fetus. It may antagonize the action of insulin in the mother, decreasing maternal glucose use and making it available to the fetus. The hormone also stimulates the growth of the breasts in preparation for lactation. Levels of hPL rise progressively throughout pregnancy.

Estrogen and progesterone

Three types of estrogen are produced by the placenta: estrone, estradiol, and estriol. Estrogen production (primarily estriol) and estrogen urinary output increase throughout pregnancy. Progesterone production also increases; progesterone is excreted in the urine as the metabolite pregnanediol.

Fetal circulation

In the fetus, blood is oxygenated via the placenta. Fetal circulation differs from neonatal circulation in that three shunts—ductus venosus, foramen ovale, and ductus arteriosus—bypass the liver and lungs and separate the systemic and pulmonary circulations. Therefore, the umbilical vein carries oxygenated blood to the fetus and the umbilical arteries carry unoxygenated blood from the fetus to the placenta.

PHYSIOLOGIC AND PSYCHOSOCIAL CHANGES DURING NORMAL PREGNANCY

Physiologic changes that occur during pregnancy are among the most dramatic that the human body can undergo. Some of these changes begin even before the woman becomes aware that she is pregnant. Furthermore, pregnancy and childbirth are psychosocial events that deeply affect the lives of parents and families. Nothing defines the self-concept of many women and men more than the challenge of bearing and raising a child. Both physiologic and psychosocial changes help the woman adapt to pregnancy, maintain health throughout pregnancy, and prepare for childbirth. The nurse's role is extremely important in helping parents to understand that pregnancy and childbirth will change their lives irrevocably, presenting them with a long-term commitment that will benefit from intellectual, physical, and emotional preparation.

PHYSIOLOGIC CHANGES IN BODY SYSTEMS

Physiologic changes associated with pregnancy may range from subtle to overwhelming. Although these changes are normal and necessary, they may be uncomfortable and—especially for the primigravid woman—even frightening. To care for a pregnant woman properly, the nurse must understand the physiologic changes of normal pregnancy and when they occur, and how they are likely to affect her.

Early pregnancy produces a constellation of physiologic changes (signs and symptoms) that the health care provider must evaluate before reaching a tentative diagnosis of pregnancy. (For more details see *Presumptive, probable, and positive signs of pregnancy.*) Physiologic changes that help diagnose pregnancy make up only a small number of the changes that occur in a pregnant woman. As the fetus grows and hormones shift,

(Text continues on page 34.)

Presumptive, probable, and positive signs of pregnancy

The following chart describes typical presumptive and probable signs of pregnancy, their pregnancy-related causes and other possible causes, and positive signs of pregnancy.

SIGN	DESCRIPTION	PREGNANCY-RELATED CAUSES	OTHER POSSIBLE CAUSES
Presumptive: Signs and symptoms that make a woman assume she is pregnant.			
Amenorrhea	Absence of menses. This is usually the first indication of pregnancy in a woman with regular menstrual periods.	• Rising levels of human chorionic gonadotropin (hCG) hormone	• Anovulation, blocked endometrial cavity, endocrine changes (early menopause, lactation, glandular dysfunction), medications (phenothiazines), metabolic changes (anemia, malnutrition, long-distance running), psychological disorder, systemic disease
Nausea and vomiting	Onset is typically at 4 to 6 weeks, continuing through first trimester or occasionally longer.	• Rising levels of hCG • Emotional stress • Reduced gastric motility, reflux • Altered metabolism	• Gastric disorders, infections, psychological disorders (pseudocyesis, anorexia nervosa)

(continued)

Presumptive, probable, and positive signs of pregnancy *(continued)*

SIGN	DESCRIPTION	PREGNANCY-RELATED CAUSES	OTHER POSSIBLE CAUSES
Presumptive *(continued)*			
Urinary frequency	Begins during first trimester when enlarging uterus exerts pressure on urinary bladder; resolves during second trimester when uterus rises out of pelvis; and resumes during third trimester when fetus descends into pelvis.	• Enlarging uterus exerts pressure on urinary bladder	• Emotional stress, pelvic tumor, renal disease, urinary tract infection
Breast changes	Enlargement begins early in first trimester. Breasts become tender and may tingle or throb. As pregnancy progresses, nipples enlarge, become more erectile, and may darken. The areolae widen. Veins become more visible beneath breast skin.	• Hormonal changes • Growth of secretory ductal system • Increase in glandular tissue	• Hyperprolactinemia induced by tranquilizers, infection, prolactin-secreting pituitary tumor, pseudocyesis, premenstrual syndrome
Fatigue	Malaise, general discomfort, lethargy with no apparent cause.	• Unexplained, although progesterone may play a role	• Anemia, chronic illness

Presumptive, probable, and positive signs of pregnancy *(continued)*

SIGN	DESCRIPTION	PREGNANCY-RELATED CAUSES	OTHER POSSIBLE CAUSES
Presumptive *(continued)*			
Quickening	Woman's first awareness of active movements of fetus, usually felt as fluttering movements in lower abdomen at 16 to 20 weeks.	• Movement of fetus	• Excessive flatus, increased peristalsis
Skin changes	May include linea nigra, chloasma, vascular markings, and striae. Because pigment changes may persist, they are not a reliable sign in multigravidas.	• Increase in melanocyte-stimulating hormone • Increased estrogen • Stretching and atrophy of connective tissue	• Cardiopulmonary disorders, estrogen-progestin oral contraceptives, obesity, pelvic tumor, lupus erythematosus
Probable: Signs and symptoms that strongly suggest pregnancy.			
Braun von Fernwald's sign (also called Piskacek's sign)	Fullness and irregular softness of fundus occurs near area of implantation. Can be felt at 5 to 6 weeks of pregnancy.	• Local reaction to implantation; increased blood flow to pelvic organs	• Uterine tumor
Hegar's sign	Softening of uterine isthmus may be felt at 6 to 8 weeks via vaginal or rectovaginal examination.	• Increased blood flow to pelvic organs	• Excessively soft uterine walls

(continued)

Presumptive, probable, and positive signs of pregnancy (continued)

SIGN	DESCRIPTION	PREGNANCY-RELATED CAUSES	OTHER POSSIBLE CAUSES
Probable (continued)			
Goodell's sign	Softening of cervix occurs at 6 to 8 weeks.	• Increased blood flow to pelvic organs	• Estrogen-progestin oral contraceptives
Chadwick's sign	Bluish coloration visible in mucous membranes of cervix, vagina, and vulva at 6 to 8 weeks.	• Engorgement caused by increased blood flow to pelvic organs	• Hyperemia of cervix, vagina, vulva
Abdominal enlargement	Softening of uterus and fetal growth cause uterus to enlarge and stretch abdominal wall.	• Enlarging uterus	• Ascites, obesity, uterine or pelvic tumor
Braxton Hicks contractions	Uterine contractions begin early in pregnancy and become more frequent after 28 weeks.	• Possibly from enlargement of uterus to accommodate growing fetus	• Hematometra, uterine tumor
Ballottment	Passive movement of fetus felt during pelvic examination; typically identified at weeks 16 to 18.	• Rebounding of fetus in response to pressure exerted on uterus	• Ascites, uterine tumor, or polyps
Funic souffle	Sharp, blowing sound detected, synchronous with fetal pulse as blood flows through umbilical cord.	• Increased vascularity as blood flows through umbilical cord	• Aneurysm of abdominal aorta, iliac artery, or renal artery

Presumptive, probable, and positive signs of pregnancy *(continued)*

SIGN	DESCRIPTION	PREGNANCY-RELATED CAUSES	OTHER POSSIBLE CAUSES
Probable *(continued)*			
Fetal outline	Fetus may be palpated through uterine wall after 24 weeks.	• Growing fetus	• Subserous uterine myoma
Positive pregnancy test	Levels of hCG secreted by chorionic villi begin to increase 6 to 8 days after conception, peak at 8 to 12 weeks, and gradually decline during second and third trimesters.	• Increased levels of hCG	• Luteinizing hormone is similar to hCG and may cross-react in some pregnancy tests
Positive: Definitive signs and symptoms caused solely by pregnancy.			
Fetal heartbeat	May be detected as early as week 5 using ultrasound, week 10 using Doppler ultrasound, week 12 using fetal electrocardiography, and week 16 using a standard fetoscope.	• Fetal cardiovascular development	• None
Fetal movement on palpation	May be felt as thump or flutter through abdomen after week 18; may be visible after week 20.	• Fetal growth	• None

the woman's body undergoes physiologic adjustments in each body system, primarily to adapt to the fetus and to prepare for childbirth.

Reproductive system

External reproductive structures affected by pregnancy include the labia majora, labia minora, clitoris, and vaginal introitus. These structures enlarge because of increased vascularity; the labia majora and labia minora also enlarge because of fat deposits. Although the structures reduce in size after childbirth, they may not return to their prepregnant state because of loss of muscle tone or perineal injury. For example, the labia majora remain separated and gape slightly after childbirth. In addition, varices may be caused by pressure on vessels in the perineal and perianal areas.

Internal reproductive structures change dramatically to accommodate the developing fetus. Like their external counterparts, these internal structures may not regain their prepregnant states after childbirth.

Ovaries

Once fertilization occurs, ovarian follicles cease to mature and ovulation stops. The chorionic villi, which develop from the fertilized ovum, begin to produce human chorionic gonadotropin (hCG) to maintain the ovarian corpus luteum. The corpus luteum produces estrogen and progesterone until the placenta is formed and functioning. At 8 to 10 weeks of pregnancy, the placenta assumes production of these hormones and the corpus luteum—no longer needed—undergoes involution

Uterus

The nonpregnant uterus is smaller than the size of a fist, measuring approximately $3'' \times 2'' \times 1''$ ($7.5 \times 5 \times 2.5$) cm. It weighs approximately 2 to $2\frac{1}{2}$ oz (60 to 70 g) in the nulliparous woman and $3\frac{1}{2}$ oz (100 g) in the parous woman. In its nonpregnant state, the uterus can hold no more than $\frac{1}{3}$ oz (10 cc) of fluid. Its walls are composed of several overlapping layers of muscle fibers that adapt to the developing fetus and aid in expulsion of the fetus and placenta during labor and childbirth.

The uterus retains the developing fetus for approximately 280 days, or 9 calendar months, and undergoes progressive changes in size, shape, and position in the abdominal cavity.

Enlargement. In the first trimester, the pear-shaped uterus lengthens and enlarges in response to elevated levels of estrogen and progesterone. This hormonal stimulation primarily causes hypertrophy and minimal hyperplasia. These changes increase the amount of fibrous and elastic tissue to more than 20 times that of the nonpregnant uterus, resulting in stronger and more elastic uterine walls.

During the first few weeks of pregnancy, the uterine walls remain thick and the fundus rests low in the abdomen. The uterus cannot be palpated through the abdominal wall. After 12 weeks of pregnancy, however, the uterus typically reaches the level of the symphysis pubis and then may be palpated through the abdominal wall.

In the second trimester, the corpus and fundus become globe-shaped, and as pregnancy progresses the uterus lengthens to become oval in shape. The uterine walls become thinner as the muscles stretch; the uterus rises out of the pelvis, shifts to the right, and rests against the anterior abdominal wall. At 20 weeks of pregnancy, the uterus may be palpated just below the umbilicus and reaches the umbilicus at 22 weeks. As uterine muscles stretch, Braxton Hicks contractions may occur, helping to move blood more quickly through the inter-villous spaces of the placenta.

In the third trimester, the fundus reaches nearly to the xiphoid process. Between 38 and 40 weeks of pregnancy, the fetus begins to descend in the pelvis (lightening), which causes fundal height to de-crease. The uterus remains oval in shape. Its muscular walls become progressively thinner as it enlarges, finally reaching a muscle wall thickness of 5 mm or less. At term (40 weeks), the uterus typically weighs approximately 39 oz (1,100 g), holds 5 to 10 L of fluid, and has stretched to approximately 11″ × 9″ × 8″ (28 × 24 × 21 cm).

Progressive abdominal enlargement is the most observable sign of pregnancy, although posture and previous pregnancies will influence the type and amount of enlargement. Enlargement typically is more pronounced in the multigravid patient because the uterus assumes a more forward position after previous pregnancies reduce abdominal muscle tone. (See *Measuring fundal height*, page 59.)

Endometrial development. During the menstrual cycle, progesterone stimulates increased thickening and vascularity of the endometrium, preparing the uterine lining for implantation and nourishment of a fertilized ovum. After implantation, menstruation ceases and the en-dometrium becomes the decidua, which is divided into three layers: decidua capsularis, decidua basalis, and decidua vera. The decidua capsularis covers the blastocyst. The decidua basalis lies directly un-der the blastocyst and forms part of the placenta. The decidua vera lines the remainder of the uterus.

Vascular growth. As the fetus grows and the placenta develops, uter-ine blood vessels and lymphatics increase in number and size. Vessels must enlarge to accommodate the increased blood flow to the uterus and placenta. By the end of pregnancy, an average of 600 ml of blood may flow through the maternal side of the placenta each minute. Maternal arterial pressure, uterine contractions, and maternal posi-tion affect uterine blood flow throughout pregnancy.

Elongation and softening of the isthmus. After 6 to 8 weeks of pregnancy, the isthmus softens and can be compressed during a vaginal or rectovaginal examination. This compression, known as Hegar's sign, offers one of the most important early signs of pregnancy. As pregnancy advances, the isthmus becomes part of the lower uterine segment. During labor, it expands further.

Cervical changes. In addition to softening (Goodell's sign), the cervix takes on a bluish color (Chadwick's sign) during the second month of pregnancy, becomes edematous, and may bleed easily upon examination or sexual activity.

Hormonal stimulation causes the glandular cervical tissue to increase in cell number and become more hyperactive, secreting a thick, tenacious mucus. This mucus thickens into a mucoid, weblike structure, eventually forming a mucus plug that blocks the cervical canal and erects a protective barrier against bacteria and other substances that might enter the uterus.

Perhaps the outstanding characteristic of the cervix is its ability to stretch during childbirth, which is possible because of increased connective tissue, elastic fiber, and enfoldings in the endocervical lining.

Vagina

Estrogen stimulates vascularity, tissue growth, and hypertrophy in the vaginal epithelial tissue. Vaginal secretions—white, thick, odorless, and acidic—increase. The acidity of vaginal secretions helps prevent bacterial infections, but it fosters yeast infections, a common occurrence during pregnancy. This change in pH arises with increased production of lactic acid from glycogen in the vaginal epithelium; increased lactic acid results from the action of *Lactobacillus acidophilus*.

Other vaginal changes include:
- development of the same bluish color as the cervix and vulva due to increased vascularity
- hypertrophy of the smooth muscles and relaxation of connective tissues, which combine to allow the vagina to stretch during childbirth
- lengthening of the vaginal vault
- possible heightened sexual response.

Breasts

During the first trimester, increased levels of estrogen and progesterone enlarge the breasts and cause tenderness. They may tingle or throb. The nipples enlarge, become more erectile, and—along with the areolae—darken in color. Sebaceous glands in the areolae become hypertrophic, producing small elevations known as Montgomery's tubercles. Areolae widen from a diameter of less than 1 ¹/₂″ (3 cm) to 2″ or 3″ (5 or 6 cm) in the primigravid patient. Rarely, patches of brownish discoloration may appear on the skin adjacent to the areolae. These patches, known as secondary areolae, may be a sign of pregnancy if the woman has never breast-fed an infant.

As blood vessels enlarge, veins beneath the skin of the breasts become more visible and may appear as intertwining patterns over the anterior chest wall. Breasts become fuller and heavier as lactation approaches. They may throb uncomfortably. Increasing hormones cause the secretion of a yellowish, viscous fluid from the nipples known as colostrum. High in protein, antibodies, and minerals but low in fat and sugar as compared with mature human milk, colostrum may be secreted as early as the first several months of pregnancy, but it is most common during the last trimester. It continues for two to four days after delivery and is followed by mature milk production.

Breast changes are more pronounced in the primigravid than in the multigravid woman. In the latter, changes are even less significant if the woman has breast-fed an infant within the preceding year because her areolae will still be dark and her breasts enlarged.

Endocrine system

Together with the nervous system, the endocrine system controls metabolic functions that promote maternal and fetal health throughout pregnancy. Estrogen stimulates and temporarily enlarges the pituitary, thyroid, and parathyroid glands. The placenta is a major source of hormones that maintain the pregnancy and support the growth of the fetus.

Pituitary gland

Anterior pituitary hormones help to maintain the corpus luteum in early pregnancy. Two hormones secreted by the anterior pituitary, thyrotropin and adrenocorticotropic hormone (ACTH), alter maternal metabolism so that pregnancy can progress. Prolactin, another anterior pituitary hormone, increases throughout pregnancy in preparation for lactation.

The posterior pituitary releases two hormones important in pregnancy. Vasopressin (antidiuretic hormone or ADH) helps regulate water balance through its antidiuretic action, and oxytocin stimulates labor and aids in lactation through its effect on breast tissue.

Thyroid gland

As early as the second month of pregnancy, thyroxine (T_4)-binding protein increases and total T_4 rises correspondingly. Because the amount of unbound T_4 does not increase, the patient does not develop hyperthyroidism. However, thyroid changes do produce a slight increase in basal metabolic rate (BMR), cardiac output, pulse rate, vasodilation, and heat intolerance. The BMR increases about 15% during the second and third trimesters as the growing fetus places additional demands for energy on the woman's system. By term, the woman's BMR may have increased 25%. It returns to the prepregnant level within one week after childbirth.

In addition, elevated chorionic gonadotropin levels are associated with thyroid stimulation. Because much of the resulting increase in hormone is bound to proteins, its elevation does not lead to a hyperthyroid condition during pregnancy.

Parathyroid gland

As pregnancy progresses, fetal demands for calcium and phosphorus increase. The parathyroid gland responds by increasing hormones during the third trimester to as much as twice the level before pregnancy.

Adrenal gland

Increased estrogen raises the levels of cortisol and aldosterone. However, increased cortisol does not significantly increase the metabolism of carbohydrates, fats, and proteins (as it normally would) because much of the cortisol is bound by the cortisol-binding globulin transcortin. Elevated aldosterone minimizes the sodium-wasting effect of progesterone by promoting sodium resorption in the renal tubules.

Pancreas

Although the pancreas itself undergoes no changes during pregnancy, maternal insulin, glucose, and glucagon levels change. As pregnancy advances, fetal growth and development require increased glucose. For example, after ingesting oral glucose, the pregnant woman has prolonged hyperglycemia, hyperinsulinism, and reduced glucagon levels. Although the reason for these level shifts is unknown, they probably provide a sustained supply of glucose to the fetus.

The placenta secretes a hormone—human placental lactogen (hPL)—that promotes lipolysis and provides the patient with an alternate source of energy. However, hPL has a complicating effect. Along with estrogen, progesterone, and cortisol, hPL inhibits the action of insulin, which results in an increased need for insulin throughout pregnancy.

Respiratory system

Throughout pregnancy, biochemical and mechanical changes occur in the respiratory system in response to hormonal alterations. As pregnancy advances, these changes facilitate gas exchange, providing the woman with increased oxygen.

Anatomic changes

The diaphragm rises by approximately 1 1/2" (4 cm) during pregnancy, which prevents the lungs from expanding as much as they normally do. The diaphragm compensates by increasing its excursion ability, and the rib cage compensates by flaring from approximately 68 degrees before pregnancy to about 103 degrees in the third trimester. In addition, the anteroposterior and transverse diameters of the rib cage increase by about $3/4''$ (2 cm) and the circumference increases by $2''$ to $2^3/4''$ (5 to 7 cm). This expansion is possible because increased progesterone relaxes the ligaments that join the rib cage. As the uterus enlarges, thoracic breathing replaces abdominal breathing.

The upper respiratory tract vascularizes in response to increasing levels of estrogen. The woman may develop respiratory congestion, voice changes, and epistaxis as capillaries become engorged in the nose, pharynx, larynx, trachea, bronchi, and vocal cords. Increased vascularization also may cause the eustachian tubes to swell, leading to such problems as impaired hearing, earaches, and a sense of fullness in the ears.

Functional changes
Changes in pulmonary function improve gas exchange in the alveoli and facilitate oxygenation of blood flowing through the lungs. The respiratory rate typically remains unaffected in early pregnancy. By the third trimester, however, increased progesterone may increase the rate by approximately 2 breaths/minute.

Tidal volume and minute volume. Tidal volume (the amount of air inhaled and exhaled) rises throughout pregnancy as a result of increased progesterone and increased diaphragmatic excursion. In fact, the pregnant woman will breathe 30% to 40% more air than she does when not pregnant. Minute volume (the amount of air expired per minute) increases by approximately 50% by term. The difference between changes in tidal volume and minute volume creates a slight hyperventilation, which decreases carbon dioxide in alveoli. The resulting lower $PaCO_2$ in maternal blood leads to a greater partial pressure difference of carbon dioxide between fetal and maternal blood, which facilitates diffusion of carbon dioxide from the fetus.

Lung capacity. An elevated diaphragm decreases functional residual capacity (the volume of air remaining in the lungs after exhalation), and decreased functional residual capacity contributes to hyperventilation. Vital capacity (the largest volume of air that can be expelled voluntarily after maximum inspiration) increases slightly during pregnancy. These changes, along with increased cardiac output and blood volume, provide adequate blood flow to the placenta.

Acid-base balance. During the third month of pregnancy, increased progesterone sensitizes respiratory receptors and increases ventilation, leading to a drop in carbon dioxide levels. This increases pH, which might cause mild respiratory alkalosis, except that a decreased bicarbonate level partially or completely compensates for this tendency.

Cardiovascular system

Pregnancy alters the cardiovascular system so profoundly that, outside of pregnancy, the changes would be considered pathological and even life-threatening. During pregnancy, however, these changes are vital to a positive outcome.

Anatomic changes

The heart enlarges slightly during pregnancy, probably because of increased blood volume and cardiac output. This enlargement is not marked and reverses after childbirth.

As pregnancy advances, the uterus moves up and presses on the diaphragm, displacing the heart upward and rotating it on its long axis. The amount of displacement varies depending on the position and size of the uterus, the firmness of the abdominal muscles, the shape of the abdomen, and other factors.

Auscultatory changes

Changes in blood volume, cardiac output, and the size and position of the heart alter heart sounds during pregnancy.

During pregnancy, S_1 tends to exhibit a pronounced splitting, and each component tends to be louder. An occasional S_3 sound may occur after 20 weeks of pregnancy. Definite changes tend not to occur in either the aortic or pulmonic components of S_2. Many pregnant women exhibit a systolic ejection murmur over the pulmonic area.

Cardiac rhythm disturbances, such as sinus arrhythmia, premature atrial contractions, and premature ventricular systole, may occur. In the pregnant woman with no underlying heart disease, these arrhythmias do not require therapy, nor do they indicate development of myocardial disease.

Hemodynamic changes

Pregnancy affects heart rate and cardiac output, venous and arterial blood pressure, circulation and coagulation, and blood volume.

Heart rate and cardiac output. During the second trimester, heart rate increases gradually until it may reach 10 to 15 beats/minute above the prepregnant rate. During the third trimester, heart rate may increase 15 to 20 beats/minute above the prepregnant rate. The woman may feel palpitations occasionally throughout pregnancy. They may result from sympathetic nervous stimulation.

Increased tissue demand for oxygen and increased stroke volume raise cardiac output by up to 50% by the 32nd week of pregnancy. The increase is highest at rest when the woman is lying on her side and lowest when she is lying on her back. The side-lying position reduces pressure on the great vessels, which increases venous return to the heart. Cardiac output peaks during labor, when tissue demands are greatest.

Venous and arterial blood pressure. When the woman lies on her back, femoral venous pressure increases threefold from early pregnancy to term. This occurs because the uterus exerts pressure on the inferior vena cava and pelvic veins, retarding venous return from the legs and feet. Because of this orthostatic hypotension, the woman may feel light-headed if she rises abruptly after lying on her back. Edema in the legs and varicosities in the legs, rectum, and vulva may occur.

Early in pregnancy, increased progesterone levels relax smooth muscles and dilate arterioles, resulting in vasodilation. Systolic and diastolic pressures may decrease 5 to 10 mm Hg. Blood pressure reaches its lowest during the second half of the second trimester and then gradually returns to first trimester levels during the third trimester. By term, arterial blood pressure approaches prepregnant levels.

Brachial artery pressure is highest when the patient lies on her back, which causes the enlarged uterus to exert the greatest pressure on the vena cava, and lowest when she lies on her left side, which relieves uterine pressure on the vena cava.

Circulation and coagulation. Venous return decreases slightly during the 8th month of pregnancy and at term increases to normal levels. Blood clots more readily during pregnancy and the postpartal period because of an increase in clotting factors VII, IX, and X.

Blood volume. Total intravascular volume increases during pregnancy, beginning between the 10th and 12th weeks and peaking with approximately a 40% increase between the 32nd and 34th weeks. Volume decreases slightly in the 40th week and returns to normal several weeks postpartum. The increase consists of two-thirds plasma and one-third red blood cells. The increased blood volume supplies the hypertrophied vascular system of the enlarging uterus, provides nutrition for fetal and maternal tissues, and serves as a reserve for blood loss during childbirth and puerperium.

Hematologic changes
Pregnancy affects red and white blood cells and fibrinogen levels. It is important to monitor these levels to ensure that neither the woman nor the fetus is in danger.

Red blood cell mass. The increase in plasma volume is disproportionately greater than the increase in erythrocytes, which lowers the patient's hematocrit and hemoglobin, causing physiologic anemia of pregnancy. A hematocrit below 35% and a hemoglobin level below 11.5 g/dl indicate pregnancy-related anemia.

Bone marrow becomes more active during pregnancy, and can produce up to a 30% excess in red blood cells if sufficient iron is available. The woman may require an iron supplement to increase this hemoglobin synthesis.

White blood cell count. Leukocytes increase for unknown reasons during pregnancy, and the white blood cell count rises, ranging from 10,000 to 12,000 µl. The count may increase to 25,000 µl or more during labor, childbirth, and the early postpartal period.

Fibrinogen levels. Fibrinogen is converted to fibrin by thrombin and is known as coagulation factor I. In the nonpregnant woman, levels average 250 mg/dl. In the pregnant woman, levels average 450 mg/dl, increasing as much as 50% by term. This increase plays an important role in preventing maternal hemorrhage during childbirth.

Urinary system

The kidneys, ureters, and bladder undergo profound changes in structure and function during pregnancy.

Anatomic changes

Significant dilation of the renal pelves, calyces, and ureters begins as early as the 10th week of pregnancy, probably caused by increased estrogen and progesterone. As pregnancy advances and the uterus becomes dextrorotated, the ureters and renal pelvis become more dilated above the pelvic brim, particularly on the right side. In addition, the smooth muscle of the ureters undergoes hypertrophy and hyperplasia. Muscle tone decreases, primarily because of the muscle-relaxing effects of progesterone.

These changes retard the flow of urine through the ureters and result in hydronephrosis and hydroureter, predisposing the pregnant patient to urinary tract infection. In addition, because of the delay between urine formation in the kidneys and its arrival in the bladder, inaccuracies may occur during clearance tests.

Hormonal changes cause the bladder to relax during pregnancy, permitting it to distend to hold approximately 1,500 ml of urine. However, in the first trimester, hormonal changes and pressure from the growing uterus cause bladder irritation, manifested as urinary frequency and urgency, even if the bladder contains little urine. Bladder vascularity increases and the mucosa bleeds easily. In the second trimester, when the uterus rises out of the pelvis, urinary symptoms abate. As term approaches, however, the presenting part of the fetus engages in the pelvis—again exerting pressure on the bladder—and symptoms return.

Functional changes

Pregnancy affects renal plasma flow, glomeruler filtration rate, renal tubular resorption, and nutrient and glucose excretion.

Renal plasma flow. Early in pregnancy, renal plasma flow (RPF) increases, rising to 40% to 50% above the prepregnant level by the third trimester. RPF then declines slightly.

Glomerular filtration rate. By the beginning of the second trimester, glomerular filtration rate (GFR) increases as much as 50% associated with the increase in renal plasma flow. It remains elevated to term. This increase in GFR produces a consequent decrease in some laboratory test values, including blood urea nitrogen and creatinine.

Renal tubular resorption. Renal tubular resorption increases as much as 50% during pregnancy as it acts to maintain sodium and fluid balance. The sodium requirement increases because the patient needs more intravascular and extracellular fluid. Total body water also increases to a total of about 7 L more than in the prepregnant state. The amniotic fluid and placenta account for about half of this amount; increased maternal blood volume and enlargement of the breasts and uterus account for the rest.

Late in pregnancy, changes in posture affect sodium and water excretion. The woman will excrete less when lying on her back because the enlarged uterus compresses the vena cava and aorta, causing decreased cardiac output. This decreases renal blood flow, which in turn decreases kidney function. The woman will excrete more when lying on her left side.

Nutrient and glucose excretion. The pregnant woman loses increased amounts of some nutrients, such as amino acids, water-soluble vitamins, folic acid, and iodine. Glycosuria may occur as GFR increases without a corresponding increase in tubular resorptive capacity. Proteinuria is considered abnormal in pregnancy. It may occur occasionally during and after difficult labors as a result of mild trauma to the bladder and urethra during labor and delivery. (For more information, see Chapter 8, Physiology of labor and childbirth, and Chapter 9, Fetal assessment).

Gastrointestinal system

Changes during pregnancy affect anatomic elements in the gastrointestinal system and alter certain functions. These changes are associated with many of the most discussed discomforts of pregnancy. (See *Minimizing the discomforts of pregnancy,* pages 63 to 67.)

Anatomic changes

The mouth and teeth, stomach and intestines, and gallbladder and liver are affected during pregnancy.

Mouth and teeth. The salivary glands become more active, especially in the latter half of pregnancy. The gums become edematous and bleed easily because of increased vascularity. The teeth are unaffected; they lose no minerals to the developing fetus.

Stomach and intestines. As progesterone increases during pregnancy, gastric tone and motility decrease, slowing the stomach's emptying time and possibly causing regurgitation and reflux of stomach contents. Therefore, the woman may complain of heartburn.

The enlarging uterus displaces the stomach upward. In late pregnancy, the uterus displaces the small intestine as well. Hormonal changes and mechanical pressure reduce motility in the small intestine. Reduced motility in the colon leads to greater water absorption, which may predispose the patient to constipation. The enlarging uterus displaces the large intestine and puts increased pressure on veins below the uterus, which may predispose the woman to hemorrhoids.

Gallbladder and liver. As smooth muscles relax, the gallbladder empties more sluggishly. This prolonged emptying time, along with increased excretion of cholesterol in the bile caused by increased hormone levels, may lead to bile that is supersaturated with cholesterol and predispose the woman to cholesterol crystal formation and gallstone development.

The liver does not enlarge or undergo any major changes during pregnancy. However, hepatic blood flow may increase slightly, and the liver's workload increases as the basal metabolic rate increases. Factors within the liver and increased estrogen and progesterone decrease bile flow.

Some liver function studies show drastic changes, possibly caused in part by increased estrogen levels. These following changes would suggest hepatic disease in a nonpregnant woman:

- Alkaline phosphatase nearly doubles, caused in part by increased alkaline phosphatase isozymes from the placenta.
- Serum albumin levels decrease.
- Plasma globulin levels increase, causing decreases in albumin globulin ratios.
- Plasma cholinesterase levels decrease.

Functional changes

Nausea and vomiting may affect appetite and food consumption, even while energy demand increases.

Appetite and food consumption. The woman's appetite and food consumption fluctuate. Many women experience nausea and vomiting early in pregnancy. Nausea typically is more pronounced in the morning, beginning at 4 to 6 weeks and subsiding by the end of the first trimester. Some women experience this morning sickness at other hours and beyond the first trimester. Severity ranges from a slight distaste for food to severe vomiting. Certain odors and the sight of food can trigger an occurrence. Peculiarities in taste and smell also may develop. Although uncomfortable for the woman, morning sickness has no deleterious effects on the fetus. Morning sickness should be considered abnormal if accompanied by fever, pain, or weight loss.

In addition to the appetite reduction caused by nausea and vomiting, the woman's appetite may be reduced by increased hCG levels and changes in carbohydrate metabolism, which are suspected appetite suppressants. Once nausea and vomiting cease, the woman's appetite increases along with increasing metabolic needs. However, the old adage of "eating for two" is erroneous.

Carbohydrate, lipid, and protein metabolism. The woman's carbohydrate needs rise to meet increasing energy demands. The woman needs more glucose, especially during the second half of pregnancy. Plasma lipid levels increase starting in the first trimester, rising at term to 40% to 50% above the prepregnant level. Cholesterol, triglyceride, and lipoprotein levels increase as well. The total concentration of serum proteins decreases, especially serum albumin and perhaps gamma globulin. The primary immunoglobulin transferred to the fetus—IgG—is lowered in the woman's serum.

Musculoskeletal system
The woman's musculoskeletal system changes in response to hormones, weight gain, and the growing fetus. These changes may affect the woman's gait, posture, and comfort.

Skeleton
The enlarging uterus tilts the pelvis forward, shifting the woman's center of gravity. The lumbosacral curve increases, accompanied by a compensatory curvature in the cervicodorsal region. The lumbar and dorsal curves become even more pronounced as breasts enlarge and their weight pulls the shoulders forward, producing a stoop-shouldered stance. Increasing sex hormones (and possibly the hormone relaxin) relax the sacroiliac, sacrococcygeal, and pelvic joints. These changes cause marked alterations in posture and gait. Symphyseal separation causes significant discomfort for a few women. Shoe and ring sizes tend to increase because of weight gain, hormonal changes, and dependent edema. Although these changes may persist after childbirth, they often return close to their prepregnant states.

Muscles
In the third trimester, the prominent rectus abdominis muscles separate, allowing the abdominal contents to protrude at the midline. The umbilicus may flatten or protrude. After childbirth, abdominal muscles regain tone but typically do not return to their prepregnant state.

Integumentary system
Skin changes vary greatly among pregnant women. Of those who experience skin changes, Blacks and brunette Whites typically show more

marked changes than blondes. Because some skin changes may remain after childbirth, they are not considered an important sign of pregnancy in the multigravida. The woman may need the nurse's help to integrate these skin changes into her self-concept. Skin changes associated with pregnancy include striae gravidarum, pigment changes, and vascular markings.

Striae gravidarum

The woman's weight gain and enlarging uterus, combined with the action of adrenocorticosteroids, lead to stretching of the underlying connective tissue of the skin, creating striae gravidarum in the second and third trimesters. Better known as stretch marks, striae on light-skinned women appear as pink or slightly reddish streaks with slight depressions; on dark-skinned women, they appear lighter than the surrounding skin tone. They develop most often in skin covering the breasts, abdomen, buttocks, and thighs. After labor, they typically grow lighter until they appear silvery white on light-skinned women and light brown on dark-skinned women.

Pigment changes

Pigmentation begins to change at approximately the 8th week of pregnancy, partly from the melanocyte-stimulating hormone and ACTH and partly from estrogen and progesterone. These changes are more pronounced in such hyperpigmented areas as the face, areolae, axillae, abdomen, anal region, inner thighs, and vulva. Specific changes may include linea nigra and chloasma.

Linea nigra refers to a dark line that extends from the umbilicus or above to the mons pubis. In the primigravida, this line develops at approximately the 3rd month of pregnancy. In the multigravid patient, linea nigra typically appears before the 3rd month.

Called the mask of pregnancy, chloasma refers to irregular, brownish blotches that appear on the cheek bones and forehead. Chloasma appears after the 16th week of pregnancy and gradually becomes more pronounced until childbirth; then, it typically fades.

Vascular markings

Tiny, bright-red angiomas may appear during pregnancy from increased subcutaneous blood flow as a result of estrogen release. They are called vascular spiders because of the branching pattern that extends from each spot. Occurring mostly on the chest, neck, arms, face, and legs, they disappear after childbirth.

Palmar erythema, commonly seen along with vascular spiders, are well-delineated, pinkish areas over the palmar surface of the hands. Once pregnancy ends and estrogen levels decrease, these changes reverse.

Epulides, also known as gingival granuloma gravidarum, are raised, red, fleshy areas that appear on the gums as a result of increased estrogen. They may increase in size, cause severe pain, and bleed profusely. An epulis that grows rapidly may require excision.

Other integumentary changes

Nevi may develop on the face, neck, upper chest, or arms during pregnancy. Oily skin and acne from increased estrogen may occur. Hirsutism may occur; it reverses when pregnancy ends. By the 6th week of pregnancy, fingernails may soften and break easily, a problem that may be exacerbated by nail polish removers.

Immune system

Ordinarily, a mature immune system rejects implanted tissue within 2 weeks. During pregnancy, however, the fetus and placenta are protected from the maternal immune system by a mechanism that is not fully understood. The cell layer covering the fetus and placenta may mask antigens, thus preventing detection by sensitized lymphocytes. The placental hormones progesterone and hCG may suppress cellular immunity. This suppression may also be responsible for the increased occurrence of colds and other viral infections.

Neurologic system

Changes in the neurologic system are poorly defined and incompletely understood. For most women, neurologic changes are temporary and cease once pregnancy is over. Functional disturbances called entrapment neuropathies occur in the peripheral nervous system from mechanical pressure. Examples of entrapment neuropathies are described below.

- Meralgia paresthetica is a tingling and numbness in the anterolateral portion of the thigh that occurs when the lateral femoral cutaneous nerve becomes entrapped in the area of the inguinal ligaments. This is more pronounced in late pregnancy, as the gravid uterus presses on these nerves and as vascular stasis occurs.
- Carpal tunnel syndrome may occur in the third trimester when the median nerve of the carpal tunnel of the wrist is compressed by edematous surrounding tissue. The woman may notice tingling and burning in the dominant hand, possibly radiating to the elbow and upper arm. Numbness or tingling in the hands also may result from pregnancy-related postural changes, such as slumped shoulders that pull on the brachial plexus.
- Hypocalcemia and muscle cramps may occur if the woman ingests insufficient calcium. Increased metabolism creates the need for greater calcium intake.

- Light-headedness, faintness, and syncope may be caused by vasomotor changes, hypoglycemia, and orthostatic hypotension.

PSYCHOSOCIAL CHANGES

The parents' response to pregnancy and childbirth is affected by psychological, social, economic, and cultural factors and by self-concept and attitudes toward sex-specific and family roles. All of these aspects of childbearing can affect their health and that of their children. Therefore, care of the expectant family presents the nurse with special responsibilities and challenges.

The nurse must promote the family's normal adaptation to and integration of the new family member. To achieve these goals, the nurse should perform the steps below and proceed based on expertise and experience.

- Promote each family member's self-esteem. Listen attentively, elicit questions and concerns, identify preferences and cultural influences, provide anticipatory guidance about emotional and psychological family changes, discuss as fully as needed each family member's necessary roles and tasks, affirm their efforts, inquire about and show concern for each family member's health care needs, and make referrals as needed.
- Deliver culturally sensitive nursing care. Gather information about the family's customs and beliefs to add to assessment data and to individualize care. Identify personal attitudes and feelings about childbearing. Avoid imposing personal values, feelings, and emotional reactions on others. Also, avoid making assumptions about the woman and her preferences. Allow her to share her feelings freely. (See *Cultural considerations of the pregnant woman.*)
- Involve all family members in prenatal visits, facilitate communication among family members, offer anticipatory guidance about family changes during pregnancy and the postpartal period, help mobilize the family's resources, offer sexual counseling, help the woman maximize her family's positive contributions and assist her in working through the negative ones, praise the family's efforts, and offer books and other materials that address all family members.
- Promote the family's prenatal bonding with the fetus. During prenatal visits, share information about fetal development; help the family identify fetal heart tones, position, and movements; and reinforce bonding behaviors—such as patting the abdomen or talking to the fetus—by asking the woman or her partner to note and report fetal movements.

Cultural considerations of the pregnant woman

Although each woman has personal beliefs and values, her cultural background may influence her psychosocial adaptation during pregnancy, self-care and health promotion measures, health-seeking behaviors, and interactions with health care professionals. The nurse must remember that no matter what the woman's background is, she may or may not follow the same beliefs as another woman of the same ethnicity or cultural background. When caring for a woman from a different culture, the nurse should keep the following considerations in mind.

North American culture

Because the North American culture encompasses various ethnic and cultural backgrounds, no typical view of childbirth exists in America. However, widespread access to medical care and the movement toward family-centered childbirth permit a few generalizations about American attitudes toward pregnancy and childbirth.

In the United States, doctors typically manage a woman's pregnancy. Americans tend to rely heavily on medical intervention to ensure a healthy outcome for the mother and neonate. They usually emphasize technological intervention, including ultrasonography and other tests, to track fetal growth and health.

Americans consider health promotion activities an indication that the woman has accepted her pregnancy. They encourage the woman to get early prenatal care, to monitor her diet carefully, and to eliminate unhealthy practices, such as drinking alcohol and smoking. A pregnant woman who engages in unhealthy practices may meet with disapproval or disdain and may experience guilt and self-doubt.

American men participate in pregnancy and delivery to a greater extent than do men in many other cultures. A large percentage of American men attend childbirth education classes and are present during delivery. Many American men also are taking an increased role in infant care at home.

Asian culture

In the United States, Chinese, Japanese, and Korean patients may practice traditional beliefs or may adopt American customs and practices regarding childbirth.

The Chinese culture values maintaining a balance between the physical and spiritual aspects of life, especially during pregnancy. To help achieve this balance, a pregnant woman may avoid certain foods and drink herbal teas. After delivery, the woman may stay home and rest for 40 days, avoiding strenuous activity. She also may avoid contact with water for 40 days after delivery, believing that a postpartal chill can cause arthritis or body aches.

(continued)

Cultural considerations of the pregnant woman *(continued)*

Japanese-Americans, who have the highest median income and educational level of any American minority group, tend to accept American practices. They view pregnancy as a normal state that requires few changes in the pregnant woman's daily routine. After delivery, the woman controls the neonate's care, although the extended family may participate.

Korean-American women believe that the pregnant woman or a family member experiences a *Tae Mong* (a dream that predicts pregnancy). After she becomes pregnant, the Korean woman may read classical literature, view beautiful artworks, and adopt an optimistic and serene attitude to promote health and an easy delivery. Dietary restrictions include balancing hot and cold foods and restricting salty, spicy, or sour foods. Other restrictions include barring men and childless women from the delivery area and keeping the neonate's father away from the mother and neonate for seven days after delivery.

The birth of a first child, especially a son, is an important event in a Korean family, integrating the mother into her partner's family and giving her status and economic security. In traditional Korean families, the mother-in-law is responsible for the pregnant woman's health and care. If she desires a grandson, the Korean mother-in-law will view care of her daughter-in-law as service to Samshin, the goddess of childbirth. Health care professionals should be aware that the Korean patient may wish to involve her mother-in-law in decision-making discussions.

Southeast Asian culture

Southeast Asian (Vietnamese, Cambodian, and Laotian) women may hold what many Americans consider to be superstitious beliefs, such as the belief that sitting on a step in a door frame can cause labor and delivery complications, or that a bath after sundown will result in an oversized neonate. Some Southeast Asian women may see an herbalist or an acupuncturist before seeking Western health care and may refrain from expressing doubts about medications or procedures out of respect for authority. If the health care professional's advice conflicts with traditional beliefs, the Southeast Asian patient may deal passively with this conflict, missing appointments or neglecting to fill prescriptions. The health care professional who is alert to such indirect messages can approach the patient with an alternative plan.

Filipino culture

Filipino women share many traits with Southeast Asian women. They are taught to respect elders, defer to their partners, and avoid confrontation. The nurse who provides care to a Filipino patient should be aware that she may wish to deal with issues indirectly and involve the family in health care planning.

- Facilitate resolution of conflicts related to pregnancy and childbirth. Help identify underlying conflicts through reflective communication, validation of feelings, and discussion of the woman's dreams and fantasies. Promote conflict resolution by teaching personal affirmation and by suggesting literature that helps identify and resolve conflicts. Refer for counseling any woman who cannot resolve conflicts.
- Support adaptive coping patterns through realistic education of the family about pregnancy, childbirth, and the postpartal period. Discuss childbirth and human responses accurately and realistically. Frankly discuss the challenges of parenting.
- Act as an advocate for the expectant family in the health care facility, community, and society. In the facility, suggest more family-centered policies, such as sibling and grandparent visiting hours. In the community, expand childbirth options for expectant families by working to establish a birth center. At the national level, lobby for the health of poor mothers and neonates and for necessary changes in health care by writing to state representatives about laws that fund maternal-neonatal health care and other family services.

5 THE NORMAL ANTEPARTAL PERIOD

During the antepartal period, members of the health care team strive to ensure the health of the woman and her fetus. This period begins with conception and ends with the onset of labor. The nurse will use the steps of the nursing process to continually update the health team on the pregnant woman's status.

ASSESSMENT

Ideally, antepartal assessment begins when a woman seeks health care to confirm a suspected pregnancy and begin prenatal care. During the initial antepartal meeting, the nurse gathers subjective and objective data pertinent to the woman's pregnancy and general health. (See *Documenting previous pregnancies*.) An extensive history is done at that initial visit and a smaller, interim history is done at each prenatal visit.

Assessment should continue regularly throughout the antepartal period. The woman may schedule a routine examination every four weeks until the 28th week, every two weeks until the 36th week, and then every week until delivery. However, the number of scheduled examinations depends on the woman's overall condition: women at lower risk are scheduled for fewer routine visits and those at higher risk for more frequent visits.

Repeated contact between nurse and woman enables the nurse to monitor the woman's well-being, the fetus's development, and the onset of any problems. It also provides an opportunity for patient teaching.

Besides a health history and physical examination, antepartal assessment includes selected laboratory tests. Follow-up care focuses on maintaining the health and well-being of the woman and fetus throughout pregnancy.

Documenting previous pregnancies

The TPAL system is a method commonly used to document previous pregnancies. The first letter, T, stands for the number of term neonates born (after 37 weeks' gestation). The second letter, P, stands for the number of preterm neonates born (before 37 weeks' gestation). The third letter, A, stands for the number of pregnancies ending in spontaneous or therapeutic abortion. The fourth letter, L, stands for the number of children currently living.

TPAL

This four-digit system is often confused with the two-digit system, gravida, para. In the two-digit system, para refers to the number of pregnancies that terminated in a birth of a baby or a fetus that reached the point of viability. The point of viability is 28 weeks gestation or a weight of 1000 g. For example, a woman who was pregnant twice, with one of those pregnancies ending in the birth of viable full-term twins and the other ending in a full-term live birth, would be gravida 2, para 3. Using the four-digit classification, the woman would be described as gravida 2, para 3003. The four-digit system is a more precise method of describing a woman's past pregnancy history.

Be aware that some institutions use T to refer to the number of term pregnancies, not the number of term neonates; refer to your institution's policy for further clarification.

Health history

The health history interview should address all pertinent areas of the woman's health—past, present, and potential. Always begin with the least sensitive areas of information to be collected and finish with the most sensitive areas. (For further information see *Performing a health history*, pages 54 and 55.) The nurse should consider the woman's physical appearance and nonverbal communication as well as her verbal responses to questions. Always remember that the purpose of the health history is to evaluate the woman's health and risk status at a given time. This information is a vital, integral part of comprehensive maternity care.

Physical assessment

After collecting complete history data, the nurse assists with or continues the physical assessment. The initial examination provides base-

ASSESSMENT TIP

Performing a health history

The health history is one of the most important tools used in the medical field. Few other tools yield the same type of information as an accurate, complete health history that is carefully documented. The following items should be included in a health history for the maternity patient.

Biographical data

- ❏ Name
- ❏ Age
- ❏ Address
- ❏ Telephone number(s)
- ❏ Preferred language
- ❏ Religion
- ❏ Ethnicity

Family history (patient, spouse, and extended family)

- ❏ Anemia or hemoglo-binopathies
- ❏ Blood dyscrasias
- ❏ Congenital disorders
- ❏ Convulsive disorders
- ❏ Diabetes mellitus
- ❏ Gastrointestinal problems
- ❏ Genetic disorders
- ❏ Genitourinary abnormalities
- ❏ Heart disease
- ❏ Hepatitis
- ❏ Hypertension
- ❏ Infectious disease(s)
- ❏ Infertility
- ❏ Malignancies
- ❏ Mental retardation
- ❏ Metabolic or endocrine disorders
- ❏ Multiple births
- ❏ Occupational hazards
- ❏ Psychiatric disorders
- ❏ Pulmonary disease
- ❏ Radiation exposure
- ❏ Renal disease
- ❏ Sexually transmitted disease(s) (STDs)
- ❏ Social habits
- ❏ Weight disorder(s)
- ❏ Other

Patient's medical history

- ❏ Accidents
- ❏ Allergies
- ❏ Blood transfusions
- ❏ Environmental exposure(s)
- ❏ Exercise habits
- ❏ Hospitalizations or operations
- ❏ Medical treatments
- ❏ Migraines or headaches
- ❏ Nutritional assessment
- ❏ Phlebitis or varicosities
- ❏ Rheumatic fever
- ❏ Social habits: tobacco use, al-cohol intake, caffeine intake, drug use

Performing a health history *(continued)*

Gynecologic history

❏ Menstrual history: onset, last menstruation, last normal menstruation, cycle frequency, length and amount of bleeding

❏ Birth control history: type, use, success vs. failure, satisfaction with methods

❏ STDs: trichomonas, gonorrhea, syphillis, HIV or AIDS, hepatitis (A, B, or C), group B streptococcus, chlamydia, herpes, pelvic inflammatory disease

❏ Sexual preference(s) and number of partners

Obstetric history

❏ Previous pregnancies and outcomes, gravida and parity, TPAL

❏ Present pregnancy: last menstrual period, viral exposures

(such as TORCH, Parvo Virus), change in sexual activity, nausea, vomiting, concerns, fetal activity including quickening

Other

❏ Socioeconomic status, occupation, employment status, educational level

❏ Domestic violence indicators or history of abuse

❏ Travel within the past year, trips planned in the next year

❏ Concerns woman may have regarding any of the history

line data against which subsequent changes can be evaluated. (See *Nurse's guide to pregnancy assessment*, pages 56 and 57.) Follow-up visits at regular intervals throughout pregnancy allow the nurse to monitor those changes and detect potential abnormalities.

Conduct all physical examinations in a private and comfortable room, and encourage the woman to relax. Begin with the least sensitive areas of the examination, such as vital signs, height, weight, and work toward the most sensitive areas, such as abdominal palpation and pelvic examination. Work efficiently but without rushing. Drape the woman as appropriate to respect her modesty; remain alert for signs of discomfort. Explain pertinent examination steps before performing them and again as they occur.

At the initial prenatal visit a complete physical examination is done by the nurse-midwife, nurse practitioner, or doctor. A complete examination includes vital signs and a total body system check, in-

(Text continues on page 58.)

ASSESSMENT TIP

Nurse's guide to pregnancy assessment

This guide provides an overview of normal changes during pregnancy from weeks 1 through 40. The nurse can conduct ongoing, anticipatory teaching with the woman regarding all of the changes discussed below.

First trimester

Weeks 1 to 4
- Amenorrhea occurs.
- Breast changes begin. These include increased vascularization, increased size, and increased size and pigmentation of the areolae.
- Immunologic pregnancy tests are positive; radioimmunoassay test is positive a few days after implantation of fertilized ovum; urine human chorionic gonadotropin test is positive a few days after amenorrhea occurs.
- Nausea and vomiting may begin between the 4th and 6th week.

Weeks 5 to 8
- Cervical mucus plug forms.
- Uterine shape changes from pear to globular.
- Urinary frequency and urgency occur.

Weeks 9 to 12
- Leukorrhea occurs due to hyperplasia of vaginal mucosa and increased mucus production by the endocervical glands.
- Fetal heartbeat may be detected using ultrasonic stethoscope.
- Nausea, vomiting, and urinary frequency and urgency lessen.
- Uterus becomes palpable just above symphysis pubis by 12 weeks.
- Woman gains approximately 3 lb (1.4 kg) in the first trimester.
- Nasal stuffiness due to elevated estrogen levels, which cause mucosal hyperplasia.

Second trimester

Weeks 13 to 17
- Woman gains about 10 to 12 lb (4.5 to 5.4 kg) during second trimester.
- Placental souffle heard on auscultation.
- Woman's heartbeat increases approximately 10 beats between 14 and 30 weeks' gestation. Rate is maintained until 40 weeks' gestation.
- By week 16, the woman's thyroid gland enlarges by approximately 25%, and the uterine fundus is palpable halfway between the symphysis pubis and umbilicus.
- Woman recognizes fetal movements, or quickening, between 16 and 20 weeks' gestation, depending on gravidity and obesity.

Nurse's guide to pregnancy assessment (continued)

Second trimester (continued)

Weeks 18 to 22
- Uterine fundus is palpable just below the umbilicus at 20 weeks and is at the umbilicus at 22 weeks.
- Fetal heartbeats are heard with fetoscope at 20 weeks' gestation.
- Fetal rebound or ballottement is possible.
- Woman may experience heartburn, constipation, hemorrhoids, backache, leg cramps, or shortness of breath.

Weeks 23 to 27
- Umbilicus appears level with abdominal skin.
- Striae gravidarum usually become apparent.
- Uterine fundus shows evidence of increasing growth.
- Shape of uterus changes from globular to ovoid.
- Braxton Hicks contractions begin.

Third trimester

Weeks 28 to 31
- Woman gains approximately 8 to 10 lb (3.6 to 4.5 kg) in third trimester.
- Uterine fundus is one-third of the way between the umbilicus and xiphoid process.
- Fetus's outline becomes palpable.
- Fetus is very mobile and may be found in any position.

Weeks 32 to 35
- Woman may experience heartburn.
- Striae gravidarum become more evident.
- Fundal height no longer indicates gestational age.
- Uterine fundus is palpable about two-thirds of the way between the umbilicus and xiphoid process at term.
- Braxton Hicks contractions increase in frequency and intensity.
- Woman may experience shortness of breath.

Weeks 36 to 40
- Umbilicus protrudes.
- Varicosities, if present, become pronounced.
- Ankle edema becomes evident.
- Urinary frequency recurs.
- Engagement occurs.
- Mucus plug is expelled.
- Cervical effacement and dilation begin.

cluding a pelvic examination and documentation of estimated date of delivery. At each return visit, check the vital signs, take abdominal and uterine measurements, and check fetal auscultation, activity, and position. (See *Performing Leopold's Maneuvers*, pages 239 and 240.) However, each woman will have a different history and needs and the examination must be tailored to the individual pregnant woman.

Monitor uterine growth to check the correlation between fetal growth and estimated gestational age. Fundal height is the characteristic used most commonly to monitor uterine growth. (See *Measuring fundal height*.)

The nurse practitioner uses several measurements to help estimate the capacity of the woman's pelvis. Pelvimetry measurements are taken during the first physical examination; they indicate whether vaginal delivery will be possible. Typically, a pregnant woman undergoes a pelvic examination during the initial assessment and at least once during the final 4 weeks of pregnancy. Late in the pregnancy, the cervix will be soft and cervical dilation may have begun.

The nurse should continue to use the *Nurse's guide to pregnancy assessment* chart (pages 56 and 57) to determine what needs to be done, which evaluations to conduct, and the instructions to teach the patient during each particular visit.

Diagnostic studies

Diagnostic tests that reflect the woman's history and physical findings may include a variety of studies. (See *Common laboratory studies*, pages 60 and 61.) Each institution and practice has standard tests that are done on each pregnant woman. Other tests may be done based on the individual needs of a particular patient. By no means is it appropriate or cost effective to perform all of these tests for every woman.

NURSING DIAGNOSIS

After completing the health history and physical assessment, the nurse analyzes the data and formulates appropriate nursing diagnoses. As much as possible, involve the woman in determining appropriate nursing diagnoses because participation creates a sense of responsibility, retains the woman's freedom of choice, and fosters her problem-solving ability.

PLANNING AND IMPLEMENTATION

The planning phase of the nursing process begins after nursing diagnoses are made. Together, the nurse, other health care team members,

PSYCHOMOTOR SKILLS

Measuring fundal height

To monitor progressive fetal growth after 16 weeks, the practitioner can use a measuring tape to determine fundal height. This measurement is most accurate when taken the same way each time. The woman should be supine with the practitioner standing at her side. With one hand, the practitioner places the zero end of the measuring tape at the superior edge of the symphysis pubis and with the other hand pulls the tape to the top of the fundus, along the abdominal midline. The length in centimeters approximately equals gestational age in weeks.

WEEKS OF GESTATION	EXPECTED LOCATION OF FUNDAL HEIGHT
12	Level of the symphysis pubis
16	Halfway between the symphysis pubis and umbilicus
20	One to two fingerbreadths below umbilicus
24	One to two fingerbreadths above umbilicus
28 to 30	One-third of the way between umbilicus and xyphoid process (three fingerbreadths above umbilicus)
32	Two-thirds of the way between umbilicus and xyphoid process (three to four fingerbreadths below xyphoid process)
36 to 38	One fingerbreadth below xyphoid process
40	Two to three fingerbreadths below xyphoid process if lightening occurs

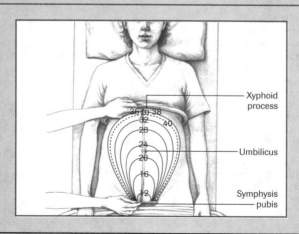

Common laboratory studies

Complete assessment data for a pregnant woman include the results of various laboratory studies. The chart below lists commonly ordered studies and describes their significance.

Blood tests

Complete blood count (CBC)
Hemoglobin and hematocrit: Screens for anemia, which may have resulted from a menstrual disorder (such as menorrhagia) or a nutritional deficiency before or during pregnancy (such as anemia).

White blood cell (WBC) count with differential: Identifies infection, which may be caused by a sexually transmitted disease (STD).

Blood type, ABO group, and antibody screens
Identifies risk of isoimmune hemolytic disease.

Rubella antibody test
Determines if the patient has antibodies to the disease because rubella infection in early pregnancy may cause fetal anomalies.

VDRL test or rapid plasma reagin (RPR) test
Screens for syphilis, which can cause congenital abnormalities if it is transmitted to a fetus.

HIV-III antibody test
Detects antibodies to the AIDS virus. Currently, the Centers for Disease Control and Prevention recommendations suggest that health care facilities offer this test to all pregnant women.

TORCH screen
Determine fetus's or mother's exposure to or status of TORCH (toxoplasmosis, other infections [chlamydia, group B beta-hemolytic streptococcus, syphilis, and varicella zoster], rubella, cytomegalovirus, and herpesvirus type 2 infections).

Urine tests

Urinalysis
Evaluates the woman's urine for infection and kidney function. Glucose, protein, and ketone evaluation is done routinely in many settings.

Urine culture and sensitivity
Identifies the organism responsible for urinary tract infection and its susceptibility to antibiotics.

Common laboratory studies *(continued)*

Other tests

Papanicolaou (Pap) test
Identifies preinvasive and invasive cervical cancer.

Wet smear
May detect infection with *Candida albicans*, *Trichomonas vaginalis*, or organisms that cause bacterial vaginosis.

Cervical culture
May detect infection with *Neisseria gonorrhoeae* or *Chlamydia trachomatis*. Confirmation of either of these STDs requires treatment for the patient and her partner.

Group B strep culture
B-strep has been implicated in preterm labor and premature rupture of membranes (PROM).

Tuberculin skin test (PPD)
Used to determine exposure to or status of virus. Do not test a woman who has active signs of TB or has been vaccinated with bacille Calmette Guérin.

Ultrasound of uterus and fetus
Used in determining gestational age, placental position and integrity, amniotic fluid volume, and fetal size, movement, and position.

Tests for hereditary disease
Used to determine if offspring are likely to have the disease. Sickle cell test helps prepare patients of African-American, Hispanic and Mediterranean descent. Tay-Sachs test is indicated for patients of Jewish or Mediterranean descent.

and the woman set goals and determine how to implement the plan of care to meet those goals.

While setting goals for the patient, the nurse has an excellent opportunity to teach the pregnant woman about pregnancy and many other self–health care activities, thus dispelling fears, empowering the patient, and increasing her sense of self-worth. During the normal antepartal period, nursing goals typically include comfort promotion for the patient, family adaptation to the addition of a new member, promoting maternal and fetal well-being, and relieving discomfort caused by physiologic changes associated with pregnancy.

Encourage family adaptation

Depending on experiences and coping abilities, family relationships may be strengthened or weakened by pregnancy. Family members may require confirmation that change is healthy or that interventions may be needed to maintain a sense of balance in the family. The nurse can help the family deal with the crisis by being supportive and by providing necessary education for childbirth and parenting.

Minimize antepartal risks

The nurse has the opportunity and responsibility to teach the patient and her family about the potential risks during the antepartal period and the care required to promote maternal and fetal well-being. In addition, without alarming the patient, the nurse should urge the patient to report immediately any of the following signs and symptoms:

- fever above 101°F (38.3°C)
- severe headache
- dizziness, blurred or double vision, spots before the eyes
- abdominal pain or cramps
- epigastric pain
- repeated vomiting
- absence of or marked decrease in fetal movement
- vaginal spotting or bleeding (brown or red)
- rush or constant leakage of fluid from the vagina
- painful urination or decreased urine output
- edema of the extremities and face
- muscle cramps or convulsions.

Nutrition

Because pregnancy depletes nutrient stores, urge the woman to maintain an adequate intake of essential nutrients during pregnancy. Assess the woman's prenatal weight and compare it to her antepartal weight; together, set up a plan to follow regarding the best dietary intake. A nutritionist can create a diet specific to the woman's particular likes and dislikes as well as specific needs for that pregnancy. Many practices use guidelines as discussed in Appendix 3, Nutritional guidelines and weight table. Remember that these are basic guidelines only. Frequently, a woman is prescribed oral multivitamins and iron supplementation to enhance a well-balanced diet and to decrease the effects of hemodilution.

Exercise

A patient should not start a new exercise regimen during pregnancy. However, a patient who exercises regularly may continue if she

(Text continues on page 71.)

Minimizing the discomforts of pregnancy

You may find that you suffer from various discomforts as your pregnancy progresses. The following list provides preventive measures that may help relieve these discomforts.

DISCOMFORT	POSSIBLE RELIEF
First trimester	
Nausea and vomiting	• Avoid smelling or eating foods that trigger nausea. • If early morning nausea occurs, eat plain crackers, dry toast, or other dry carbohydrates before getting out of bed. • Keep hard candy at the bedside. • Rise slowly from a lying or sitting position to avoid nausea. • Eat a small meal every two to three hours. • Avoid fatty or highly seasoned foods. • Eat a bedtime snack high in protein, such as cheese and crackers. • If you arise at night to urinate, drink 8 oz (237 ml) of a sweet beverage such as apple juice. • Wait for 30 minutes after a meal to drink beverages. • Consult your doctor or certified nurse-midwife (CNM) if vomiting occurs more than once daily or if it continues beyond the 16th week.
Urinary frequency and urgency	• Restrict fluids in the evening to reduce having to urinate during the night (daily intake should not be below eight 8-oz glasses). • Void every 2 to 3 hours during the day to reduce urgency and minimize the risk of urine staying in your bladder, which can lead to infection. • Consult your doctor or CNM if signs and symptoms of urinary tract infection arise, such as pain, burning, or blood in the urine.

(continued)

This teaching aid may be reproduced by office copier for distribution to women.
© 1998, Springhouse Corporation.

Minimizing the discomforts of pregnancy *(continued)*

DISCOMFORT	POSSIBLE RELIEF
First trimester *(continued)*	
Urinary frequency and urgency *(continued)*	• Perform Kegel's exercises (tightening the muscles used to control urine flow) in sets of 10 several times a day to maintain perineal tone and control over urination.
Breast tenderness or tingling	• Wear a well-fitting support bra.
Fatigue	• Rest periodically during the day. • Allow more time for sleep at night.
Increased vaginal discharge	• Clean the perineum daily. • Wear cotton-crotch underwear, which allows air circulation. • Avoid douching, which can lead to infection.
Nasal stuffiness or bleeding	• Use a cool-air vaporizer, especially while sleeping.
Excessive saliva production	• Use an astringent mouthwash regularly.
Second and third trimesters	
Heartburn	• Eat smaller meals at shorter intervals. • Avoid fried or spicy foods. • Avoid lying down immediately after eating. • Maintain adequate fluid intake (six to eight 8-oz glasses daily, 30 minutes after meals). • Avoid citrus juices. • Avoid sodium bicarbonate (baking soda) because it disrupts the sodium-potassium balance. • Use an antacid as recommended.

Minimizing the discomforts of pregnancy *(continued)*

DISCOMFORT	POSSIBLE RELIEF
Second and third trimesters *(continued)*	
Ankle edema (swelling) and varicose veins	• Avoid sitting or standing for long periods. • Avoid garters, knee-highs, or other restrictive bands around your legs. • Avoid crossing your legs. • Wear support or elastic stockings. • Exercise regularly to promote blood flow in your legs. • Elevate your feet and legs whenever possible; support your entire leg rather than simply propping up your feet. Put a telephone book under the foot of your mattress at night to elevate feet and reduce edema. • Lie down with your feet elevated several times daily.
Enlarged veins in the groin	• Support your perineum with two sanitary pads worn inside your underpants. • When elevating your legs, elevate your pelvis as well to avoid pooling of blood in the pelvic area.
Hemorrhoids	• Avoid straining when having a bowel movement. • Use ice packs, warm soaks, and topical ointments and anesthetics. • Eat foods high in fiber to avoid constipation. • Maintain adequate fluid intake (six to eight 8-oz glasses daily, preferably water). • Insert hemorrhoids and lie on one side with your knees drawn up for several minutes. • Consult your doctor or CNM if hemorrhoids feel hard, are painful, or if rectal bleeding (more than a few spots) develops.

(continued)

PATIENT TEACHING

Minimizing the discomforts of pregnancy *(continued)*

DISCOMFORT	POSSIBLE RELIEF
Second and third trimesters *(continued)*	
Constipation	• Increase fluid intake to more than eight 8-oz glasses daily, preferably water. • Increase dietary fiber by eating more fruits and vegetables. • Eat prunes, which are a natural laxative. • Exercise daily. • Take time for regular bowel movements. • Take laxatives only as prescribed by your doctor or CNM.
Backache	• Use proper body mechanics and good posture. • Perform exercises aimed at restoring body alignment. • Use leg muscles when lifting objects. • Avoid lifting heavy objects. • Recline on a bed or lounge chair to rest back muscles.
Leg cramps	• Stretch the calf muscle by standing up, pressing your foot firmly on the ground, and straightening your knee. • Stretch the calf muscle by facing a wall and doing a gentle, controlled lunge toward the wall, placing your palms flat on the wall. The calf muscle of the posterior leg will stretch slowly. Remain in this position for 30 to 60 seconds and stand up straight. Repeat the exercise on the other side. Repeat as many times as desired. • Use a warm towel to relieve discomfort.
Faintness	• Avoid sudden changes in position (lying to sitting, for example). • Avoid crowds and standing for long periods.

Minimizing the discomforts of pregnancy *(continued)*

DISCOMFORT	POSSIBLE RELIEF
Second and third trimesters *(continued)*	
Faintness *(continued)*	• Lie on one side rather than on your back. • When feeling faint, sit down and place your head between your knees.
Shortness of breath	• Use proper posture when standing. • Use pillows to support your back when sitting. • Stretch your abdomen by standing with your hands over your head and deep breathing.
Insomnia	• Lie on your left side with pillows supporting your back, under your abdomen, and between your legs. • Have a warm, caffeine-free drink or a back rub. • Perform relaxation techniques. • Attempt to alleviate distracting discomforts, such as lower back pain.
Abdominal discomfort, Braxton Hicks contractions	• Lightly massage the abdomen with a slow, circular motion. • Apply cream or lotion for dry skin. • Take a warm shower. *Caution:* Excessive heat may be harmful to the fetus.

Increasing nipple protractility

A woman who has inverted nipples can help them protrude by performing Hoffman's exercises or by wearing a special breast shield prenatally or postpartally.

Hoffman's exercises
Teach the woman to perform Hoffman's exercises by positioning her thumbs or index fingers on opposite sides of one areola, near the edge. She should then stretch the areola while pressing into the breast to help free any adhesions that could be causing the inversion. Instruct the woman to repeat the exercise on the other breast.

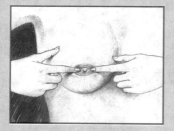 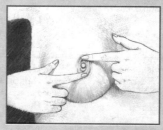

Breast shields
Breast shields, typically more successful than Hoffman's exercises, employ constant gentle pressure on the areola, gradually pushing the nipples out through a hole on the inside of each shield. Used during the third trimester and the postpartal period if necessary, breast shields should not be worn for more than a few hours at a time to minimize their drying effect.

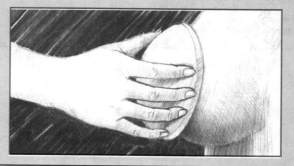

Prenatal exercises

Abdominal muscles

These exercises will strengthen your abdominal muscles, which support your back, assist with pushing during childbirth, and promote recovery after childbirth. Before doing any abdominal exercises, however, check with your doctor, nurse-midwife, or nurse practitioner.

Caution: After the 4th month of pregnancy, avoid doing exercises while lying flat on your back. Resume these exercises after your baby's birth.

Resisted knee to chest
Lie flat on your back with your knees bent and your feet flat on the floor. Start with a pelvic tilt and then lift your head toward your chest as you raise one knee toward your abdomen. Grab your leg just below the knee using both hands. Using your leg muscles, try to push the knee toward your feet while your hands pull the knee toward your abdomen. Hold for a count of 5, then release. Repeat on the opposite knee. Do this exercise 5 times at first. Build up to 10 repetitions.

Straight curl up
Lie flat on your back with your knees bent and feet flat on the floor. Bring your chin to your chest as you exhale, continuing forward for about 8˝ (20 cm). Be sure to curl your back without raising your waist. Then roll back down. Repeat this curl up 5 times at first. Build up to 10 repetitions.

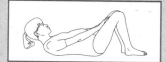

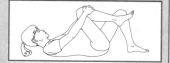

Pelvic muscles

Pelvic exercises can relieve lower back strain and promote good posture. They also will improve abdominal muscle tone, which helps support your growing uterus, deliver your baby, and protect your lower back during pregnancy and throughout life.

Pelvic floor muscles support your pelvic organs (the intestines, bladder, and uterus) and help control your urethra, vagina, and anus. During

(continued)

Prenatal exercises *(continued)*

Pelvic muscles *(continued)*

pregnancy, exercise of pelvic floor muscles can increase their strength, giving you greater control and ability to relax during delivery. They can improve healing, strength, and bladder control after childbirth.

Pelvic tilt on all fours

Position yourself on your hands and knees with your head and back parallel to the floor. Tighten your stomach muscles and tuck your buttocks under to round the lower back. Hold for a slow count of 5, then release. Do not hold your breath. Repeat this pelvic tilt 5 times at first. Build up to 10 repetitions.

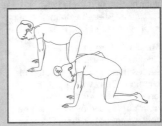

Pelvic floor or Kegel exercises

Tighten your pelvic floor muscles by squeezing the urethral and vaginal openings. (You can identify these muscles by trying to stop your urine flow.) You should feel the pelvic floor rise. Hold for a count of 5 and release. Repeat 5 times for a set, and perform a set 8 to 10 times each day.

Lower back and thigh muscles

Exercises for these muscles will help improve your posture and back stability and increase comfort during childbirth. During these exercises, be careful not to stretch too far because pain may result from separation of the pelvic joints. Because of this potential problem, the tailor stretch and extended leg stretch are optional.

Tailor (Indian style or cross-legged) sit and stretch

Sit on the floor with your knees out and ankles crossed. Hold your back erect to avoid slouching. While in this position, place your hands under your knees. Then press your knees toward the floor while resisting this movement with your hands. Hold for a count of 5, then release. Do this stretch 5 times at first. Build up to 10 repetitions.

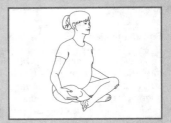

modifies her regimen. Recommendations include:
- Warm up and stretch to help prepare the joints for activity.
- Exercise for shorter intervals.
- Decrease the intensity of the exercise as pregnancy progresses.
- Avoid prolonged overheating.
- Avoid high-risk activities that require balance and coordination.
- After exercise, cool down with a period of mild activity.
- After cooling down, lie on the left side for 10 minutes to improve venous return from the extremities and promote placental perfusion.
- Wear appropriate sports shoes and a support bra.
- Stop exercising and contact the health care practitioner if any of the following occur: dizziness, shortness of breath, tingling, numbness, vaginal bleeding, or abdominal pain.

Minimize discomforts
Discomforts of pregnancy can cause varying amounts of distress for the patient and her family. Discuss the patient's comfort level at each antepartal visit and recommend appropriate interventions if she reports problems. (See *Minimizing the discomforts of pregnancy*, pages 63 to 67.)

Provide education
The nurse instructs the pregnant patient on antepartal care measures to enhance patient and fetal well-being. Education topics should include rest during and after pregnancy, breast preparation (see *Increasing nipple protractility*, page 68) clothing, personal hygiene, childbirth exercises (see *Prenatal exercises*, pages 69 and 70), fetal activity monitoring, childbirth and parenting, and sexual activity.

This information can increase a woman's compliance with and involvement in her health care. The nurse can also act as a facilitator by assisting the woman to get help as needed from a social worker or nutritionist.

EVALUATION

In this step of the nursing process, evaluate whether nursing diagnoses have been resolved and goals met. Unmet goals may require modification.

Evaluation should take place during each antepartal visit. Observe the woman and ask her about previously identified problems. Evaluation statements should reflect actions performed or outcomes achieved for each goal.

HIGH-RISK ANTEPARTAL PATIENTS

Although pregnancy is a normal biological event for most women, it represents a high-risk situation for those with conditions that threaten maternal or fetal health or conditions that interfere with normal fetal development, childbirth, or the transition to parenthood.

High-risk conditions include medical problems, such as diabetes and anemia; socioeconomic factors, such as poverty, domestic violence, and substance abuse; and age-related concerns such as childbearing during adolescence or maturity. These may be conditions that exist before conception, such as cardiac disease or infection; conditions that occur suddenly during pregnancy such as those related to trauma; or an acute condition that requires immediate surgery such as appendicitis. Other complications of pregnancy can also place the mother and fetus at risk. These include premature rupture of membranes, preterm labor and delivery, hypertensive disorders of pregnancy, and Rh incompatibility.

The high-risk antepartal patient is typically identified during an office visit. Depending on her condition, she may be followed in the home. (See *Home assessment of the high-risk prenatal patient.*)

AGE-RELATED CONCERNS

Most women give birth between ages 20 and 34. Various age-related factors can place an adolescent female (under age 19) or a mature woman (over age 35) at risk during pregnancy. (See *Age-related risks during pregnancy*, page 74 and 75.)

Adolescent female

Pregnancy poses risks to adolescents because of their physical and psychological immaturity, potential for pregnancy complications, lack of prenatal care, and lack of social and economic support systems. The pregnant adolescent may not finish school, which can eventually affect her quality of life, job opportunities and advancements, and economic stability.

Home assessment of the high-risk prenatal patient

With the changes in health care today, high-risk patients are often sent home with instructions on care and encouraged to keep scheduled visits with health care providers, a home nurse, or visiting nurse.

Because each pregnancy is different, the home care nurse must be well-versed in all areas that will be evaluated. Home visits can then be customized to evaluate a patient's obstetric and medical condition.

The following list can be used as a guide to the key areas and physical changes that should be evaluated during a home-based assessment. It can also be used to supplement any assessment tools already in use. All pertinent observations and findings should be recorded. In addition, an immediate referral system should be available if the patient's condition should warrant transfer to the office or hospital.

- ❏ Mental status, including level of orientation
- ❏ Interim history as related by the patient, including complaints and concerns
- ❏ Vital signs: temperature, pulse, respirations, and blood pressure
- ❏ Fetal status: fetal movement 8 to 10 times every three hours and fetal heart rate
- ❏ Edema: severity and degree of pitting
- ❏ Deep tendon reflexes and clonus
- ❏ Headaches: presence, severity, duration, comfort and relief measures used by patient
- ❏ Visual disturbances (such as flashing lights or spots in front of eyes), sleeping disturbances (such as increasing nightmares or inability to feel rested after sleeping), respiratory disturbances (such as shortness of breath)
- ❏ Contractions: tightening, low back pain, or vaginal pressure; gauge timing and duration
- ❏ Bleeding: location (such as vaginal or nasal), severity, duration
- ❏ Vaginal discharge vs. premature rupture of membranes
- ❏ Nausea and vomiting vs. appetite
- ❏ Exercise: evaluate when, where, and how much
- ❏ Test results: urine dipstick for glucose, ketones, and protein

Mature patient

An older woman who is healthy before pregnancy can reasonably expect a healthy pregnancy, as long as she receives appropriate antepartal care. She also may want genetic counseling and special antepartal testing for certain physiologic and psychosocial risks. Mature women are at significantly higher risk for medical problems that complicate

(Text continues on page 76.)

Age-related risks during pregnancy

The following chart compares the physical and psychosocial risks of pregnancy and their nursing considerations for adolescent and mature patients.

Adolescent

Physical risks
- Inadequate intake of protein, calories, vitamins, and minerals (especially calcium and iron) for fetal development
- Increased risk of maternal, fetal, and neonatal morbidity: pregnancy-induced hypertension (PIH), iron-deficiency anemia, cephalopelvic disproportion, sexually transmitted diseases, premature birth, low-birth-weight neonate
- Increased maternal, fetal, and neonatal mortality rate

Psychosocial risks
- Arrested psychosocial development or identity confusion
- Denial of pregnancy, leading to inability to cope
- Avoidance of visits to health care professionals
- Late or no prenatal care
- Lack of adequate information about pregnancy and health care in general
- Increased desire to sever parent or family ties caused by mistaken beliefs about pregnancy and stressors associated with pregnancy
- Difficulty assuming an adult identity
- Failure to complete the tasks of adolescence, such as finishing school
- Failure to establish a stable family
- Failure to become self-supporting
- Failure to bear a healthy neonate
- Lack of social, physical, psychological, and financial assistance during and after pregnancy and birth
- Lack of parental support
- Usurpation of mother role by maternal grandmother, producing role confusion

Nursing considerations
- Provide prenatal education about pregnancy, fetal development, birth, and infant care, preferably in a setting that makes the patient comfortable.
- Emphasize the importance of early and continual prenatal care.
- Discuss other options, such as adoption and abortion.
- Encourage the adolescent to continue formal schooling to help her mature and increase her career opportunities.
- Help the adolescent adjust to parenting through individual counseling sessions that identify and plan ways to meet her parenting needs.
- Suggest that the adolescent join in peer group discussions to seek help and suggestions from others in similar circumstances.

Age-related risks during pregnancy (continued)

Adolescent (continued)

- Help the adolescent obtain financial aid from federal and state programs, such as the Special Supplemental Food Program for Women, Infants, and Children and Aid to Families with Dependent Children.
- Promote the adolescent's self-esteem and assist with decision making and problem solving as necessary.
- Teach the adolescent to recognize and report signs of complications.
- Teach about tests that should be performed during pregnancy, their purpose, and the results.
- Arrange for counseling to discuss problems and maintain family unity.
- Arrange for other appropriate support systems, such as nutrition counseling and education counseling.
- Teach about postpartal period, birth control, and general health care follow-up.

Mature patient

Physical risks
- Increased risk of placental abruption and previa
- Increased risk of PIH
- Increased risk of diabetes
- Increased risk of thromboembolitic problems
- Increased risk of cesarean delivery
- Increased risk of fetal and neonatal mortality
- Increased risk of trisomies

Psychosocial risks
- Increased stress level as the pregnancy advances
- Difficulty adjusting to work restrictions for a career woman whose identity and self-worth are strongly tied to her work
- Isolation from family, friends, and fellow professionals
- Potential loss of support from peers, which may threaten self-esteem and satisfaction with personal and professional decisions

Nursing considerations
- Encourage the woman to maintain her health before and during the pregnancy.
- Inform the woman and her partner about genetic counseling and the availability, benefits, and risks of prenatal tests, such as amniocentesis, chorionic villus sampling, and alpha-fetoprotein testing.
- Identify the woman's concerns about the antepartal, intrapartal, postpartal, and parenting periods. Reduce her anxiety about these periods by teaching about expected changes and counseling her, as appropriate.
- Teach the woman to recognize and report signs of pregnancy complications such as PIH.

pregnancy secondary to their age. (See *Chorionic villus sampling and amniocentesis*.)

Advanced paternal age

Paternal age over 40 years old can be a factor in various chromosomal abnormalities of the fetus. For example, it can increase the relative risk for birth defects and autosomal dominant mutations (although it does not contribute to Down syndrome).

Chorionic villus sampling and amniocentesis

As a part of antepartal care, a woman may elect to have certain tests to detect genetic and other fetal abnormalities. Two commonly performed tests—chorionic villus sampling and amniocentesis—are illustrated here. Women who are Rh-negative typically receive $Rh_o(D)$ immune globulin to prevent sensitization from either procedure.

Chorionic villus sampling
Transcervical aspiration of a chorionic villus sample, as pictured at right, may also be performed transabdominally. With ultrasound as a guide, the examiner passes a sterile plastic catheter through the cervical canal into the uterus. Tissue aspirated from the developing placenta may undergo chromosomal analysis, biochemical testing, or DNA studies.

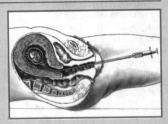

Amniocentesis
The procedure for aspirating a sample of amniotic fluid is shown here. Using ultrasound, the examiner passes a needle through the abdomen into the uterus and removes 25 to 35 ml of fluid. If fetal bleeding occurs, fetal blood cells may enter the maternal circulation, possibly causing Rh isoimmunization.

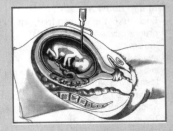

CARDIAC DISEASE

Preexisting cardiac disease is thought to place about 1% of pregnant women at risk. (See *Functional classifications for patients with cardiac disease*.) Common cardiac diseases affecting pregnant women include rheumatic heart disease, congenital heart defects, mitral valve prolapse, and peripartum cardiomyopathy. (See *Common cardiac diseases*, page 78 and 79.)

With any cardiac disorder, cardiac decompensation may occur, challenging maternal and fetal health. Rarely, it may lead to maternal or fetal death. Careful medical, obstetric, and nursing care before and during pregnancy can minimize maternal and fetal risks.

Functional classifications for patients with cardiac disease

This classification system from the New York Heart Association identifies the woman's physical response to her cardiac disease. Before conception, if possible, the woman's functional capacity should be assessed by a cardiologist to serve as a baseline. After conception, it should be reassessed and compared to the baseline to evaluate the effect of pregnancy on the woman's heart.

CLASS	DESCRIPTION
Class I Uncompromised	No limitation of physical activity; no symptoms of cardiac insufficiency; no anginal pain
Class II Slightly compromised	Slight limitation of physical activity; comfortable at rest; may experience excessive fatigue, palpitations, dyspnea, or anginal pain when engaging in ordinary physical activity
Class III Markedly compromised	Marked limitation of physical activity; comfortable at rest; experiences excessive fatigue, palpitations, dyspnea, or anginal pain with minor activity
Class IV Severely compromised	Inability to perform any physical activity without discomfort; possible symptoms of cardiac insufficiency or angina at rest; increased discomfort during activity

Common cardiac diseases

The chart below lists the clinical findings and treatments for common cardiac diseases that may affect a pregnant patient.

Rheumatic heart disease

Clinical findings
- Inadequate cardiac functioning
- Possible signs of right-sided heart failure, such as pitting dependent edema, weight gain, decreased urine output, and jugular vein distention
- Possible signs of left-sided heart failure, such as crackles, dyspnea, coughing, tachycardia, tachypnea, and decreased urine output

Treatment
- If needed, surgical correction before pregnancy through valvular repair or replacement
- After surgery, warfarin (Coumadin) or heparin (for the pregnant patient) to prevent emboli at the valve prosthesis site
- Close monitoring of the pregnant patient if functional limitations remain after surgery because pregnancy will further strain her body
- Daily supplementation with 300 mg of ferrous sulfate and 0.2 to 0.4 mg of folic acid
- Restriction of sodium intake to 2 g daily
- Depending on the patient's status, revise her medical regimen

Congenital heart defect

Clinical findings
- Minor functional limitations after mandatory surgical correction

Treatment
- Surgical repairs early in life to improve cardiac functioning
- If minor functional limitations remain after surgery, close monitoring of the patient during pregnancy
- Depending on the patient's status, revision of her medical regimen, which includes digitalis glycoside preparations, diuretics, resting in semi-Fowler's position, and proper nutrition

Mitral valve prolapse

Clinical findings
- Typically asymptomatic, but may cause arrhythmias, palpitations, light-headedness, dizziness, and fatigue

Common cardiac diseases (continued)

Mitral valve prolapse (continued)

Treatment
- Lifestyle adjustments as necessary, such as paced activity and rest periods
- Propranolol (Inderal) to treat associated tachyarrhythmias
- Close monitoring for signs of complications

Peripartum cardiomyopathy

Clinical findings
- Similar to heart failure
- Fatigue, weakness, dyspnea, orthopnea, angina, chest pain, palpitations, cough, hemoptysis, and abdominal pain

Treatment
- Digitalis glycoside preparations, diuretics, anticoagulant (heparin), furosemide (Lasix), and bed rest

Assessment

If the woman's heart maintains adequate output through all the physiologic changes of pregnancy and delivery, she should be free from cardiac complications. If she maintains her health and prevents complications, her functional classification should not change during pregnancy.

However, physiologic changes of pregnancy may cause cardiac stress, especially during the second trimester. These changes include increased plasma volume and expanded uterine vascular bed, which increase heart rate 10 to 15 beats per minute by the end of pregnancy and boost cardiac output by about 30% between 28 and 32 weeks' gestation. A woman who experiences this cardiac stress needs weekly evaluation and may require bed rest, fluid restrictions, or such drugs as digitalis glycoside preparations, diuretics, antiarrhythmics, antibiotics, or anticoagulants. Heparin is the preferred anticoagulant in pregnant women because coumadin passes through the placental barrier and may cause fetal hemorrhage and birth malformations.

Cardiac stress may intensify in the third trimester and may be severe enough to cause persistent pulmonary effects, such as crackles, tachycardia, tachypnea, dyspnea, or orthopnea. A woman who experiences severe cardiac stress should adhere to prescribed treatments and should be monitored weekly for changes in pulmonary effects. To prevent complications, she may need to be placed on bed rest.

For a woman with cardiac disease, expect to monitor the results of the complete blood count, electrolyte levels, and, if complications arise, cardiac enzyme levels.

Nursing diagnoses

After considering all the assessment findings, formulate appropriate nursing diagnoses for the patient. (See Appendix 1, NANDA taxonomy of nursing diagnoses.)

Planning and implementation

The high-risk antepartal patient may have a nursing diagnosis of *decreased cardiac output related to valvular dysfunction*. To monitor her status, obtain her vital signs and weight at each prenatal visit. Obtain an electrocardiogram periodically, as prescribed. Monitor fluid intake and output. If a patient develops pulmonary complications, be aware that a pulmonary artery catheter may be inserted to provide pulmonary pressure measurements.

Teach the patient to monitor herself and report significant changes, especially signs and symptoms of potential complications. Inform the patient of the need for regular examinations and tests. Advise her of all test results. (See *Fetal testing for high-risk antepartal patients*.)

Additionally, when caring for the high-risk antepartal patient with a cardiac condition, the nurse should:
- advise the patient to use a semi-Fowler's position to promote fetal oxygenation
- administer oxygen to the hospitalized patient as needed
- stress the importance of obtaining adequate rest and limiting sodium and fluid intake
- encourage the patient to obtain sufficient rest and recommend that she avoid crowds, drafts, and people with viral infections to decrease her risk of infection
- emphasize the importance of healthful nutrition and adherence to prescribed vitamin and iron supplementation.

Evaluation

To evaluate nursing care, determine if specific goals were achieved. The following examples illustrate some appropriate evaluation statements:
- The patient accurately described her condition and its limitation on her health.
- The patient correctly listed the signs and symptoms of complications in her condition and pregnancy.
- The patient endorsed a care regimen that affords her optimum health and functioning.

(*Text continues on page 85.*)

Fetal testing for high–risk antepartal patients

The high-risk pregnant patient may benefit from antepartal testing, which may be noninvasive or invasive. The chart below describes various antepartal tests, their purposes, timing, and nursing considerations.

Noninvasive Tests

Ultrasonography

Description

The examiner applies conducting gel to the woman's abdomen and moves a transducer across the area. The transducer transmits high-frequency sound waves to a screen, where they are displayed as images.

Purpose

- To determine position of the uterus and cervix, size and position of the developing fetus, area of placental formation, and cord insertion site
- To determine number of fetuses, congenital abnormality, ectopic pregnancy, amniotic fluid volume, and fetal organ structures
- To diagnose fetal death through absence of fetal heart sounds and fetal movements or by identifying overlapping of fetal skull sutures
- To estimate gestational age by measuring crown-rump length (CRL), fetal skull biparietal diameters (BPD), and femur length, calculating the ratios between them, and comparing these measurements and ratios to those expected for various gestational ages
- To provide a baseline that allows meaningful interpretation of fetal growth during the pregnancy

Timing

This examination may occur as early as 5 weeks after the first day of the woman's last menstrual period (LMP) to confirm pregnancy or at 20 to 24 weeks' gestation (if patient's first visit takes place at this time) to correlate the pregnancy dates with fetal gestational age and size.

Fetal movement count

Description

The woman identifies the presence and frequency of fetal movements. According to one researcher, fetal movements normally average 200/day at 20 weeks' gestation, 575/day at 32 weeks' gestation, and 282/day at term. Usually, normal fetal movement counts suggest a healthy fetus; decreased counts could indicate possible fetal compromise.

Purpose

- To provide a rough index of fetal health

Timing

At 27 weeks' gestation and later

(continued)

Fetal testing for high-risk antepartal patients *(continued)*

Noninvasive Tests *(continued)*

Biophysical profile (BPP)

Description

Through ultrasonography, the BPP evaluates fetal health by assessing five variables: fetal breathing movements, gross body movements, fetal muscle tone, reactive fetal heart rate (nonstress test [NST]), and qualitative amniotic fluid volume. Each variable receives 2 points for a normal response and 0 points for an abnormal response. A fetus scoring 8 to 10 points is considered normal with a low risk of oxygen deprivation. One scoring 6 or fewer points is at risk for asphyxia and premature birth.

Purpose
• To predict perinatal asphyxia
• To assess fetal risks
• To detect fetal anomalies

Timing
At 28 weeks' gestation or later

Nonstress test

Description

The examiner places a tocodynamometer (Toco) over the uterine fundus to record fetal movements while a Doppler ultrasound attachment, placed over the fetus's back, records the fetal heart rate (FHR). Both devices are connected to an electronic fetal monitoring machine, which records a tracing of the FHR and fetal movement. The heart rate tracing is evaluated for accelerations during fetal movement. This test may be used immediately before, after, or independently of the BPP.

Purpose
• To assess fetal well-being

Timing
At 28 weeks' gestation or later. May be repeated weekly if results are normal and daily if they are abnormal or can't be interpreted.

Nipple stimulation contraction stress test (NSCST)

Description

For the NSCST, the nurse places the Toco and Doppler as described for the NST. Warm, moist towels may be applied to nipples for several minutes to increase suppleness and blood supply. Then the woman brushes her palm across one nipple (through her clothes) until uterine contractions begin (up to 2 minutes). She stops this stimulation until the uterus relaxes, then repeats the stimulation for 2 minutes and rests for 5 minutes. Provide sufficient privacy for the woman.

Fetal testing for high-risk antepartal patients *(continued)*

Noninvasive Tests *(continued)*

Nipple stimulation contraction stress test (NSCST) *(continued)*

She repeats this cycle for 40 minutes. If no contractions occur, she brushes both nipples. An electric breast pump may be used for nipple stimulation. The FHR is monitored as for the NST, because contractions may cause changes in the FHR.

Purpose
• To evaluate the FHR in response to uterine contractions

Timing
At 30 weeks' gestation or later, usually after an NST

Fetal acoustic stimulation (FAS)
Description
This antepartal test evaluates FHR acceleration during fetal movement. An acoustical stimulus is applied to the patient's uterus several times to stimulate the fetus while the patient undergoes an NST. The FHR is recorded on an electronic fetal monitor and evaluated for accelerations.

Purpose
• Same as NST

Timing
Same as NST

Invasive Tests

Chorionic villus sampling
Description
For this early antepartal test, a sample of placental material is obtained and analyzed to detect fetal abnormalities.

Purpose
• To diagnose fetal karyotype, hemoglobinopathies (sickle cell anemia, alpha and some beta thalassemias), alpha-antitrypsin deficiency, phenylketonuria, Down syndrome, and Duchenne muscular dystrophy

Timing
From 10 to 12 weeks' gestation

Alpha-fetoprotein (AFP) test
Description
A fetal serum protein, AFP may be tested in maternal serum (MSAFP) or in amniotic fluid (AFAFP). The examiner performs venipuncture for MSAFP testing. An amniocentesis is required to determine AFAFP.

(continued)

Fetal testing for high-risk antepartal patients *(continued)*

Invasive Tests *(continued)*

Alpha-fetoprotein (AFP) test *(continued)*
Purpose
• To predict open neural tube defects (NTD), such as spina bifida, encephalocele, and anencephaly

Timing
Some researchers indicate the test should be conducted between 16 and 18 weeks after the LMP, when AFP levels are most stable. If AFP levels are elevated, another sample should be taken and tested.

Amniocentesis
Description
This test evaluates a sample of amniotic fluid aspirated transabdominally from the amniotic sac.

Purpose
• To detect genetic disorders
• To determine fetal sex and diagnose various fetal defects, including chromosomal anomalies, skeletal disorders, infections, central nervous system disorders, blood disorders, inborn errors of metabolism, miscellaneous metabolic disorders, and porphyrias
• To assess fetal health through lung maturity during the third trimester by evaluating the lecithin/sphingomyelin (L/S) ratio in the amniotic fluid

Timing
At 16 weeks' gestation to detect genetic disorder; at 30 weeks' gestation or later to assess L/S ratio

Percutaneous umbilical blood sampling (PUBS)
Description
PUBS requires intrauterine aspiration of a fetal blood sample from the umbilical artery or vein. It allows fetal transfusions in utero and access to fetal circulation for diagnostic tests and treatments.

Purpose
• One expert advises using this test to diagnose fetal blood disorders, such as coagulopathies, hemoglobinopathies, and hemophilias; fetal infections, such as rubella and toxoplasmosis; chromosomal abnormalities; isoimmunization; and metabolic disorders; also used for fetal karyotyping, fetal hypoxia evaluation; fetal therapy via transfusion or to monitor fetal drug therapy. Other experts advise using this test to treat Rh isoimmunization through blood transfusions.

Timing
After 15 weeks' gestation

Fetal testing for high–risk antepartal patients *(continued)*

Invasive Tests *(continued)*

Oxytocin contraction test

Description
Oxytocin (Pitocin) stimulates uterine contractions to evaluate FHR. The nurse applies the Toco and the Doppler as for the NST. As prescribed, the nurse performs an NST first and then begins an I.V. solution of 1,000 ml of dextrose 5% in water with 5 to 10 units of oxytocin (5 to 10 milliunits per 1 ml). An infusion pump regulates the solution, which is increased as prescribed, until three contractions occur in 10 minutes. A main I.V. line without oxytocin should also be infusing, per protocol.

Purpose
• To evaluate the FHR in response to uterine contractions

Timing
Around 30 weeks' gestation

DIABETES MELLITUS

The most common endocrine disorder in obstetrics, diabetes mellitus has seen tremendous changes in its management since the use of insulin began in the 1920s. Although the introduction of insulin therapy for diabetes has reduced fetal morbidity and mortality, the risk of congenital anomalies remains high in women with insulin-dependent diabetes mellitus (IDDM). However, strict control of maternal serum glucose levels before conception and especially during the first trimester can help reduce this risk. Careful medical and nursing care can also help the woman manage her disorder successfully and deliver a normal, healthy neonate.

Classifications
The National Diabetes Data Group classifies diabetes and other types of glucose intolerance into three groups:
• Diabetes mellitus. This disorder may take three forms: type I, insulin-dependent diabetes mellitus (IDDM); type II, non-insulin-dependent diabetes mellitus; and secondary diabetes, or diabetes resulting from another condition, such as a pancreatic, hormonal, or insulin-receptor disorder.
• Impaired glucose tolerance (IGT). Formerly called latent or borderline diabetes, this asymptomatic disorder is characterized by

normal or slightly elevated fasting levels of plasma glucose but abnormal glucose tolerance test values.
- Gestational diabetes mellitus (GDM). This disorder begins or is first diagnosed during pregnancy. A woman with GDM may be asymptomatic except for impaired glucose tolerance. GDM has great implications for pregnancy because even mild diabetes increases the risk of fetal or neonatal morbidity and mortality. GDM may resolve after childbirth or may become IGT or type I or II diabetes mellitus.

Assessment

All pregnant women experience dramatic changes in carbohydrate, lipid, and protein metabolism. Pregnancy also affects insulin needs in all women. A pregnant diabetic woman is particularly susceptible to hypoglycemia and hyperglycemia. In some women, the growing fetus stresses maternal glucose production and use, disrupting normal carbohydrate metabolism and causing GDM. Look for these four classic signs and symptoms of diabetes:
- polyuria, which develops because the renal tubules do not reabsorb water
- polydipsia, which is caused by the dehydration of polyuria
- polyphagia, which results from tissue catabolism and inadequate cellular use of glucose
- weight loss, which occurs when the body burns fat and muscle tissues for energy.

Maternal effects

The severity of the diabetes determines the degree to which the mother is affected. Uncontrolled diabetes or diabetes associated with vascular damage increases the risk of complications. However, comprehensive health care can control and lessen these risks.

Maternal effects include:
- hyperglycemia
- ketosis
- diabetic ketoacidosis
- hydramnios
- hypertension
- retinal vascular changes
- infection.

Fetal and neonatal effects

Maternal diabetes may have many adverse effects on the fetus and neonate. It increases the incidence of fetal anomalies and neonatal morbidity and predisposes the neonate to diabetes. Without careful management, it increases the risk of fetal or neonatal death.

Fetal and neonatal effects include:

- intrauterine growth retardation
- macrosomia leading to cephalopelvic disproportion, uterine dystocia, and shoulder dystocia
- lack of fetal nutrition
- hypotension leading to fetal distress
- hyperbilirubinemia
- hypoglycemia.

Diagnostic studies

Because it is believed that selective screening may miss previously undiagnosed diabetes, all pregnant women should be screened for glucose intolerance with a 1-hour (50-gram) diabetes screening test. If screening reveals glucose intolerance, further testing should be done and treatment should begin as indicated.

Urine glucose testing. Using chemically treated strips (Clinistix or Diastix), test the woman's urine for glucose and ketones at each visit. This test should not be used to determine dietary management or insulin administration. However, it should be used as a general guide to determine how well the woman's entire course is regulating her gestational diabetes.

1-hour (50-gram) diabetes screening test. This oral glucose screening test is recommended for each pregnant woman at 24 to 28 weeks' gestation. Earlier testing—and, therefore, diagnosis—may benefit a woman with a previous history of gestational diabetes. Advise the woman that she does not need to fast before the test. Inform her that a blood sample for glucose testing will be drawn 1 hour after she ingests 50 g of glucose solution. If her plasma glucose level exceeds 130 mg/dl, expect to prepare her for a 3-hour oral glucose tolerance test.

3-hour oral glucose tolerance test (OGTT). The OGTT may be used to diagnose gestational diabetes. Advise the patient to eat a high-carbohydrate diet (more than 200 g daily) for 2 days before this test. Also tell her to fast from midnight until the test time. When she arrives for her test, explain that a blood sample will be drawn to obtain a fasting glucose level. Then after she ingests 100 g of oral glucose solution, blood samples for plasma or whole blood glucose levels will be drawn at 1, 2, and 3 hours. Whole blood glucose levels are lower than plasma glucose levels, making it important to know which type of test your laboratory uses. Different professional groups use slightly different values for diagnosis with this test, but most agree that two abnormally high levels indicate that the woman has gestational diabetes mellitus. (For additional information, see *Glucose tolerance test values*, page 88.)

Glucose tolerance test values

The following are the typical normal glucose levels found in the blood at various intervals during a 3-hour glucose tolerance test.

TIME OF MEASUREMENT	WHOLE BLOOD GLUCOSE LEVEL	PLASMA GLUCOSE LEVEL
Fasting	90 mg/dl	105 mg/dl
1 hour	165 mg/dl	190 mg/dl
2 hours	145 mg/dl	165 mg/dl
3 hours	125 mg/dl	145 mg/dl

Glycosylated hemoglobin. Used to evaluate diabetic control, this test measures the percentage of glycohemoglobin in the blood, reflecting the blood glucose level during the previous 6 to 8 weeks. When performed monthly, it assists in diabetic management. Elevated glycohemoglobin levels indicate uncontrolled diabetes.

Blood glucose levels. In gestational and insulin-dependent diabetes, this test can be used to manage diabetes. It measures the blood glucose level, which is used to determine dietary changes and insulin dosage. This can often be performed with fingerstick blood samples drawn by the woman in her home. An obstetrician and endocrinologist frequently co-manage women with advanced diabetes in pregnancy along with other team members, such as a nutritionist, nurse, and social worker.

Nursing diagnoses

After considering all the assessment findings, formulate appropriate nursing diagnoses. (See Appendix 1, NANDA taxonomy of nursing diagnoses.)

Planning and implementation

For a woman with diabetes, nursing diagnoses may include ***knowledge deficit related to the effects of diabetes on pregnancy.*** For such a patient, provide information about diabetes, its effects on her and her fetus and neonate, and the treatment. Reassure her that careful management during pregnancy can prevent fetal and neonatal problems.

Also, advise her to avoid smoking because of its vasoconstrictive effects on the fetus and herself.

Teach the woman and her partner about diabetes mellitus, home glucose monitoring, and insulin, highlighting the drug's purpose, types, dosage, and administration. Also review the signs and symptoms of hypoglycemia and hyperglycemia.

Reinforce the doctor's recommendations for home glucose monitoring, insulin administration, and dietary management. Teach the patient about acceptable glucose values, and encourage her to record these levels accurately along with the amount of insulin she self-administers. A visiting nurse can help with this and act as a liaison between the woman and the obstetric team.

For the woman with gestational diabetes with a fasting plasma glucose level <105 mg/dl and a 2-hour postprandial glucose level <120 mg/dl, diabetes is typically controlled by diet. Insulin therapy is used for a woman with gestational diabetes with a fasting plasma glucose level >105 mg/dl and a 2-hour postprandial glucose level >120 mg/dl. Insulin therapy is also used when a woman has a preexisting history of diabetes controlled by an oral hyperglycemic agent or insulin. If blood glucose cannot be regulated with intermittent insulin administration, a continuous infusion pump may be used or the woman may be hospitalized during pregnancy for adjustment of insulin dosages.

Diet

A pregnant woman with IDDM should ingest 35 calories/kg of her ideal body weight, or 2,200 to 2,400 calories daily. A pregnant woman with gestational diabetes should ingest 2,000 to 2,200 calories daily. Of these calories, 20% should be from proteins, 50% to 60% from complex carbohydrates, and 25% to 30% from fats. She should divide her daily intake into three meals and three snacks, with 25% of calories ingested at breakfast, 30% at lunch, 30% at dinner, and 15% in snacks, especially at bedtime to prevent hypoglycemia during sleep. The goal of this diet is to regulate blood glucose levels, knowing that protein, carbohydrates, and fats are metabolized at different rates; prevent starvation ketosis; and provide the nutrients necessary for the mother and fetus. This can be further enhanced by having a nutritionist as an active member of the obstetric team.

Exercise and rest

A diabetic pregnant woman should exercise because it helps reduce the need for insulin and helps regulate postmeal glucose levels. If she exercised before pregnancy, she should continue her usual program. If she did not exercise before pregnancy, she should ease into nonstressful activities under her doctor's guidance.

Because muscles use glucose for energy, exercise can decrease blood glucose levels. To correct any glucose deficiencies, the patient must report pre- and post-exercise glucose levels to her doctor, who can suggest compensatory dietary or insulin dosage changes.

Encourage the diabetic woman to obtain adequate rest, including 8 to 10 hours of sleep each night and daily rest periods. To help manage the woman's condition, provide guidelines for effectively incorporating exercise into her daily regimen. The diabetic patient may have a nursing diagnosis of *altered nutrition: Less than body requirements, related to inadequate intake and excessive exercise.* Suggest that she exercise about 1 hour after meals, when her blood glucose level is elevated, and inform her that she may need the added sugar in hard candy during exercise.

Home glucose monitoring

Home glucose monitoring is an accurate, convenient way to determine the diabetic woman's response to treatment. The nurse should provide the patient with guidelines for acceptable blood glucose ranges and instruct her to report abnormal values to her doctor.

An insulin-dependent diabetic woman should monitor her glucose level four times a day, usually after fasting and meals. A woman with any other type of diabetes should monitor her blood glucose as prescribed by her doctor.

Insulin administration

The goal in diabetes treatment is to keep blood glucose levels within the normal range for pregnancy. If diet management cannot accomplish this goal, insulin therapy should be initiated. Results of home glucose monitoring enable the doctor to prescribe insulin dosages that will meet the woman's needs. Oral hypoglycemic agents cause prolonged hypoglycemia in the fetus if exposed near term and should not be used during pregnancy.

Insulin is administered subcutaneously. Typically, the woman needs a mixture of NPH and regular insulin in the morning and evening. Usually, two-thirds of the total insulin dosage is taken at breakfast, with the remaining third at dinner. Some doctors may prescribe continuous insulin therapy using an insulin pump and regular insulin to maintain blood glucose levels throughout pregnancy.

Fetal evaluation

For a diabetic woman, regular fetal evaluations are particularly important. Tests for fetal well-being typically include ultrasonography, biophysical profile, fetal movement counts, nonstress test, nipple stimulation contraction stress test, and oxytocin contraction test.

Monitor the fetus. During each prenatal visit, monitor fetal status by assessing fetal movement and fetal heart rate. A nonstress test and nipple stimulation contraction stress test may be ordered.

In addition, inform the woman and her partner about other diagnostic tests to determine fetal health, including ultrasonography, biophysical profile, oxytocin contraction test, and amniocentesis. Careful examination of the fetus assures the couple that optimum care is being provided and may relieve a patient with a nursing diagnosis of *anxiety related to maternal, fetal, and neonatal effects of diabetes*. Allow time for questions and discussion of test results.

Prevent infection

The pregnant diabetic woman is likely to have a nursing diagnosis of *risk for infection related to metabolic and vascular abnormalities*. Teach her to watch for signs of infection, such as redness, warmth, swelling, and fever. Also instruct her to look for broken skin, slow healing, bleeding, or bruises, and to report these findings to her doctor. Advise her to trim her fingernails and toenails carefully to avoid accidental cuts. Adequate circulation, especially to the lower extremities, helps decrease the risk of ulceration and infection. Teach her to maintain adequate peripheral circulation by avoiding constricting clothing on her legs.

Provide support

The high-risk antepartal patient may have a nursing diagnosis of *anxiety related to possible maternal, fetal, and neonatal effects of diabetes.* To help such a woman, identify her concerns; an experienced nurse clinician should provide psychological support and counseling during and after the pregnancy.

Clearly inform the woman of the risks for delivering a stillborn or abnormal neonate if this is anticipated. Maintain honesty and confidentiality throughout pregnancy testing and discussion of results. Initiate counseling sessions to discuss the patient's concerns and fears and provide guidance for future care. If necessary, refer her to a support group or mental health professional.

Promote compliance

To promote compliance with the medical regimen, invite the woman to participate in her health care planning. Help her identify her needs throughout the pregnancy, and encourage her to become a member of the health care team. Consider her educational level and daily schedule. Respect her judgments and incorporate her prescribed regimen into a workable daily plan.

Evaluation

To evaluate nursing care, determine if specific goals were achieved. These include maintaining safe maternal blood glucose levels, adequate assessment of fetal well-being, and good communication within the health care team.

IRON DEFICIENCY ANEMIA

This form of anemia results from an inadequate supply of iron for optimal formation of red blood cells (RBCs), producing microcytic cells. Insufficient iron stores lead to a depleted RBC mass and to a decreased concentration of hemoglobin, which normally transports oxygen throughout the body. (See *Maternal, fetal, and neonatal effects of anemias.*)

Pregnancy greatly increases the body's need for iron, and a woman may not have adequate iron stores to meet the greater need. Without iron supplementation and proper nutrition, the woman may develop iron deficiency anemia.

Assessment

A woman with iron deficiency anemia may be easily fatigued and be susceptible to infection. Other signs and symptoms may include weakness, headache, shortness of breath on exertion, anorexia, pica, irritability, and pallor. Even minimal blood loss during childbirth or postpartally may cause an already anemic person to experience difficulty, such as decreased blood pressure and dizziness.

Anemia is diagnosed by blood tests after a thorough health history and physical examination. When iron deficiency anemia is present, the hemoglobin level is below 11 g/dl, and the hematocrit drops below 32%. For an anemic woman, expect to monitor the results of hemoglobin electrophoresis, complete blood count, folic acid levels, and serum iron measurements.

Nursing diagnoses

After considering all assessment findings, formulate appropriate nursing diagnoses. (See Appendix 1, NANDA taxonomy of nursing diagnoses.)

Planning and implementation

Supplemental iron should be administered to an anemic woman before conception to maintain normal hemoglobin concentration. It should be continued during pregnancy. Daily oral doses of 200 mg of elemental iron, supplied in 1 g of ferrous sulfate or 2 g of ferrous gluconate, provide the necessary requirements for a pregnant woman

Maternal, fetal, and neonatal effects of anemias

Iron deficiency anemia, folic acid deficiency anemia, and sickle cell anemia can increase the risks of the conditions below in the mother, fetus, and neonate.

ANEMIA	MATERNAL EFFECTS	FETAL AND NEONATAL EFFECTS
Iron deficiency anemia	• Poor tissue integrity with possible damage at delivery • Antepartal or postpartal infection with impaired healing • Excessive bleeding after delivery • Fatigue, dizziness, shortness of breath, skin and mucous membrane pallor, tachycardia on exertion, pica	• Spontaneous abortion, stillbirth, or small-for-gestational-age (SGA) neonate • Intact fetal iron stores • Fetal distress from hypoxia during later pregnancy and labor, when hemoglobin fails to carry sufficient oxygen to the mother and fetus
Folic acid deficiency anemia (megaloblastic anemia, pernicious anemia)	• Fatigue, shortness of breath, dizziness, malaise, pica, skin and mucous membrane pallor, sore tongue, tachycardia on exertion • Urinary tract and other infections • GI distress, fatigue, pallor, weakness • Bleeding complications during delivery • Pancytopenia resulting from immature red blood cell production	• Spontaneous abortion and abruptio placentae complications • Possible increase in neural tube defects • Fetus may not be deficient even when the mother is severely deficient

(continued)

Maternal, fetal, and neonatal effects of anemias (continued)

ANEMIA	MATERNAL EFFECTS	FETAL AND NEONATAL EFFECTS
Sickle cell anemia (SS disease, SC disease, and S-Beta thalassemia disease)	• Pregnancy-induced hypertension • Pulmonary emboli • Pneumonia, upper respiratory infection • Urinary tract infection • Intrauterine infection • Sickle cell crises increase in frequency in pregnancy	• Abruptio placentae complications • Increased incidence of spontaneous abortions • Intrauterine growth retardation • Prematurity • SGA neonate • Compromised fetal safety that can cause stillbirth and neonatal death when patient's crises interfere with general vascular supply

with anemia. Divided doses help prevent or decrease adverse GI effects, such as nausea and constipation. Occasionally, a stool softener and high-fiber diet may be given to reduce constipation. An adequate diet, well-balanced in proteins, minerals, and vitamins, is also necessary to decrease anemia.

Teach about the disorder and its effects

Depending on the woman's disorder or problem, provide information about its treatment and care and about the effects they should produce.

This is particularly important for a woman with a nursing diagnosis of **knowledge deficit related to the effects of anemia on pregnancy.** Inform her that she should report any evidence of bleeding, especially vaginal bleeding or any exacerbated signs or symptoms of anemia. Identify special needs for the anemic woman during pregnancy, such as compliance with iron supplementation and a referral to a nutritionist.

Promote adequate nutrition

The high-risk antepartal woman may have a nursing diagnosis of **altered nutrition: Less than body requirements, related to increased need for intake of iron-rich foods.** To help such a person, evaluate her food preferences, needs, and restrictions, and estimate the nutritional value of the foods she eats. Incorporate these evaluations into a balanced diet that is economical, fulfills nutritional requirements, and meets food preferences. For any patient, outline a pattern of ideal weight gain during pregnancy.

Depending on the patient's underlying disorder, make specific dietary recommendations. To prevent or correct iron deficiency or folic acid deficiency anemia, suggest foods that are rich in these nutrients. Foods high in iron include: organ meats, dried fruits, enriched grains, egg yolk, and leafy, green vegetables. Refer the patient to a nutritionist as needed.

Evaluation

Evaluation should include patient follow-up at regular intervals during pregnancy, interim history taking to assess any changes in signs and symptoms, answering questions the woman might have, and referring the patient to a nutritionist or other team members as needed. The nurse must then decide whether the plan of care for the woman meets her needs at that time or if alterations are needed.

FOLIC ACID DEFICIENCY ANEMIA

Also known as megaloblastic anemia, or macrocytic anemia, folic acid deficiency anemia is rare in the United States. Women with multiple pregnancies and those with hemoglobinopathies or other hemolytic disorders are especially susceptible to developing folic acid deficiency anemia. Other women prone to this disorder include those with Crohn's disease, alcohol abuse, and inflammatory dermatologic disorders. (See *Maternal, fetal, and neonatal effects of anemias.*)

During pregnancy, the need for folic acid increases because of tremendous cell multiplication and accelerated erythropoiesis and deoxyribonucleic acid synthesis by the fetus and placenta. This places the pregnant woman at risk for folic acid deficiency.

Assessment

Folic acid deficiency anemia gradually produces such clinical findings as decreased hemoglobin levels despite sufficient iron intake, GI distress (including anorexia, nausea, and vomiting), fatigue, weakness, and pallor. In advanced stages, dyspnea and edema may appear.

Nursing diagnoses

After considering all assessment findings, formulate appropriate nursing diagnoses. (See Appendix 1, NANDA taxonomy of nursing diagnoses.)

Planning and implementation

To prevent folic acid deficiency anemia, the woman should take 400 mcg of folic acid daily during pregnancy. To treat anemia, she should receive 1 mg of folic acid three times daily. Because iron deficiency anemia almost always coexists with folic acid deficiency anemia, the woman also should receive iron supplements.

The nurse should encourage the woman to eat foods high in folic acid, such as legumes, nuts, whole grains, liver, yeast, and leafy, green vegetables. The nurse also should teach her to use little or no water in cooking because folic acid is a water-soluble vitamin that can be removed from foods as they cook.

Evaluation

Evaluation should include following up with the patient at regular intervals during pregnancy, interim history taking to assess any changes in signs and symptoms, answering questions the woman might have, and referring the patient to a nutritionist or other health care team members as needed. The nurse must then decide whether the plan of care for the woman meets her needs at that time or if alterations are needed.

SICKLE CELL ANEMIA

Sickle cell anemia is characterized by recurring, acute, painful, vaso-occlusive attacks known as crises. The most common types are sickle cell anemia (SS disease), sickle cell–hemoglobin C disease (SC disease), and sickle cell–beta-thalassemia disease (S-thalassemia disease). These disorders can cause organ damage and death.

Some pregnant patients with sickle cell anemia can carry to term safely if they receive careful management. However, nearly one-half of pregnancies of patients with sickle cell anemia end in spontaneous abortion (20%) or perinatal death (5.5%). Since 1972, maternal mortality from sickle cell anemia has decreased from approximately 6% to 1% because of better understanding of the disease and subsequent better care. However, many of these women do not reach childbearing age or are unable to conceive because of the disease.

Assessment

A pregnant woman with sickle cell anemia is likely to experience crises during the second half of her pregnancy, although they may occur at any time. Sickle cell crises are characterized by acute, painful, recurring vaso-occlusive attacks that affect the extremities, abdomen, chest, and vertebrae. The woman also may experience fever, dehydration, debilitation, hypertension, anemia, pulmonary problems, and osteomyelitis.

Sickle cell anemia is diagnosed through laboratory testing with hemoglobin electrophoresis, which can distinguish between sickle cell anemia and sickle cell trait.

Nursing diagnoses

After considering all assessment findings, formulate appropriate nursing diagnoses. (See Appendix 1, NANDA taxonomy of nursing diagnoses.)

Planning and implementation

Teach the patient with sickle cell anemia about precipitating factors. Advise her to maintain proper nutrition and hydration. Also instruct her to avoid crowds and individuals with colds or infections to decrease the risk of infection. Stress the importance of noting and reporting signs and symptoms of impending infection to the doctor.

During a crisis, the patient may need hydration, analgesics, and treatment for infection. Acetaminophen relieves mild pain; meperidine with a sedative controls severe pain. She also may need a transfusion of RBCs.

During a sickle cell crisis, fetal status should be monitored. Unless the woman is in labor or has an arterial oxygen level below 70 mm Hg, antepartal oxygen administration is not necessary.

For a woman with sickle cell anemia, emphasize rest and pain-relief measures, such as hot showers or warm baths.

Evaluation

To evaluate nursing care, determine if specific goals were achieved. The following examples illustrate appropriate evaluation statements:
- The woman correctly listed the signs and symptoms of complications in her condition or pregnancy.
- The woman reported a change in her condition as it occurred.

INFECTION

Throughout pregnancy, the woman should avoid infection. If infection occurs, she should be evaluated and treated promptly to prevent maternal and fetal complications. The most common or potentially harmful infections during pregnancy are TORCH (toxoplasmosis, other infections [Chlamydia, group B beta-hemolytic Streptococcus, syphilis, and varicella zoster], rubella, cytomegalovirus, and herpesvirus type 2 infections), human immunodeficiency virus (HIV), and genitourinary infections. For infection's causes, signs and symptoms, and effects, see *Maternal, fetal, and neonatal effects of infections*, pages 98 to 110.

(Text continues on page 110.)

Maternal, fetal, and neonatal effects of infections

The following chart compares the causes and maternal, fetal, and neonatal effects of TORCH, human immunodeficiency virus (HIV), and selected genitourinary infections as well as their nursing considerations. Remember that the woman's partner generally must be treated concomitantly to prevent her reinfection.

TORCH

Toxoplasmosis

Cause
Toxoplasma gondii infection is transmitted through contact with oocytes in feline feces, by eating undercooked meat that has encysted organisms, or can be acquired transplacentally only if mother is infected during pregnancy.

Signs and symptoms
Fatigue, muscle pains, sometimes lymphadenopathy; generally no signs or symptoms are present; most cases are subclinical

Possible effects
Maternal: Spontaneous abortion (with widely disseminated infection in early pregnancy) and possibly fatal complications (in an immunosuppressed patient)
Fetal and neonatal: Stillbirth, premature birth, microcephaly (abnormally small head), hydrocephaly (abnormally large head with accumulation of cerebrospinal fluid in the brain), hypotonia, seizures, coma, mental retardation, blindness, deafness, or chorioretinitis (choroidal and retinal inflammation)

Nursing considerations
- Evaluate each patient at risk for the disease to ensure prompt identification.
- Instruct the patient to cook meat thoroughly to kill bacteria.
- Teach the patient to avoid contact with cat box filler if the cat is permitted outdoors.
- Advise the patient to wear gloves while gardening and wash hands thoroughly after possible contacts. Infected cat box filler or soil may come into contact with hand cuts or contaminate food during preparation.

Other—*Chlamydia*

Cause
Chlamydia trachomatis genital infection is one of the most common sexually transmitted diseases.

Maternal, fetal, and neonatal effects of infections *(continued)*

TORCH *(continued)*

Other—*Chlamydia* *(continued)*
Signs and symptoms
Urethritis, salpingitis, mucopurulent cervicitis

Possible effects
Maternal: Pelvic inflammatory disease, dysuria, spontaneous abortion, placental inflammation, and postpartal endometritis
Fetal and neonatal: Stillbirth, premature birth, neonatal mortality; pneumonia, conjunctivitis (7 to 15 days after birth), or otitis media

Nursing considerations
- Advise the infected patient that she and her partner must be examined and treated during the same time period.
- Teach patient that chlamydia risk increases with the number of sexual partners and decreases with use of barrier contraceptives.

Other—group B beta-hemolytic *Streptococcus* infection
Cause
Group B *Streptococcus* (GBS)

Signs and symptoms
Generally asymptomatic

Possible effects
Maternal: Increased risk of septic abortion, chorioamnionitis, premature rupture of membranes (PROM), postpartal endometritis, arthritis, pyelonephritis, pneumonia, meningitis, and endocarditis
Fetal and neonatal: Stillbirth or fetal infection; group B *Streptococcus* is the leading infection associated with illness and death among newborns in the United States including neonatal infection, such as pneumonia and septicemia; invasive disease within 7 days of birth, which can lead to death; meningitis within about 24 days, which can lead to death

Nursing considerations
- Be aware that risk factors include premature labor, PROM, and a prolonged period of time between rupture of membranes and labor.
- Remind patient that failure to report signs and symptoms or to appear for prenatal visits increases the risk of undiagnosed infection.
- The Centers for Disease Control and Prevention (CDC) recommends that women who develop PROM or premature labor before 37 weeks' gestation be offered intrapartal antibiotic prophylaxis or that the women who develop one or more risk factors for GBS at the time of labor onset or rupture of membranes be provided with prophylaxis.
- Be aware that treatment before delivery significantly reduces maternal and neonatal infections.

(continued)

Maternal, fetal, and neonatal effects of infections *(continued)*

TORCH *(continued)*

Other—group B beta-hemolytic *Streptococcus* infection *(continued)*
• Be alert for signs of neonatal infection. Be prepared to notify the pediatrician and prepare for blood transfusion and I.V. antibiotic administration.

Other—syphilis
Cause
Syphilic spirochete with an incubation period of 10 to 90 days

Signs and symptoms
Chancre; nontender, enlarged inguinal lymph nodes; skin rash 6 to 8 weeks after chancre heals

Possible effects
Maternal: Second trimester spontaneous abortion, progression of disease if untreated
Fetal and neonatal: Stillbirth, premature labor and birth, congenital infection, and possible anomalies

Nursing considerations
• Treatment includes benzathine penicillin G (Bicillin). If the patient is allergic to penicillin, she may be referred for desensitization.
• Erythromycin is not used because it seldom cures fetal infection. Tetracycline is not advised due to effects on fetal teeth and bones, increased fetal inguinal hernias, and increased maternal liver toxicity.
• Advise the woman to return every month to be checked for reinfection. Expect to use quantitative nontreponemal serologic tests, such as Venereal Disease Research Laboratories and rapid plasma reagin tests.
• Advise the woman that if she receives adequate antibiotic treatment during pregnancy, the risk to her neonate is low.
• Instruct the woman to observe for signs and symptoms of premature labor. Use nonstress tests as indicated.

Other—varicella-zoster (herpes zoster, chickenpox) infection
Cause
Varicella-zoster virus

Signs and symptoms
Generally more pronounced in adults than children: fever, skin rash with vesicular and maculopapular lesions, pruritus

Possible effects
Maternal: Secondary bacterial infection of skin lesions; possible death from severe varicella pneumonia
Fetal and neonatal: Varicella in the first trimester may result in congenital abnormalities, including limb deformity, cerebral cortical atrophy, eye

Maternal, fetal, and neonatal effects of infections *(continued)*

TORCH *(continued)*

Other—varicella-zoster (herpes zoster, chickenpox) infection *(continued)*

abnormalities, cutaneous scars, mental retardation, growth retardation, and pneumonia; neonatal varicella may lead to pneumonia, encephalitis, and possibly death

Nursing considerations

- Be aware that maternal infection in the last 4 days of pregnancy and within 48 hours after delivery can cause neonatal varicella. (During its incubation period, the infection is contagious.)
- Be aware that vaccines usually are not given during pregnancy. However, varicella-zoster vaccine to pregnant women is under investigation.
- Know that 95% of adult women are immune to varicella.
- Be aware that varicella-zoster immune globulin may be given prophylactically to a pregnant woman within 3 days of exposure.

Rubella—German measles

Cause
Rubella virus

Signs and symptoms
Fever, lymphadenopathy, erythematous rash, arthralgia

Possible effects
Maternal: Possible spontaneous abortion
Fetal and neonatal: Congenital anomalies, including cardiac defects (pulmonary artery stenosis and patent ductus arteriosus), intrauterine growth retardation, deafness, cataracts, hepatitis, hepatosplenomegaly, jaundice and mental retardation; delayed effects (possibly for decades), such as insulin-dependent diabetes mellitus, sudden hearing loss, glaucoma, and encephalitis

Nursing considerations

- Advise patient to avoid contact with anyone known to have rubella.
- Be aware that a negative antibody titer indicates that the woman is not immune to rubella. An antibody titer of 1:16 or greater indicates immunity; of less than 1:8, susceptibility to rubella infection; between 1:16 and 1:8, low resistance to infection. A nonpregnant woman with low resistance should be vaccinated.
- Advise the woman to obtain rubella vaccination after she has delivered. Advise her not to become pregnant for at least 3 months after receiving the vaccine, which contains the live, attenuated virus.
- Know that infants born with congenital rubella may shed virus for months; contact threatens susceptible adults and children.

(continued)

Maternal, fetal, and neonatal effects of infections *(continued)*

TORCH *(continued)*

Cytomegalovirus infection

Cause
Cytomegalovirus (CMV)

Signs and symptoms
Generally patient is asymptomatic; 10% to 15% of cases may present a mononucleosis-like illness, including fever, lymphadenopathy, pharyngitis, and polyarthritis.

Possible effects
Maternal: Lymphocytosis, abnormal liver function tests, transplacental transmission of disease to the fetus or transmission to the neonate during vaginal delivery
Fetal and neonatal: Neonatal hepatosplenomegaly, jaundice, thrombocytopenia, microcephaly, hearing loss, mental retardation, cerebral palsy, epilepsy, blindness, microcephaly, hydrocephaly and possibly death; severe, permanent damage reported in about 10% of infected neonates

Nursing considerations
- Be aware that cytomegalovirus can be transmitted by any close contact, including kissing, breast-feeding, and sexual intercourse.
- Advise the infected woman that she should not breast-feed her neonate because the virus can be transmitted through breast milk.
- Be aware that the disease may be fatal to a fetus, although it usually is innocuous in adults and children.
- Accurate diagnosis in a pregnant woman is made by detecting cytomegalovirus in urine, noting a rise in immunoglobulin M (IgM) levels, and identifying cytomegalovirus antibodies in a serum IgM fraction.
- Advise the woman that, although no treatment exists for this infection, her doctor may prescribe immunotherapy or an antiviral agent.

Herpesvirus type 2 infection

Cause
Herpes simplex virus type 2 is transmitted generally via sexual contact

Signs and symptoms
Papular eruption with tingling, pruritus, and occasionally pain after 3- to 6-day incubation period; inguinal adenopathy; transient, flulike symptoms: occasionally, pneumonia, hepatitis, encephalitis.

Possible effects
Maternal: Discomfort from lesions during the pregnancy, increased incidence of secondary infection, and increased likelihood of cesarean delivery because virus can be transmitted to neonate during vaginal delivery

Maternal, fetal, and neonatal effects of infections (continued)

TORCH (continued)

Herpesvirus type 2 infection (continued)

Fetal and neonatal: Premature labor if virus becomes active later in pregnancy; local infection of the skin, eyes, or mucous membranes; microcephaly and other central nervous system lesion symptoms that develop after birth, such as fever or hypothermia; poor feeding, seizures, and jaundice

Nursing considerations

- Be aware that the safety of systemic acyclovir (Zovirax) in pregnant women has not been established. Therefore, acyclovir should be used only with extreme prudence in a pregnant patient.
- Expect a vaginal delivery for a woman with genital herpes but no lesions. On the day of delivery, obtain a herpesvirus culture from the woman and the neonate.
- Expect a woman with active genital lesions at the time of labor or rupture of membranes to have a cesarean section to reduce the risk of virus transmission to the neonate. Although cesarean delivery should be performed within 6 hours of membrane rupture, it may prevent neonatal herpes regardless of the duration of membrane rupture.
- For a woman with genital lesions at or near term (but before labor or membrane rupture), collect cultures every 3 to 5 days to monitor viral activity and assess appropriateness of vaginal delivery, as prescribed.
- Know that mother and neonate need not be isolated from each other, although intimacy carries a small risk (about 0.1%) of neonatal infection.
- Allow the infected mother to care for her neonate as long as she washes her hands thoroughly before and after touching the neonate.
- Reassure the woman that she may safely breast-feed her neonate because herpesvirus type 2 is not present in breast milk.
- Be aware that the incubation period is 2 to 12 days. A neonate who is symptom-free at birth may display symptoms later.
- Have patient avoid sexual activity with partner when she has lesions.

HIV infection

Cause

Human immunodeficiency viruses 1 and 2 are transmitted via sexual intercourse, blood and blood products, and breast-feeding by an infected mother to her infant

Signs and symptoms

Multiple opportunistic infections, such as herpes, tuberculosis, candidiasis, cytomegalovirus, toxoplasmosis, pneumocystis; neurologic disease is common; patient may become aware of infection through prenatal

(continued)

Maternal, fetal, and neonatal effects of infections *(continued)*

HIV infection *(continued)*

testing; may or may not have symptoms (AIDS); should not breast-feed as virus may be transmitted to neonate via breast milk

Possible effects
Maternal: Transplacental transmission of HIV to the fetus may occur or mother may transmit virus to neonate through breast-feeding; anticipate maternal grieving

Fetal and neonatal: Possibility that parents may permanently abandon the neonate in the health care facility; 25% to 50% rate of contracting HIV infection prenatally; infected neonates die within a few years

Nursing considerations
- Identify the woman at risk for HIV infection and expect serum HIV studies. Risk factors include sexual intercourse with an HIV-positive individual or a bisexual or promiscuous partner; contact with HIV-infected blood, blood products, body fluids, or used needles.
- Offer all women testing for HIV infection with the possibility of Zidovudine therapy to reduce the risk of perinatal transmission to fetus.
- Counsel the woman about disease transmission to her fetus and partner whether or not she is HIV positive so she can better understand the disease and protect herself, her baby, and her partner.
- Teach patient and staff about disease transmission to reduce its spread.
- Advise the woman not to breast-feed; virus can be transmitted to neonate via breast milk.
- Take precautionary measures to prevent contamination from infected body fluids and blood during testing and hospitalization. Alert caregivers to blood and body fluid precautions according to CDC recommendations.
- Be aware that diagnosis may be made during pregnancy. Provide support and referrals to counseling for the woman faced with the devastating information that she has a terminal illness and referral for treatment of herself and her fetus.
- Expect cord blood tests for maternal HIV antibodies at delivery, which indicate maternal infection. Also expect the neonate's blood to be tested for HIV antibodies after delivery and regularly thereafter. If the neonatal titer decreases after delivery, the neonate has not been infected. If it increases, the neonate is infected.

Hepatitis

Cause
Hepatitis viruses of various types and transmissions:
- Type A: transmitted by ingestion of contaminated food

Maternal, fetal, and neonatal effects of infections *(continued)*

Hepatitis *(continued)*

- Type B: transmitted by sexual contact
- Type C: transmitted by sexual contact
- Type D: transmitted by sexual contact
- Type E: transmitted by contact with contaminated enteric substances

Signs and symptoms
Many cases are subclinical; symptoms may include vomiting, malaise, headache, occasional low-grade fever; all precede jaundice by 1 to 2 weeks

Possible effects
Maternal: Varies with type, including: fulminant hepatitis, cirrhosis, esophageal varices with chronic hepatitis, hepatocellular carcinoma
Fetal and neonatal: Possible transplacental transmission depending on type; may need hepatitis vaccine after birth depending on type of hepatitis

Nursing considerations
- Be aware that infant may contract infection via breast-feeding, depending on type of hepatitis mother has.
- Use CDC standards on bodily secretion precautions; teach patient about transmission prevention, testing, and long-range follow-up.
- Offer support services as needed.

Genitourinary Infection

Trichomoniasis

Cause
Trichomonas vaginalis protozoan, transmitted via sexual contact

Signs and symptoms
Yellowish-greenish, foul-smelling ("fishy") vaginal discharge or pruritus; patient is frequently asymptomatic

Possible effects
Maternal: Possible PROM, postpartal endometritis
Fetal and neonatal: Neonatal pneumonia

Nursing considerations
- Know that trichomoniasis occurs in 10% to 25% of childbearing women.
- Advise the woman to avoid sexual intercourse or to use condoms.
- Reevaluate the couple to assess treatment effectiveness.
- Test for gonorrhea and chlamydia, as prescribed, which commonly accompany this infection.
- Tell the woman to practice thorough perineal hygiene.
- Inform the woman that unless her partner has been treated effectively, the infection may recur.

(continued)

Maternal, fetal, and neonatal effects of infections *(continued)*

Genitourinary Infection *(continued)*

Trichomoniasis *(continued)*

- Treat with metronidazole, but not during the first trimester, as it may be teratogenic. Metronidazole may be used later in pregnancy but only for cases unrelieved by topical clotrimazole cream.

Gonorrhea

Cause
Neisseria gonorrhoeae transmitted via sexual contact or neonatally during passage through birth canal

Signs and symptoms
Vaginal discharge, dysuria, abnormal uterine bleeding

Possible effects
Maternal: Dysuria, urinary frequency and urgency; PROM associated with peripartal fever and chorioamnionitis; possible sterility or infertility
Fetal and neonatal: Neonatal sepsis, meningitis, or arthritis; ophthalmia neonatorum (from vaginal delivery); anal, vaginal, and nasopharyngeal infection; intrauterine growth retardation (IUGR)

Nursing considerations
- Expect to conduct laboratory tests to rule out other sexually transmitted diseases (STDs) and to retest late in the third trimester.
- Treat the woman as prescribed, usually with ceftriaxone I.M., followed by erythromycin for 7 days. Also treat her partner, typically with ceftriaxone and doxycycline. Reevaluate them to assess treatment effectiveness.
- Teach about transmission prevention and the need for follow-up care.

Condylomata acuminata

Cause
Human papilloma virus is transmitted via sexual contact

Signs and symptoms
Genital warts with soft, round, pebbled surfaces (flat or mushroom-like)

Possible effects
Maternal: Increased reproduction of genital warts; possible obstruction of birth canal by warts; increased possibility of tissue laceration during delivery due to poor tissue integrity at sites
Fetal and neonatal: Epithelial tumors of mucous membranes on larynx, genital warts, and respiratory papillomatosis appear by 5 years of age

Nursing considerations
- Expect to prepare patient for cryosurgery or laser treatments to remove warts because topical podophyllum resin can be toxic to fetus.

Maternal, fetal, and neonatal effects of infections *(continued)*

Genitourinary Infection *(continued)*

Condylomata acuminata *(continued)*

- Expect vaginal delivery except when condylomata obstruct the birth canal. Because the route of transmission of the infection is unknown, routine cesarean delivery has no preventive value.
- Instruct the woman to report recurrence of warts after treatment.
- During incubation (3 to 8 months), teach patient to keep area dry and clean, prevent transmission, and treat partners as needed.

Pediculosis pubis
Cause
Phthirus pubis, the crab louse is transmitted generally via sexual contact

Signs and symptoms
Genital pruritus causing intense itching; lice or nits seen occasionally; malodorous ("fishy") vaginal discharge

Possible effects
Maternal: Skin irritation
Fetal and neonatal: Neurotoxicity if maternal condition is treated with lindane (Kwell) during pregnancy or breast-feeding

Nursing considerations
- Substitute permethrin 1% creme rinse for lindane to treat pediculosis pubis in a pregnant or breast-feeding woman.
- Teach patient about disease's high level of contagiousness.
- Incubation period is 30 days; wash clothing and bed linens appropriately.
- Treat partner(s) and household members.

Vaginitis (candidiasis)
Cause
Candida albicans yeast

Signs and symptoms
Vaginal and vulvar inflammation, pruritus, and edema; itching can lead to excoriation; white to yellow adherent vaginal plaques; vaginal discharge with occasional water ring around it on the woman's underpants

Possible effects
Maternal: Increased discomforts from vaginal itching and discharge
Fetal and neonatal: Thrush from delivery if vaginal organisms enter neonate's mouth

Nursing considerations
- Be aware that candidiasis commonly occurs in pregnant diabetic women.
- Teach the woman about candidiasis and support her during occurrences.

(continued)

Maternal, fetal, and neonatal effects of infections *(continued)*

Genitourinary Infection *(continued)*

Vaginitis (candidiasis) *(continued)*

- Expect to provide local anticandidal preparations for the woman and her partner if he has candidal balanitis.
- Tell the woman to practice thorough perineal hygiene.
- Reevaluate the woman and her partner to assess treatment effectiveness and to detect recurrence.
- Assess the neonate after delivery for signs of thrush, such as creamy, white, slightly elevated plaque inside the mouth, primarily on inner cheeks and tongue.

Scabies
Cause
Sarcoptes scabiei, a mite that burrows into the skin to lay its eggs; is transmitted generally via sexual contact or close person-to-person contact such as within very close living quarters

Signs and symptoms
Pleomorphic, pruritic rash, presence of burrows

Possible effects
Maternal: Insidious onset of pruritus that worsens at night; pleomorphic lesions and burrows on wrists, finger webs, elbows, axillae, genitals, and buttocks
Fetal and neonatal: No specific effects

Nursing considerations
- Treat with crotamiton 1% (Eurax) applied to entire body from neck down for 2 days at bedtime; wash thoroughly 24 hours after each application. Partners and close household members must be treated.
- Wash linens and clothes at 122° F (50° C) for at least 10 minutes.
- Teach woman about high level of contagiousness, treatment, and transmission prevention.

Bacterial vaginosis (BV)
Cause
Maldistribution of bacteria that compromise normal vaginal flora

Signs and symptoms
Vaginal discharge, offensive odor, presence of "clue" cells; increased risk of postpartal infection, such as metritis and chorioamnionitis; increased risk of preterm labor

Possible effects
Maternal: Increased risk of postpartal infection such as metritis and chorioamnitis; increased risk of preterm labor

Maternal, fetal, and neonatal effects of infections *(continued)*

Genitourinary Infection *(continued)*

Bacterial vaginosis *(continued)*

Fetal and neonatal: Teratogenic effects if the mother is treated with metronidazole (Flagyl) during the first trimester

Nursing considerations
- Instruct the woman to practice thorough perineal hygiene.
- Do not use metronidazole during first trimester; use prudently in the later trimesters. Evaluate patient for possibility of pregnancy before treatment begins. Ampicillin or erythromycin may be used in pregnancy. Topical metronidazole and clindamycin cream may be effective.
- Be aware that treatment of the woman's partner is not necessary because concomitant treatment does not decrease recurrence.

Pelvic inflammatory disease (PID)
Cause
Prolonged or untreated sexually transmitted diseases; intrauterine device may be a predisposing factor

Signs and symptoms
Salpingitis, fever, abdominal pain

Possible effects
Maternal: Sterility from tubal infection and scarring; other effects, depending on the infecting organism
Fetal and neonatal: Various effects, depending on the infecting organism

Nursing considerations
- Be aware that PID is rare in pregnancy because the cervical mucus plug prevents infection from ascending into the uterus. However, it may occur in the first weeks of pregnancy.
- Instruct the woman to receive antibiotic treatment and take precautions to prevent reinfection.
- Test the patient for chlamydia, herpes, and other STDs commonly associated with PID, as indicated.
- Provide additional nursing care and support referrals as needed, depending on the infecting organism.

Pyelonephritis and urinary tract infection
Cause
Predisposing factors include asymptomatic bacteriuria and renal calculi; can be caused by multiple bacteria types

Signs and symptoms
Fever, dysuria, protienuria, hematuria, flank pain, urinary frequency

(continued)

Maternal, fetal, and neonatal effects of infections *(continued)*

Genitourinary Infection *(continued)*

Pyelonephritis and urinary tract infection *(continued)*
Possible effects
Maternal: Increased genitourinary and abdominal discomfort, possible premature labor, flank pain, dysuria
Fetal and neonatal: Possible teratogenic effect if the mother is treated with sulfonamides (evidence is inconclusive); sulfonamides can cause increased free bilirubin and kernicterus if given to a neonate: do not administer to a pregnant woman near term

Nursing considerations
- Be aware that the incidence of pyelonephritis increases because of the urinary stasis that occurs during pregnancy. Those at highest risk are primigravid patients, women with difficult labors, diabetic women, and women with sickle cell anemia and sickle cell trait.
- Encourage the woman to maintain bed rest, drink plenty of fluids, and report worsening of symptoms.
- Reevaluate the woman to assess the effectiveness of treatment with antibiotics, fluids, and rest, and to detect recurrence.
- Teach the patient about need for treatment and recurrence prevention.
- Recommend urologic consultation after delivery to assess for permanent genitourinary changes caused by the infection.
- Evaluate for preterm labor and expect tocolytics, if needed.
- Assess the neonate for elevated bilirubin levels after birth.

Assessment

For a woman with an infection, laboratory data reveal antibody titers and immune status. An abnormally high white blood cell count signals infection. Cultures taken from lesions or drainage samples can be used to identify a specific infecting organism.

Nursing diagnoses

After considering all assessment findings, formulate appropriate nursing diagnoses. (See Appendix 1, NANDA taxonomy of nursing diagnoses.)

Planning and implementation

Teach the pregnant woman about the causes of infections, transmission routes, and prevention techniques. Describe the signs and symptoms of common infections and help her identify predisposing factors. Encourage her to seek medical help if she suspects infection.

Care for the woman with an infection involves all family or household members in controlling the infection, assures satisfactory health for these individuals, and protects the family caregivers. To accomplish these goals, educate the family about the infection, its risks, and preventive measures. These measures may include:

- sexual abstinence during the active phases of the disease
- use of a condom during sexual intercourse as recommended by health care professionals
- simultaneous treatment of the woman and her partner
- evaluation for reinfection, as indicated by health care professionals
- careful adherence to perineal hygiene measures
- careful attention to proper disposal of body fluids and contaminated needles
- thorough handwashing after contact with infected areas and before contact with the neonate and others.

The woman with an infection may have a nursing diagnosis of **knowledge deficit related to disease transmission and prevention.** Encourage the woman and her partner to obtain information about the disease so they can prevent transmission, and help them identify the neonate's needs as a member of their family. Also, help the couple identify ways to handle societal fears of disease transmission as applicable. Refer them for counseling as needed.

Evaluation

When evaluating the patient with an infection, appropriate evaluation statements include:

- The woman correctly described the potential effects of her condition on herself and her fetus or neonate.
- The woman and family demonstrated correct infection control measures.

DOMESTIC VIOLENCE

Domestic violence is a multifaceted social problem commonly perpetuated by ignorance, denial, social acceptance, and shame. According to recent literature reviews, half of all women in the United States will experience domestic violence in their lifetime; during pregnancy, 8% to 20% of women report abuse. In many cases, abuse increases during pregnancy or in the early postpartum period. Overall, pregnant women experience domestic violence more frequently than hypertension, gestational diabetes, or any other major antepartal complication.

In a violent relationship, the abuser sets out to slowly destroy the victim's sense of self-worth. (See *Domestic violence indicators*.) The victim feels powerless to defend herself or to change the relationship and is reluctant to discuss her fears and concerns. Additionally, health care providers are often uncomfortable asking a patient about domestic violence. The literature shows that more information will be collected about each situation if the woman is interviewed privately by a health care provider. Routine and repeated inquiry regarding domestic violence is essential. The health care provider must convey to the victim a zero tolerance attitude toward domestic violence and explain that a support network is available to help meet her needs.

Domestic violence indicators

Domestic violence is a public health problem that is only recently being implicated in poor pregnancy outcomes. It can be discovered by the alert and knowledgeable nurse who is willing to ask the correct questions in a caring, nonjudgmental way.

The three categories of domestic violence and abuse are physical abuse, emotional abuse, and financial abuse.

These can present in numerous ways; examples are listed below. Usually, there is violence or abuse in more than one category simultaneously. The one common dynamic is the need for the abuser to control the abused person in any way possible. The process is generally one that occurs slowly over time as the abuser strives to destroy the abused person's sense of self.

Physical violence can include:
- history of pushing, slapping, punching, shoving; use of weapons
- signs of battery or injury, such as bruising or burning with cigarettes
- signs of injury inconsistent with history given for a particular injury
- sexual violence including engaging in sexual acts without the woman's consent (rape); forcing the woman to watch sexual acts against her consent; making derogatory remarks about the woman's sexuality.

Emotional or psychological violence can include:
- history of emotional abuse, humiliation, or intimidation
- history of social isolation from family and friends
- history of progressive coercion and control
- reduction of patient's ego, strength, or self-worth.

Financial abuse can include:
- history of withholding money from the woman
- history of threat or loss of monetary support for woman and children
- partner's accumulation of bills in the woman's name.

Domestic violence has long been a public health problem but has only recently been implicated in poor pregnancy outcomes. Research has shown that when compared to nonabused women, abused women are twice as likely to begin prenatal care in the third trimester, four times more likely to deliver low-birth-weight babies, twice as likely to miscarry, and far more likely to abuse drugs.

Assessment
The assessment of domestic violence should be performed by a nurse educated in this area. A thorough assessment takes time, patience, and repeated inquiries for the woman to feel comfortable enough to share information about abuse. Use a nonjudgmental demeanor during this assessment.

Nursing diagnosis
After considering all assessment findings, formulate appropriate nursing diagnoses for the woman. (See Appendix 1, NANDA taxonomy of nursing diagnoses.)

Planning and implementation
The patient's choices should guide the nurse's referrals. Whether the woman decides to seek a safe house or remain with her abuser, the nurse must remain nonjudgmental and supportive. The nurse must also initiate the involvement of the entire health care team to address the violence and assist the woman and her family as necessary.

The nurse must observe for potential problems in the woman's prenatal care. These include poor maternal nutrition, poor maternal weight gain, potential low birth weight of the infant, potential intrauterine growth retardation if there is current substance abuse, and imminent physical danger to the woman. If the woman does not return for her prenatal visits, the nurse may have a visiting nurse go to the home to make an evaluation.

Evaluation
When evaluating the goals of a patient who has been diagnosed as a victim of domestic violence, appropriate evaluation statements would include:

- The woman recognizes the domestic violence in her life.
- The woman returns for follow-up appointments.
- The woman is gaining adequate weight prenatally.

SUBSTANCE ABUSE

When a pregnant woman abuses a substance such as illegal drugs or alcohol, it can affect her as well as her fetus and neonate. (See *Maternal, fetal, and neonatal effects of substance abuse.*)

Maternal risks

A pregnant substance abuser may suffer physical, psychological, social, and economic consequences. In addition, she may have a spontaneous abortion or premature delivery, or she may develop pregnancy-induced hypertension, hemorrhage, or abruptio placentae.

This patient is likely to neglect prenatal care because she fears admonishment from health care professionals, lacks the self-esteem to make personal health care a priority, or views prenatal care as unimportant and unnecessary. However, such a patient has an even greater need for care because of possible exposure to human immunodeficiency virus, sexually transmitted diseases, hepatitis, malnutrition, and infection from injection sites—as well as the risk of hypertension, antepartal bleeding, abruptio placentae, spontaneous abortion or stillbirth, and preterm labor. These factors and risks may arise from poor health, inadequate nutrition, infection, shared needles, multiple sex partners, and drug abuse and its effects.

Fetal and neonatal risks

First-trimester substance abuse has teratogenic effects on the fetus and increases the risk of spontaneous abortion. Use of cocaine may cause chromosomal abnormalities that lead to major genitourinary malformations. Cocaine has also been implicated in the occurrence of placental abruptions and neonatal withdrawal symptoms. Maternal alcohol use or abuse can lead to fetal alcohol syndrome. Maternal substance abuse also may cause problems for the neonate, including intrauterine growth retardation, premature birth, and withdrawal symptoms.

Assessment

Review the results of appropriate laboratory tests for the substance abuser. Urine drug testing provides information about the substances abused. Biophysical profile testing assists with fetal health evaluation.

Nursing diagnoses

After considering all assessment findings, formulate appropriate nursing diagnoses. (See Appendix 1, NANDA taxonomy of nursing diagnoses.)

Maternal, fetal, and neonatal effects of substance abuse

The woman who abuses controlled substances while pregnant puts her own body and that of her fetus or neonate at significant risk, as described in the chart below. The nurse should remember that illicit drug users seldom abuse just one drug. Further, the nurse should remember that these women are also at higher risk for other socioeconomic problems, such as sexually transmitted diseases, poverty, and inadequate health care.

SUBSTANCE	MATERNAL EFFECTS	FETAL AND NEONATAL EFFECTS
Depressants		
Ethanol (alcohol)	Spontaneous abortion; no safe level of intake has been determined in pregnancy	Stillbirth, intrauterine growth retardation (IUGR), short palpebral fissures, microcephaly, mild to moderate mental retardation, irritability, poor coordination, fetal alcohol syndrome
Narcotics heroin, methadone hydrochloride (Dolophine)	Spontaneous abortion, premature rupture of membranes, preterm labor, infections of the placenta, chorion, and amnion; increased risk of human immunodeficiency virus and hepatitis infections secondary to needle use (purer forms of heroin can be snorted)	Low birth weight, IUGR, withdrawal symptoms (vomiting, tremors, sneezing, increased muscle tone), seizures, respiratory distress, meconium aspiration, increased perinatal morbidity and mortality
Barbiturates phenobarbital (Luminal)	Drowsiness, lethargy, vertigo, headache, and central nervous system (CNS) depression; consider benefits and risks of use for seizure disorder in pregnancy.	CNS depression, seizures, withdrawal symptoms, hyperactivity, decreased sucking reflex, possible teratogenic effects, delayed lung maturity *(continued)*

Maternal, fetal, and neonatal effects of substance abuse *(continued)*

SUBSTANCE	MATERNAL EFFECTS	FETAL AND NEONATAL EFFECTS
Depressants *(continued)*		
Tranquilizers chlordiazepoxide (Librium), diazepam (Valium)	Overdose results in prolonged hypoxia, malnutrition, poor weight gain, cross-dependence on alcohol and barbiturates	Same as for barbiturates, plus tremors, irritability, tachypnea, poor weight gain, sudden infant death syndrome (SIDS), hypotonia, hypothermia
Mixed narcotic agonist-antagonists T's and Blues: pentazocine (Talwin) and tripelennamine (Pyribenzamine)	Addiction	Low birth weight, IUGR, withdrawal symptoms
Stimulants		
Amphetamines amphetamine sulfate (Benzedrine)	Malnutrition, possible ventricular tachycardia and asystole during obstetric anesthesia	Possible congenital abnormalities; recent studies are inconclusive
dextroamphetamine sulfate (Dexedrine)	Insufficient nutrition; serious cardiac arrhythmias, ventricular tachycardia, and withdrawal symptoms, including lethargy and profound depression	Withdrawal symptoms, low birth weight, IUGR from poor maternal nutrition, congenital heart defects
Cocaine	Vasoconstriction leading to tachycardia, arrhythmias, hypertension, dilated pupils, and muscle twitching; myocardial infarction; cardiac and respiratory arrest; increased	Stillbirth; genitourinary tract malformations including prune-belly syndrome and hydronephrosis, SIDS, depressed interactive behaviors, brain infarction, significantly

Maternal, fetal, and neonatal effects of substance abuse *(continued)*

SUBSTANCE	MATERNAL EFFECTS	FETAL AND NEONATAL EFFECTS
Stimulants *(continued)*		
Cocaine *(continued)*	spontaneous abortion, abruptio placentae, and preterm labor	increased clearing time of cocaine by fetus
Nicotine	Increased risk of neonatal mortality (20 or fewer cigarettes daily); decreased placental perfusion, abruptio placentae, placenta previa, functional anemia, premature rupture of membranes, preterm labor, spontaneous abortion (more than 20 cigarettes daily)	Reduced fetal breathing movements, small for gestational age, low birth weight, increased risk of SIDS, or possible death
Psychotropics		
Cannabis sative (marijuana)	Cross-dependence on nicotine, alcohol, and other drugs	Possible teratogenic effects, low birth weight, prematurity, potential for meconium release and for meconium aspiration
Lysergic acid diethylamide (LSD)	Possible spontaneous abortion	Possible prematurity, chromosomal damage, or anomalies

Planning and implementation

If a pregnant substance abuser seeks health care, the nurse should obtain baseline data and suggest ways to correct her health deficits. For example, the nurse may encourage her to join a drug rehabilitation program to control her substance abuse. The nurse could provide nutrition counseling and information about vitamin and iron supplements that may be prescribed. The nurse should encourage the patient to schedule appointments, as necessary, and inform her that she may have to provide a urine specimen for drug screening at each visit to identify the presence, type, and amount of the drug abused. It is imperative to try to establish a trusting, nonjudgmental and honest relationship with the woman so that she understands that the health care team wants to provide the safest and best care possible to her and her baby. The patient must also know that she is expected to play an active, honest role in her own care.

The substance abuser may have a nursing diagnosis of **knowledge deficit related to fetal effects of substance abuse.** Teach the patient about the adverse effects of various substances on her and her fetus and neonate. Inform her that her neonate will have to undergo withdrawal and will be treated as an addict after birth.

For a substance abuser with an opiate or heroin addiction, a controlled substance withdrawal method with methadone administration may be recommended. "Cold turkey" withdrawal is not recommended during pregnancy because of the risk of fetal seizures, hypoxia, and death. A patient receiving methadone also should participate in group counseling sessions. This multidisciplinary approach provides comprehensive physical, psychological, social, and economic care to the pregnant substance abuser.

Other suggestions for nursing care include:

- Teach the woman the reasons, causes, signs, and symptoms of infections related to I.V. drug abuse. Explain how such infections can harm her and her fetus.
- Promote adequate nutrition. If necessary, consult a social worker who will determine the woman's eligibility for food stamps and Women, Infants, and Children assistance.
- Provide neonatal care instruction during individual counseling sessions or peer group sessions.

Evaluation

Appropriate evaluation statements may include:

- The woman correctly described the potential effects of her condition on herself and on her fetus or neonate.
- The woman kept all appointments for prenatal care and laboratory tests.

TRAUMA OR NEED FOR SURGERY

A pregnant woman suffering from trauma or requiring surgery needs special management. The nurse must be aware of several considerations to provide appropriate patient care.

Trauma may result from accidental injury, physical abuse, or other factors. If the injury is major, it can endanger maternal and fetal health. Therefore, a pregnant woman who suffers trauma needs immediate, expert health care. (See *Effects of trauma on pregnancy*, pages 120 and 121.)

Pregnant women undergo surgery each year in the United States for such problems as ovarian cyst removal, acute appendectomy, repairs of incompetent cervix, and cholecystectomy. Surgery for nonobstetric problems can be hazardous, resulting in an increased incidence of low birth weight, preterm infants, and neonatal death within 7 days postpartum. However, the rates of congenital malformations and stillbirth do not increase.

Because of the risks, surgery should be postponed until after delivery whenever possible; instead, nonsurgical interventions should be used. These interventions may include rest, I.V. therapy, antibiotics, and gastric decompression via nasogastric tube. If these measures fail to control the woman's condition, they may be used to provide relief until further evaluation is completed and surgery can be performed.

If surgery becomes necessary, the health care team should take a multidisciplinary approach to maternal preparation. Before surgery, consultants from anesthesiology, perinatology, cardiology, and internal medicine may evaluate maternal and fetal risks to reduce the probability of complications.

Assessment

Preoperative care begins with chest X-rays and electrocardiography, which may be required if concerns exist about the woman's cardiopulmonary status. During a chest X-ray, the patient will wear a shield over her abdomen to protect the fetus from radiation.

Laboratory tests can rule out some potential problems, such as anemia and infection, and provide preoperative baseline data.

Nursing diagnoses

After considering all assessment findings, formulate appropriate nursing diagnoses. (See Appendix 1, NANDA taxonomy of nursing diagnoses.)

Planning and implementation

When surgery is needed, the risk of maternal, fetal, and neonatal morbidity and mortality depends on the stage of the pregnancy and the surgical procedure. Because controversy exists over the fetal risks of various anesthetics in the first trimester, nonemergency surgery should be postponed until the second trimester to protect against spontaneous abortion and possible teratogenic effects from medications. Even for ab-

Effects of trauma on pregnancy

Common causes of trauma during pregnancy include accidental injuries and physical injury from domestic violence and its psychological stress. The chart below details typical injuries and their effects on pregnancy.

COMMON INJURIES	EFFECTS ON PREGNANCY
Accidental injury	
• Falls resulting from too-flexible joints and a displaced center of gravity (Falls may cause fractures, but usually leave the fetus unharmed.) • Blunt abdominal trauma • Crushing injuries from vehicular accidents	• Depending on injury severity and gestational age, maternal and fetal death or fetal death from abruptio placentae • With blunt abdominal trauma during the third trimester, uterine and fetal injury • With fractured pelvis, abruptio placentae, ruptured bladder, retroperitoneal hemorrhage, and shock • With severe head trauma or internal injury hemorrhage, possible maternal death • With severe abdominal trauma sustained during a vehicular accident, uterine rupture and placental separation from the uterine wall, spontaneous membrane rupture, premature labor, and severely jeopardized fetal health or death
Physical abuse	
• Burns • Lacerations • Contusions • Fractures • Head injuries • Dislocations • Penetrating injuries, such as stab or gunshot wounds • Stress-related disorders, such as headaches, insomnia, depression, and suicidal thoughts	• In early pregnancy, possibly no fetal harm because uterus is low in abdominal cavity and protected by amniotic fluid, organs, muscles, and bony pelvis • During late pregnancy, amniotic fluid protects the fetus somewhat; however, the fetus can be harmed because the uterus is protected less by the thinner abdominal wall

Effects of trauma on pregnancy (continued)

COMMON INJURIES	EFFECTS ON PREGNANCY
Physical abuse (continued)	
	• Compromised fetal development if the woman cannot eat or has multiple areas of bleeding
• Spontaneous abortion from uterine rupture or placental abruption

dominal surgery, the second-trimester uterus should not be large enough to interfere with the operative site. Although surgery may induce premature labor, no evidence suggests that a higher incidence of fetal malformations is associated with anesthesia and surgery. (See *Nursing considerations for the pregnant patient requiring surgery*, pages 122 and 123.)

Evaluation

Appropriate evaluation statements for the patient suffering from trauma or requiring surgery may include:

- The woman correctly described the potential effects of trauma and surgery on herself and on her fetus and neonate.
- The woman's family demonstrated support and concern.
- The woman reported a change in her condition as soon as it occurred.

PREMATURE RUPTURE OF THE MEMBRANES

Premature rupture of the membranes (PROM) is rupture of the amniotic sac before onset of labor, independent of length of gestation. PROM presents a management challenge because of the divergent opinions surrounding its treatment. It is associated with maternal morbidity and mortality, primarily because of increased incidence of infection. Fetal and neonatal risks include sepsis, preterm delivery, anoxia, respiratory distress syndrome, cord prolapse, and traumatic delivery.

Nursing considerations for the pregnant patient requiring surgery

Certain physiologic changes of pregnancy may make surgery difficult. The chart below shows how to overcome these difficulties when caring for the pregnant surgical patient.

PHYSIOLOGIC CHANGE	EFFECT ON THE PATIENT	NURSING CONSIDERATIONS
Decreased gastric motility	Increased risk of gastric regurgitation and chemical pneumonitis from pulmonary aspiration of acidic gastric contents	• Expect to administer an antacid to increase gastric pH and decrease the risk of chemical pneumonitis if the patient vomits and aspirates during surgery. • Insert a nasogastric tube, as prescribed, for gastric decompression. • Assist with endotracheal intubation, rapid anesthesia induction, or use of regional anesthesia, as ordered.
Weight gain	Difficulty with endotracheal intubation	• Assist with pulmonary assessment during surgical evaluation by anesthesiologist or nurse anesthetist.
Decreased functional pulmonary residual capacity (can impair oxygenation)	Further decrease in functional capacity with general anesthesia and remaining in the supine position	• Oxygenate the patient, as ordered, before anesthesia. • Expect to place a pillow under the patient's right hip or tilt the operating room table to the left. • Expect the patient to receive regional anesthesia, which reduces hyperventilation, improves maternal oxygenation, and benefits the fetus. This is preferred in cases where increased cardiac work load is detrimental to the patient.

Nursing considerations for the pregnant patient requiring surgery *(continued)*

PHYSIOLOGIC CHANGE	EFFECT ON THE PATIENT	NURSING CONSIDERATIONS
Increased blood volume	Tolerance to blood loss during surgery	• Be aware that the pregnant patient may not need blood transfusions as readily as the nonpregnant patient.
Aortocaval compression by gravid uterus when the patient lies supine	Impaired blood circulation and perfusion	• Expect to place a pillow under the patient's right hip or tilt the operating room table to the left to displace the uterus, decreasing vessel compression and maintaining adequate perfusion to the heart, uterus, and placenta. • Use electronic fetal heart rate monitoring during and after surgery to evaluate for fetal distress, as prescribed.
Organ displacement	Difficulty in locating the appendix in a woman with appendicitis	• Be aware that after the fifth month of pregnancy the appendix lies at the iliac crest level and continues to rise above it during the last trimester.

Assessment

An in-depth, interim history can aid in the difficult diagnosis of PROM. The specific information that should be evaluated includes amount of fluid loss, inability of the woman to control loss by use of Kegel exercises, time of rupture, color of fluid, odor of fluid, and last sexual intercourse (occasionally semen is mistaken for amniotic fluid). According to some estimates, the woman who gives a history of a vaginal fluid gush that is uncontrollable is self-diagnosing PROM 90% of the time.

A pelvic examination discloses whether PROM has occurred. Using aseptic technique, a doctor, nurse-midwife, or specially prepared nurse uses a *sterile* speculum to observe the cervix. Direct observation of amniotic fluid seeping from the cervical os confirms PROM. If this fluid is not visible, the practitioner may elect to test with nitrazine paper, which will indicate an alkaline substance (such as amniotic fluid) by turning blue.

Nitrazine paper has about a 95% accuracy rate. False-negative results may occur if several hours have elapsed since rupture of the membranes or if the vaginal area has been contaminated with blood, urine, or antiseptic solutions.

Other tests to determine if fluid is amniotic include a smear on a clean slide to evaluate for ferning patterns, a study of cell structure, or a staining technique to identify fetal fat cells. However, no laboratory or clinical test is foolproof, so a combination of tests is needed for an accurate diagnosis.

Ultrasound may be useful in identifying PROM if oligohydramnios can be identified on the scan. Once a diagnosis of PROM has been confirmed, the age of the fetus must be determined. If the woman cannot remember the exact date of her last menstrual period, ultrasound can be useful in determining fetal age.

Nursing diagnoses
After gathering assessment data, the nurse reviews it carefully to identify pertinent nursing diagnoses for the patient with antepartal complications. (See Appendix 1, NANDA taxonomy of nursing diagnoses.)

Planning and implementation
An inaccurate diagnosis of PROM may lead to unnecessary induction of labor, cesarean delivery, or preterm delivery. Therefore, the doctor or nurse-midwife must make every effort to accurately diagnose the disorder. The nurse's history taking will aid significantly in this diagnosis.

Management of PROM usually involves two distinctly different approaches based on the assessment of risks to both mother and fetus. In active management, labor is induced and, if not effective, a cesarean delivery is performed. In expectant management, no action is taken to speed the onset of labor except in cases of amnionitis or fetal distress.

Because the patient may have the nursing diagnosis of *risk for infection related to PROM,* prophylactic antibiotics also may be used. Little agreement exists, however, on their value if labor begins within 24 hours after PROM.

Respiratory distress syndrome (RDS) develops in 10% to 40% of neonates born to patients with PROM. Neonatal sepsis is identified in approximately 10% of neonates and amnionitis occurs in 4% to 30%. Other neonatal complications include asphyxia, malpresentation, and cord prolapse. Maternal complications include cesarean delivery and endometritis.

Maternal mortality related to PROM is rare. Neonatal mortality is caused by RDS in 30% to 70% of cases. Anomalies account for 10% to 30% and infection for 3% to 20%.

Infections following PROM are common and potentially severe. A woman with oligohydramnios after PROM may have more clinically evident infections than one who did not have oligohydramnios. Amniocentesis for Gram stain and culture of the amniotic fluid is sometimes used to identify infection. Some problems are associated with this diagnostic tool; amniotic fluid is not always available for testing after PROM and so there can be up to a 30% false-positive rate.

Other procedures to identify infection include maternal serum C-reactive protein and fetal movement studies and frequent, accurate charting of maternal vital signs and fetal heart rate.

In cases of PROM, a neonatologist should be notified and be available at time of delivery.

Evaluation

Appropriate evaluation statements for the woman with PROM may include:

- The woman accurately describes PROM.
- The woman remained afebrile with PROM.
- The woman had spontaneous labor onset within first 24 hours after PROM.
- Fetal heart rate tracing remained reactive.

PRETERM LABOR AND DELIVERY

Preterm labor and delivery is defined as any onset of contractions or delivery, regardless of the neonate's birth weight, occurring between 20 and 37 weeks after the patient's last menses, with premature rupture of membranes or progressive cervical changes. Preterm labor and delivery has been a significant cause of perinatal morbidity and mortality for many years. Advances in technology have enhanced medical management of small neonates, but no significant decrease in low-birth-weight, preterm neonates has been documented. The problem of preterm delivery is one of the single most significant problems in obstetrical practices today. Factors relating to the patient's history, current pregnancy, and socioeconomic status can determine whether the patient is at high or low risk of preterm labor and delivery. (See *Identifying the patient at risk for preterm labor*, pages 126 and 127.)

Identifying the patient at risk for preterm labor

Several factors are reliable indicators of a patient's predisposition for preterm labor. Preterm labor starts after the beginning of the 20th week or any time thereafter until the 37th week of pregnancy. Many of these high-risk pregnancies are monitored in the home.

Any single factor from the high-risk category or any two from the low-risk category call for increased antepartal surveillance. It is important to evaluate the patient for the following criteria at the time of the initial home care visit and during follow-up care.

High-risk category

History factors

- Cone biopsy
- Uterine anomaly
- At least one therapeutic abortion during the second trimester
- Diethylstilbestrol exposure
- Preterm delivery
- Preterm labor

- Domestic violence
- Substance abuse
- Hemoglobinopathies
- One or more spontaneous abortions in the second trimester
- Incompetent cervix

Factors in current pregnancy

- Placenta previa
- Hydramnios
- Abdominal surgery or trauma
- Multiple gestation
- Urinary tract infection or pyelonephritis

- Premature rupture of membranes
- Cervical dilation
- Effacement greater than 50%
- Uterine irritability

Low-risk category

Socioeconomic factors

- Low socioeconomic status
- Age less than 19 or over 34
- Single parent
- Work outside the home

- Height: less than 5′ 3″ (160 cm)
- Weight: less than 100 lb (45 kg)
- Cigarettes: more than 10/day

History factors

- Febrile illness
- Pyelonephritis
- First trimester abortion (fewer than three)

- Less than 1 year since last delivery
- History of domestic violence or injury

HOME CARE

Identifying the patient at risk for preterm labor (continued)

Low-risk category (continued)

Factors in current pregnancy

- Bleeding after 12 weeks' gestation
- Weight gain less than 7 lb (3.2 kg) by 22 weeks
- Albuminuria
- Hypertension

- Bacteriuria
- Weight loss of 5 lb (2.3 kg)
- Febrile illness
- Fetal head engaged at 32 weeks' gestation

Assessment

The early symptoms of preterm labor are so subtle that they may be overlooked by the woman and the medical and nursing staffs. The signs and symptoms of preterm labor include:
- abdominal or menstrual-like cramps
- backache
- bleeding from vagina
- change in fetal movement
- change in urinary patterns
- change in vaginal discharge
- diarrhea
- intermittent thigh pain
- pelvic pressure
- regular uterine contractions that may be painless
- rupture of membranes.

Because the onset of preterm labor is insidious, prevention is a primary goal of obstetric care. Many of the factors contributing to preterm labor are reliable indicators and can be used to identify the woman at risk. Factors relating to the patient's history, current pregnancy, and socioeconomic status can determine whether the patient is at high or low risk for preterm labor and delivery.

Regardless of the patient's problem, assess the fundal height, weight, and vital signs and listen for the fetal heart rate. If the membranes are intact, the doctor or nurse-midwife usually will perform a digital pelvic examination of the cervix. Progressive cervical changes may indicate that labor is proceeding; nevertheless, in some cases the doctor or nurse-midwife may choose to wait for progressive cervical changes before beginning therapy.

Because urinary tract infections commonly are associated with preterm labor, a urinalysis should be performed to determine whether bacteria are present.

Nursing diagnoses

After considering all assessment findings, formulate appropriate nursing diagnoses. (See Appendix 1, NANDA taxonomy of nursing diagnoses.)

Planning and implementation

Management of preterm labor begins with bed rest in the lateral decubitus position and external uterine monitoring of fetal status.

Research has shown that hydration and sedation do not significantly reduce preterm labor. However, if the woman has an infection or is dehydrated, hydration may be indicated.

Certain hormones—serum estradiol, progesterone, and prostaglandin or its metabolites—have been studied to determine their effect on preterm labor. Serial measurements of these hormones have provided data on their fluctuation, but no relationship has been consistently demonstrated between the levels of any of these hormones and the incidence of preterm labor.

Tocolysis is a primary tool in caring for a woman with preterm labor. Tocolytic drugs are 60% to 88% effective in stopping uterine contractions; however, many of the drugs have adverse effects on both the mother and the fetus. Furthermore, little is known about the cumulative effect of tocolytic drugs used in early gestations and continued over long periods. Absolute contraindications to tocolytic drugs include severe pregnancy-induced hypertension, severe bleeding from any cause, chorioamnionitis, fetal death, a fetal anomaly that is incompatible with life, and severe fetal growth retardation. Relative contraindications include mild chronic hypertension, stable placenta previa, uncontrolled diabetes mellitus, fetal distress, and cervical dilation greater than 5 cm.

Tocolytic drugs may be used with success to inhibit labor until term, interrupt labor long enough to transport the mother to a high-risk health care facility, or inhibit labor until prenatal steroids to increase fetal lung maturity can become effective. (See *Drugs used to inhibit labor.*)

Beta-adrenergic agents inhibit the contractility of the myometrium. A woman taking one of these drugs may have a nursing diagnosis of *altered health maintenance related to skipping medication doses.* Anticipatory teaching will help the woman better understand the side effects.

Drugs used to inhibit labor

The following is a summary of the major tocolytic drugs in current clinical use.

DRUG AND MECHANISM OF ACTION	USUAL DOSAGE AND EFFICACY	NURSING IMPLICATIONS
magnesium sulfate		
Direct-acting calcium antagonist; affects uterine contractility by competing with calcium both inside and outside the cell. Recent human studies have shown no reduction in preterm labor with magnesium.	I.V. bolus of 4 g over 15 to 20 minutes followed by a constant infusion of 2 g/hour. Some physicians prescribe 4 to 5 g I.M. into each buttock in addition to the I.V. medication. Stable level is difficult to maintain because of rapid excretion through the kidneys.	• Toxicity signaled by a respiratory rate below 15 breaths/minute, hyporeflexia, and urine output below 30 ml/hr. May cause neonatal lethargy, poor sucking reflex, and delayed motility of the gastrointestinal tract. Keep 10% calcium gluconate at bedside as antidote for overdose. • Monitor respiratory rate, deep tendon reflexes, and urine output every hour.
beta-adrenergic agonists (ritodrine and terbutaline sulfate)		
Stimulate beta-adrenergic receptors, which activate an enzyme (adenylate cyclase) that converts adenosine triphosphate to adenosine monophosphate, initiating a number of reactions to prevent activation of proteins that cause myometrium to contract.	Initially, 50 to 100 mcg of ritodrine/minute by I.V. infusion, increasing by 50 mcg/minute every 10 minutes up to the minimum effective dose. Usual dose is 150 to 350 mcg/minute. Initially, 2.5 to 10 mcg of terbutaline sulfate/minute by I.V. infusion, increasing by 5 mcg/minute every 10 minutes up to a maxi-	• May cause tachycardia, hypotension, bronchial dilation, increased plasma volume, increased cardiac output, arrhythmias, myocardial ischemia, reduced urine output, restlessness, apprehension, tremulousness, hyperglycemia, hypokalemia, lactic

(continued)

Drugs used to inhibit labor (continued)

DRUG AND MECHANISM OF ACTION	USUAL DOSAGE AND EFFICACY	NURSING IMPLICATIONS
beta-adrenergic agonists (ritodrine and terbutaline sulfate) (continued)		
	mum dose of 80 mcg/minute. After contractions cease, continue the infusion for at least 12 hours.	acidosis, ketoacidosis, headache, nausea, and vomiting. • Place the patient in a left lateral position to minimize hypotension. • Monitor the maternal and fetal heart rates constantly. • Pulmonary edema is a serious but rare adverse reaction. Monitor weight and intake and output daily to detect fluid overload.
calcium antagonists (nifedipine)		
Block the flow of calcium through calcium-specific channels in the myometrial cells. Nifedipine appears to have fewer adverse effects than ritodrine and has equal or superior effect on myometrial relaxation.	Because safety and efficacy have not been established, tocolytic use of nifedipine should be limited to protocol conditions. Dangerous to use in conjunction with magnesium because it increases the toxicity rate.	• May cause facial flushing, transiently elevated heart rate, palpitations, headache, dizziness, nausea, and hypotension. *Caution:* It is not organ-specific and can affect all smooth-muscle tissue to varying degrees.

Drugs used to inhibit labor *(continued)*

DRUG AND MECHANISM OF ACTION	USUAL DOSAGE AND EFFICACY	NURSING IMPLICATIONS
prostaglandin synthetase inhibitors or nonsteroidal anti-inflammatory agents (indomethacin, salicylates, naproxen)		
Inhibit prostaglandin synthetase to decrease the amount of prostaglandins, which interfere with labor.	Dosage varies with drug used. May be used orally or rectally.	• *Fetal effects:* premature closure of ductus arteriosus. *Neonatal effects:* hyperbilirubinemia, altered platelet function, decreased urine output. *Maternal effects:* epigastric pain, rectal intolerance if suppositories are used, interference with platelet function, and increased bleeding time. • Monitor patient with ruptured membranes carefully. These drugs can mask infection through antipyretic effect.

Magnesium sulfate, used for years to treat hypertensive episodes in pregnancy, grew in popularity as a tocolytic agent. However, recent human studies have shown magnesium sulfate to have no benefits in reducing preterm labor. Absolute contraindications to magnesium sulfate include myasthenia gravis, impaired renal function, and recent myocardial infarction.

Calcium antagonists, agents that regulate the flow of calcium within the cells of the myometrium, are under investigation for use as tocolytic agents. Because calcium is the key element in uterine contractility, calcium antagonists would seem to be the perfect tocolytic agent. Multiple studies have compared their efficacy with ritodrine as a tocolytic agent and have found calcium antagonists to be successful or better than ritodrine with fewer adverse reactions to mother and fetus. However, their use for inhibiting labor continues to be experimental because of the non-specificity of the drug's absorption by all smooth muscle tissue.

Prostaglandin synthetase inhibitors—such as salicylates, indomethacin, and naproxen—relax the gravid uterus and have been linked to the incidence of postmaturity. However, their use in preventing preterm labor has been limited due to concerns about bleeding, prolonged labor, and the potential fetal and neonatal effects.

The development of a lightweight, highly sensitive tocodynamometer has allowed outpatient monitoring of uterine activity. This in-home monitoring capability is marketed by an intensive perinatal nursing service that incorporates 24-hour nurse availability, daily transmission of recorded uterine activity, weekly doctor update, and ongoing patient teaching and reinforcement of the treatment plan. An appropriate nursing diagnosis for an outpatient woman is *knowledge deficit related to at-home uterine monitoring.* These services were designed exclusively for the high-risk preterm labor group. Monitoring usually is initiated at around 20 weeks' gestation and continues until 36 weeks' gestation. It is commonly used in conjunction with tocolytic drugs. The cost of these programs varies, but many are covered under health insurance plans. The long-term cost savings may result from the decrease of intensive care nursery costs and long-term problems that may have needed intervention with a preterm delivery.

Evaluation
Examples of appropriate evaluation statements include:
- The woman has demonstrated proper use of an at-home uterine monitor.
- The woman is able to describe signs of preterm labor.

HYPERTENSIVE DISORDERS

Hypertension is the third leading cause of maternal mortality in the United States, preceded only by hemorrhage and infection. About 7% of all pregnancies are affected by hypertension; 6% to 10% of perinatal deaths are associated with hypertensive episodes. The hypertensive episode may result directly from the pregnancy itself or predate the pregnancy and result from cardiovascular or renal disease. (See *Pathophysiology of pregnancy-induced hypertension.*)

The American College of Obstetricians and Gynecologists accepts the following terms in association with gestational hypertension: chronic hypertension, preeclampsia and eclampsia, pregnancy-induced hy-

Pathophysiology of pregnancy-induced hypertension

Pregnancy-induced hypertension (PIH) initiates changes in major body systems that frequently reverse themselves postpartally. Many of the PIH-induced changes in these systems—such as tissue ischemia and fibrinogen deposits in the vessel walls—can be identified only through postmortem studies. The effects of PIH on the kidneys, liver, lungs, placenta, and cardiovascular, hematologic, and endocrine systems are described below.

Effects on kidneys
Low protein levels cause decreased plasma colloidal pressure and allow fluid to shift from intravascular to interstitial spaces, causing edema. Blood flow to the kidneys is decreased by the fluid shift. The decreased blood flow diminishes renal perfusion, triggering the release of renin that leads to the formation of angiotensin, a potent vasopressor. These work to increase the blood pressure to offset the effects of diminished renal perfusion. Renal function becomes inefficient and the glomerular filtration rate decreases. Vascular spasms also decrease glomerular blood flow and constrict glomerular capillaries. Diminished renal function results in proteinuria and increased blood urea nitrogen.

Effects on liver
Vascular spasms result in vessel compression and, in some cases, extravasation (hemorrhage under the liver and in the intra-abdominal cavity). Fibrin clots also may form from elevated plasma fibrinogen levels in gestational hypertension.

Effects on lungs
Pulmonary changes resulting from PIH include pulmonary edema and diffuse intrapulmonary bleeding, which could predispose the patient to bronchopneumonia.

Effects on placenta
Placental changes from PIH affect the uteroplacental perfusion. These changes include premature aging, degeneration and calcification of tissues, congested intervillous spaces, and arteriolar thromboses. Extensive endothelial injury has been identified in placental biopsy samples of women with PIH. The integrity of uterine vessels and coagulation capabilities were also altered in those women.

Effects on cardiovascular system
Cardiovascular changes with PIH include normal left ventricular filling pressures, high systemic vascular resistance, hyperdynamic ventricular function, increased cardiac output, and hemoconcentration. *(continued)*

Pathophysiology of pregnancy-induced hypertension (continued)

Effects on hematologic system

PIH can be complicated by hematologic changes including thrombocytopenia, a decrease in some clotting factors, and erythrocytic changes. Disseminated intravascular coagulation (DIC) may play a dominant role in the pathogenesis of PIH. Despite ongoing research, the causes of all of these problems continue to be unknown.

Effects on endocrine and metabolic systems

In PIH some endocrine levels are at normal or below prepregnant levels and do not function as effectively. For example, low aldosterone levels do not increase sodium excretion as would be assumed. Endocrine levels play an unknown role in the development of edema.

pertension (PIH), chronic hypertension with superimposed preeclampsia, and transient hypertension.

Chronic hypertension is present and observable before the pregnancy and is diagnosed by week 20 of gestation or extends 42 days after delivery. Chronic hypertensive disease may occur alone or with superimposed PIH.

PIH is characterized by hypertension, proteinuria, and edema. It has two basic forms: preeclampsia (a nonconvulsive form marked by the onset of acute hypertension after 20 weeks' gestation) and eclampsia (a convulsive form that occurs between 20 weeks' gestation and the end of the first postpartal week). This syndrome may develop at any point after 20 weeks' gestation or in the early postpartal period. Hypertension before 20 weeks' gestation is usually associated with gestational trophoblastic disease. Typically, the syndrome appears in the last trimester and disappears after 42 postpartal days. PIH may be difficult to distinguish from hypertensive states that predate the pregnancy. In addition, a definitive diagnosis of PIH may be impossible unless the woman's blood pressure returns to baseline after pregnancy. Severe preeclampsia-eclampsia may be seriously complicated by a syndrome that is given the acronym HELLP. (See *H.E.L.L.P. syndrome.*)

Assessment

Question the patient with a hypertensive disorder about the length of her pregnancy; PIH typically occurs after 20 weeks' gestation. Ask if in a previous pregnancy she had elevated blood pressure, proteinuria, or

H.E.L.L.P. syndrome

HELLP is a group of signs and symptoms that include hemolysis (H), elevated liver enzymes (EL), and low platelet count (LP). The etiology of this condition is poorly understood and there does not appear to be a precipitating cause. Both high maternal mortality rate (ranges up to 24%) and perinatal mortality rate (ranges reported from 17.7% to 60%) have been reported in patients exhibiting this syndrome.

Maternal complications resulting from this syndrome can include disseminated intravascular clotting, abruptio placentae, acute renal failure, pulmonary edema, and ruptured liver hematoma. Abruptio placentae, intrauterine asphyxia, and extreme prematurity are cited as the primary causes of perinatal death. One-third of these infants are severely growth-restricted in utero.

Signs and symptoms and predisposing factors include preeclampsia or eclampsia; severe upper right quadrant pain from hepatic subcapsular hematoma (1%); placental abruption (7%); acute renal failure (7%); pulmonary edema (6%) and intrauterine growth retardation/small for gestational age.

The only effective treatment is prompt delivery. These severely compromised women require tertiary care and aggressive medical management to ensure a successful outcome.

---

edema in her face, hands, feet, or legs. Ask her if she has vascular spasms, headaches, epigastric pain, or visual disturbances. Evaluate for factors that predispose a woman to PIH:

- Primigravidity. Most women who develop PIH are pregnant for the first time. The incidence is especially high in those under age 17 or over age 40. Women over 40 years old have a threefold incidence of PIH over women 20 to 30 years old.
- Multiple gestation. The incidence of PIH increases with the number of fetuses.
- Vascular disease. Diabetes mellitus, hypertensive renal disease, or essential hypertension are associated with PIH.
- Gestational trophoblastic disease (GTD). This can be divided into two groups: hydatidiform mole and gestational trophoblastic neoplasia. The hypertensive syndrome usually appears before 20 weeks' gestation if associated with GTD.
- PIH susceptibility. This vulnerability may be due to a single recessive gene.
- Dietary calcium deficiencies. There is a decreased incidence of PIH with calcium supplementation.

Physical examination will disclose the three classic signs of PIH: elevated blood pressure, proteinuria, and facial or generalized edema of the extremities.

Evaluate the woman for edema in her legs, hands, and face. To assess for edema, depress the woman's skin over a bony prominence, such as the shin bone. In pitting edema, a depression remains in the skin and subcutaneous tissue after the pressure has been removed. The depth of the depression indicates the degree of pitting, which is classified as 1+, 2+, 3+, or 4+. A minor depression that disappears rather quickly indicates 1+ pitting; 4+ indicates a deep depression (approximately 2 cm) that remains for an extended period.

When assessing a woman with preeclampsia, weigh her daily, measure urine output every 8 to 12 hours or more frequently as necessary, and assess for proteinuria using a reagent strip. Also assess for other indicators of PIH.

Assessment of deep-tendon reflexes may indicate hypo- or hyperreflexia. Elicit the patellar, biceps, and ankle reflexes. Reflexes should be checked every 4 to 8 hours, depending on the woman's condition.

Nursing diagnoses
After considering all assessment findings, formulate appropriate nursing diagnoses. (See Appendix 1, NANDA taxonomy of nursing diagnoses.)

Planning and implementation
Bed rest is prescribed for the woman with a hypertensive disorder. Instruct her to assume a left lateral position to increase renal and uterine perfusion. Increased renal perfusion facilitates diuresis. Other positions may compromise renal and uterine blood flow through compression of the vena cava and aorta. (See *Drugs used to treat pregnancy-induced hypertension.*)

Mild preeclampsia
Nursing care is aimed at improving or stabilizing the woman. The woman may remain at home as long as edema and proteinuria do not increase. A member of the health care team must assess the woman at least weekly to determine changes in her condition. As term approaches, data about fetal maturity and cervical status are required in case labor must be induced. For a nursing diagnosis of **knowledge deficit related to hypertensive condition**, teach the woman to keep an accurate daily record of weight and intake and output. She should report a weight gain of more than 1 lb (0.45 kg)/day. In addition, carefully explain to the woman and her family the signs that indicate a deterioration in her condition, such as severe headache, rapid rise in

Drugs used to treat pregnancy-induced hypertension

The major drugs used to treat pregnancy-induced hypertension are highlighted below.

DRUG AND MECHANISM OF ACTION	USUAL DOSAGE	NURSING IMPLICATIONS
methyldopa (Aldomet)		
Stimulates central inhibitory alpha-adrenergic receptors; reduces plasma renin activity	Oral: 250 mg b.i.d. to t.i.d., may increase to 500 mg to 2 g daily in two to four doses 250 to 500 mg every 6 hours	• Drug may cause false-positive direct Coombs' test result, sodium retention, constipation, or drowsiness.
propranolol hydrochloride (Inderal)		
Nonselective beta-adrenergic blocking agent; principally affects myocardial (beta$_1$), bronchial, and vascular smooth-muscle (beta$_2$) receptors; may block renin release	Initial oral: 40 mg b.i.d. Maintenance oral: 120 to 240 mg per day divided b.i.d. or t.i.d.	• Drug may cause bradycardia, hypotension, short-term memory loss, emotional lability, nausea, vomiting, or dry mouth. • Drug may potentiate effects of insulin; effects potentiated by furosemide.
magnesium sulfate		
Anticonvulsant; prevents and controls seizures in preeclampsia and eclampsia	I.M.: 4 to 5 g of 50% solution in alternate buttocks I.V.: 4 g in D$_5$W; follow with continuous infusion of 1 to 2 g per hour for maintenance	• Drug may cause hypotension, drowsiness, sweating, absent or diminished reflexes, oliguria, respiratory paralysis. • Observe deep tendon reflexes every 4 hours. If absent, discontinue medication and notify doctor

Drugs used to treat pregnancy-induced hypertension (continued)

DRUG AND MECHANISM OF ACTION	USUAL DOSAGE	NURSING IMPLICATIONS
magnesium sulfate (continued)		
		immediately. Check vital signs regularly, especially respiratory rate, based on health care facility protocol. • Check urine output hourly; it must be no less than 30 ml per hour.
labetolol (Trandate, Normodyne)		
Nonselective beta-adrenergic blocking agent	Initial oral: 200 mg/day in two doses Maintenance: 400 to 800 mg/day in two doses	• Drug may cause orthostatic hypotension and dizziness. • Check hourly urine output. If below 30 ml per hour, notify doctor.
atenolol (Tenormin)		
Selective inhibition of cardiac and lipolytic beta-adrenergic receptors	Oral: 25 to 50 mg/day; may increase to 100 mg/day	• Drug may cause bradycardia, hypotension, heart failure. • Teach patient to take drug at regular time every day. Monitor blood pressure frequently. • Fetal effects of drug: growth restricted fetus; fetal heart rate can have ominous pattern during labor.

blood pressure, epigastric pain, hyperreflexia, edema, decreased urine output, or visual disturbances. Instruct her to report such signs to the doctor immediately. The patient may have a nursing diagnosis of *impaired mobility related to prescribed bed rest* or *constipation related to bed rest.* She must remain on bed rest and maintain a well-balanced, adequate protein and high-fiber diet. Protein requirements are 70 to 80 g of protein/day (1 g/kg of body weight/day). The diet must contain adequate fiber and fluids because limited exercise can cause constipation.

The prescribed regimen may become boring and stressful for the woman. Family members need to be involved because home management and child care must be assumed by someone else for the remainder of the pregnancy. Diversion is necessary for both the woman and young children in the family. Preschoolers cannot understand why their mother stays in bed all day. Ensure that the woman and her family understand all aspects of the regimen and why they are necessary. A nursing diagnosis of *ineffective family coping: Compromised, related to prolonged bed rest of the mother* may be appropriate in this situation.

Severe preeclampsia

Treatment includes bed rest in a left lateral position. Keep the environment quiet, with minimal stimulation and dim lighting, and follow these procedures:

- Assess vital signs and deep-tendon reflexes at least every 4 hours but generally more often per facility protocol. Record weight daily; measure urine output every 1 to 4 hours according to the woman's status.
- Perform ocular fundoscopic examinations daily to detect arteriolar spasms, edema, and hemorrhage. Administer sedatives as prescribed. Use a fetal and uterine contraction monitor for signs of labor and fetal well-being.
- If the woman's condition improves within 3 to 5 days (for example, if urine output increases or weight decreases by 4.4 lb (2 kg) or more), further therapy will depend on the gestational age of the fetus. If the fetus is at 38 weeks' gestation or less, the woman can be discharged to home care. Instruct her to record the frequency of fetal movement for 1-hour periods, two to three times daily, and to report any decreases.

The doctor may choose delivery if the patient's condition does not improve, hyperreflexia occurs, the fetus is at 38 weeks' gestation or more, or the lecithin/sphingomyelin ratio is appropriate.

Nursing care for the woman with severe preeclampsia aims to:
- prevent eclamptic seizures
- facilitate maternal survival with minimal morbidity

- promote the birth of as mature a neonate as possible
- eliminate significant postdelivery complications.

Continue to provide the same monitoring and care that the patient received before she was hospitalized. In addition, prepare emergency equipment as soon as the woman is admitted in case eclampsia occurs. Emergency equipment should include medications, suctioning apparatus, and, in some cases, padded side rails on the patient's bed.

Keep emergency anticonvulsant and antihypertensive medications available. These include magnesium sulfate, methyldopa, hydralazine, and propranolol hydrochloride. Be aware of the mechanism of action, usual dosage, and special considerations for each of these medications.

Eclampsia

Eclampsia is a complication of PIH. Hyperreflexia is common just before seizures in the patient with preeclampsia. It is preceded by the signs of severe preeclampsia and one or both of the following:

- tonic and clonic seizures
- hypertensive crisis, in which elevated blood pressure increases the patient's chances of developing a cerebrovascular accident or shock

Tonic-clonic seizures are followed by hypotension and collapse and, in many cases, nystagmus, muscle twitching, and coma. Oliguria or anuria also may occur. Disorientation and amnesia delay immediate recovery.

The nurse's first priority during seizures is to ensure a patent airway, then to provide adequate oxygenation and alert the doctor immediately.

Evaluation

Appropriate evaluation statements include:

- The woman with mild preeclampsia shows a 2-lb (0.9 kg) weight gain, no proteinuria, and a diastolic blood pressure of 84 mm Hg this visit.
- The woman kept all appointments for prenatal care and laboratory tests.
- The woman reported a change in her condition as soon as it occurred.
- The woman's family demonstrated support and concern.

RH INCOMPATIBILITY

Hemolytic disease of the newborn, also called erythroblastosis fetalis, is a progressive disorder of the fetal blood and blood-forming organs characterized by hemolytic anemia and hyperbilirubinemia. Erythroblastosis fetalis results from the transfer of red blood cell (RBC)-destroying antibodies from the mother to the fetus. (See *Other RBC antigen incompatibilities.*)

The more severe forms of isoimmune hemolytic disease are associated with $Rh_o(D)$ group incompatibility. Before prophylactic $Rh_o(D)$ human immunoglobulin (RhIg) became available in 1968, this disease occurred in 0.5% to 1% of all term pregnancies in North America. Since immunization with RhIg began, however, the incidence of severe hemolytic disease of the newborn has been reduced drastically.

Assessment

Gather data focusing on previous pregnancies including history of previous blood transfusion, history of previous stillbirth or neonatal death of unknown cause, history of jaundiced baby needing transfusion, history of receiving RhoGAM after deliveries or abortions. (See *Monitoring Rh incompatibility in the patient and neonate*, page 142.)

The physical assessment may not be significant for a patient with Rh incompatibility, but diagnostic studies are important. Blood type for

---

Other RBC antigen incompatibilities

Fetal-maternal incompatibility of ABO groups also may cause hemolytic disease. The blood type of a person who has red blood cells (RBCs) with neither the A antigen nor the B antigen is designated as group O. Blood of individuals with group O contains anti-A and anti-B antibodies. Therefore, the group O mother who is pregnant with a fetus whose blood group is A, B, or AB has anti-A and anti-B antibodies that may be stimulated by the pregnancy and may be transferred across the placenta to her fetus. In ABO incompatibility, even the first child can be affected.

The largest percentage of neonates who are affected by ABO incompatibility have blood group A and mothers with blood group O. Black neonates are more likely to develop ABO incompatibility than Caucasian neonates.

The clinical manifestations of fetal-maternal ABO incompatibility typically are mild and short-lasting. However, severe hemolysis with resultant hyperbilirubinemia and kernicterus is possible. No preventive agent is known for use in ABO incompatibility. Treatment of affected neonates is symptomatic, involving phototherapy to breakdown the extra RBCs, and increased fluids to increase renal output thereby excreting the RBCs' waste products.

Other, less common RBC antigens also are capable of transplacental isoimmunization. Fortunately, isoimmunization related to these antigens is not common, and serious fetal injury from these factors is unlikely.

NEONATAL STATUS

Monitoring Rh incompatibility in the patient and neonate

When a patient has an Rh incompatibility, neonatal status must be monitored closely through neonatal blood studies and physical assessment, including assessment of the placenta.

Neonatal cord blood studies at delivery
- Blood type and Rh. These tests indicate the need, if any, for further assessment of maternal antibody formation.
- Direct Coombs' test on neonatal cord blood. This test determines the presence of maternal antibodies attached to the neonate's red blood cells (RBCs). A washed suspension of the neonate's RBCs obtained from the umbilical cord is mixed with Coombs' serum (serum containing antiglobulin). The test is positive—that is, maternal antibodies are present—if the neonate's RBCs agglutinate.
- Hemoglobin level and hematocrit. Progressive hemolytic anemia reflects increased production of RBCs (erythropoiesis) as indicated by shifts in hemoglobin level and hematocrit as well as by an increased number of immature RBCs.
- Blood glucose level. Increased erythropoiesis increases blood glucose use. Hypoglycemia in the neonate must be recognized and treated early.
- Indirect or direct serum bilirubin level. Elevated levels of indirect bilirubin indicate hemolysis of RBCs, which frees bilirubin in the serum.

Postdelivery assessment
- Yellow-stained vernix or umbilical cord. Evidence of edema (hydrops fetalis), respiratory distress, and alterations in heart rate or rhythm may indicate pleural or pericardial effusions. Pleural or pericardial effusions and ascites indicate cardiac failure.
- Placental enlargement. The weight of the placenta is normally one-sixth that of the neonate. In hemolytic disease, the weight of the placenta may be as much as one-half to three-quarters that of the neonate.
- Hepatosplenomegaly. Liver and spleen enlargement indicates increased demands for disposal of bilirubin and increased erythropoiesis.
- Neonatal pallor with jaundice. Pallor is caused by RBC hemolysis; jaundice, by increased bilirubin levels. Jaundice typically appears within 24 to 36 hours of birth.
- Central nervous system manifestations of kernicterus. These include twitching, irritability, and high-pitched cry.

ABO and Rh factor is established early in pregnancy to identify a woman at risk for isoimmune hemolytic disease. Maternal isoimmunization is probable when antibody screening tests on maternal serum at around

20 weeks' gestation are positive. If the first test is negative, it should be repeated at 28 weeks. For the indirect Coombs' test, maternal blood serum is mixed with Rh-positive RBCs.

In a positive test, the red cells become coated with Rh antibodies. The dilution of the blood at which this occurs determines the titer or level of maternal antibodies, and the titer indicates the degree of maternal sensitization. If the titer reaches 1:16, an amniocentesis can be performed to measure the amount of bilirubin in the amniotic fluid.

Nursing diagnoses

After considering all assessment findings, formulate appropriate nursing diagnoses. (See Appendix 1, NANDA taxonomy of nursing diagnoses.)

Planning and implementation

Prophylaxis for Rh isoimmunization requires the use of RhIg. RhIg is not a treatment for isoimmunization because it has no effect against antibodies present in the maternal bloodstream. It provides passive immunity, which is transient and therefore will not affect a subsequent pregnancy. RhIg also prepares RBCs containing the Rh antigen for destruction by phagocytes before the patient's immune system is activated to produce antibodies (active immunity). Antibodies formed by an active immune response remain within the individual's bloodstream, presumably for life. RhIg given to an $Rh_o(D)$-negative patient who already is sensitized would accomplish nothing. Therefore, RhIg is recommended only for Rh-negative women at risk for developing Rh isoimmunization.

The American College of Obstetricians and Gynecologists recommendations for RhIg are:

- RhIg is given after delivery or abortion only to a patient who is Rh negative and D^u negative, has not already developed isoimmunization, and whose fetus is $Rh_o(D)$ positive or D^u positive. (In a D^u-positive individual, RBCs display a weak positive reaction when tested with standard Rh-typing serums.) RhIg is never given to the neonate or the neonate's father.
- RhIg is not useful for a woman who has Rh antibodies.
- RhIg should be administered intramuscularly, not subcutaneously or intravenously.

Assure the Rh-negative woman with a nursing diagnosis of *fear related to unknown effect of blood incompatibility on the fetus* that in over 95% of cases, administering RhIg to the mother within 72 hours of delivery or abortion prevents isoimmunization to the Rh factor in her fetus.

Rh sensitization also is possible during pregnancy if the cellular layer separating the maternal and fetal circulations is disrupted and fetal blood enters the maternal bloodstream. The cellular layer may be disrupted during amniocentesis or by abruptio placentae.

For the woman who is $Rh_o(D)$ negative and D^u negative and who has not already formed Rh antibodies, RhIg administered at about 28 weeks' gestation and again within 72 hours after delivery can help prevent Rh isoimmunization.

Evaluation

During this step of the nursing process, the nurse evaluates the effectiveness of the plan of care against subjective and objective criteria. Evaluation findings should be stated in terms of actions performed or outcomes achieved for each goal.

7 ANTEPARTAL COMPLICATIONS

A normal pregnancy under ordinary circumstances is accompanied by multiple physiologic and psychological changes. If complications develop, however, the woman and her entire family can be negatively affected.

An antepartal complication is defined as a disorder or malfunction of the pregnancy itself that occurs by the 20th week of pregnancy. The discovery of such a complication can change a natural, joyful experience into a time of stress and anxiety. The woman and her family may no longer look forward to the birth of a child; instead, fear may alter their expectations. In addition to worrying about the future, one or more family members—typically the woman or her partner—may feel responsible for the problem.

Nursing care must meet physical, psychological, and sociocultural needs of the woman and her family. When antepartal complications arise, the woman and her family may need significant emotional support.

Antepartal complications may be caused by such reproductive system disorders as spontaneous abortion, ectopic pregnancy, gestational trophoblastic disease, and incompetent cervix, or multisystem disorders such as hyperemesis gravidarum.

SPONTANEOUS ABORTION

Abortion is the termination of a pregnancy at any time before the age of viability or 20 weeks after last menstrual period. Abortions can be classified according to weight; viability is reached at a weight of over 500 g, when the fetus is able to survive in an extrauterine environment. (See *Assessing different types of abortion*, pages 146 and 147.) An abortion may be spontaneous, or the pregnancy may be terminated for medical or therapeutic reasons or for other, elective reasons.

Assessing different types of abortion

The nurse must assess the different types of abortion accurately to provide adequate nursing care and emotional support.

TYPE AND DEFINITION	PHYSICAL FINDINGS	MANAGEMENT
Threatened		
Signs and symptoms indicate possible loss of embryo	*Bleeding:* slight *Cramping:* mild and intermittent *Expelled tissue:* none *Internal cervical os:* closed *Uterus size:* varies with length of gestation	Bed rest, sedation, decreased stress, and no sexual intercourse, douches, or cathartics. Further treatment depends on specific signs and symptoms. Blood replacement therapy, I.V. therapy, and antibiotics may be indicated.
Inevitable		
Signs and symptoms indicate certain loss of embryo	*Bleeding:* slight *Cramping:* mild and intermittent *Expelled tissues:* none *Internal cervical os:* open *Uterus size:* varies with length of gestation	Prompt termination of pregnancy by dilatation and curettage (D&C). Blood replacement therapy, I.V. therapy, and antibiotics may be indicated.
Incomplete		
Part of the products of conception retained in the uterus	*Bleeding:* heavy *Cramping:* severe *Expelled tissues:* some *Internal cervical os:* open *Uterus size:* smaller than expected for length of gestation	Prompt termination of pregnancy by D&C or suction curettage. Blood replacement therapy, I.V. therapy, and antibiotics may be indicated.

Assessing different types of abortion (continued)

TYPE AND DEFINITION	PHYSICAL FINDINGS	MANAGEMENT
Complete		
All products of conception expelled from uterus	*Bleeding:* slight to moderate *Cramping:* mild to moderate *Expelled tissues:* all products of conception *Internal cervical os:* closed *Uterus size:* smaller than expected for length of gestation	No intervention needed unless hemorrhage or infection develops
Missed		
Nonviable fetus and other products of conception retained in uterus for 2 months or longer	*Bleeding:* slight *Cramping:* none *Expelled tissues:* none *Internal cervical os:* closed *Uterus size:* smaller than expected for length of gestation	Pregnancy terminated if it does not occur spontaneously within 1 month. Termination method depends on length of gestation. Monitor patient for signs of disseminated intravascular coagulation. Teach patient signs and symptoms and reasons for immediate medical care.
Septic		
Infection of products of conception or endometrial lining of uterus, which may result from attempted interference early in pregnancy	*Bleeding:* varies; malodorous *Cramping:* varies *Expelled tissue:* depends on whether tissue fragments remain *Internal cervical os:* usually open *Uterus size:* varies *Other:* fever	Immediate termination of pregnancy by D&C; cervical cultures and sensitivities performed; broad-spectrum antibiotic administered; temperature monitored; I.V. fluid p.r.n.

The nurse should keep in mind that for many people there are negative connotations with the word "abortion." For this reason, a spontaneous abortion is commonly referred to as a "miscarriage."

An early, spontaneous abortion occurs before 12 weeks' gestation; a late abortion, between 12 and 20 weeks' gestation. Births after 20 weeks are considered preterm. Almost 80% of all spontaneous abortions occur before 12 weeks' gestation; of those, the majority occur before 8 weeks. Recurrent or habitual abortion refers to the loss of three or more pregnancies before the age of viability. Such repeated losses can be caused by chromosomal aberrations, anomalies of the woman's reproductive tract (double uterus and its variants), an incompetent cervix, endocrine imbalances (such as hypothyroidism or diabetes mellitus), or systemic disorders (such as lupus erythematosus).

Assessment

Signs and symptoms of spontaneous abortion depend on the development of the implantation site, and are determined by the length of gestation. The three stages of development of the implantation site are:

- Early (or decidual). The fertilized ovum, surrounded by decidua, is poorly attached to the uterus. This stage covers the first 6 weeks of gestation. During the early stage of placental development, the symptoms of abortion are not severe; bleeding and cramping are minimal.
- Intermediate (or attachment). Chorionic villi in the basal plate of the decidua attach moderately well to the decidua basalis. This stage extends from 6 to 12 weeks of gestation. During the intermediate stage, moderate cramping and blood loss are expected because the ovum and its surrounding tissues are larger and more firmly attached to the uterus.
- Late (or placental). After 12 weeks of gestation, the placenta is fully formed and firmly attached to the decidua basalis. Severe pain is associated with a late abortion because the fetus must be expelled. Abdominal cramping, similar to labor, is usual. The amount of bleeding, however, is less than with an intermediate-stage abortion because the placenta remains attached until after the fetus has been delivered. Bleeding is more controlled because of strong uterine contractions.

A woman who has a late-stage abortion may experience breast engorgement and lactation. Alterations in hormonal levels subsequent to pregnancy in conjunction with pregnancy loss may contribute to a labile emotional state.

A pregnancy may have been terminated for several days before signs and symptoms become definite. For this reason, the exact date of termination can be difficult to determine. The following laboratory findings are characteristic of abortion:

- Urine. A negative or weakly positive urine pregnancy test.
- Blood. If blood loss is excessive or prolonged, hemoglobin level below 10.5 g/dl or hematocrit less than 32 g/dl are probable. If sepsis occurs following a missed or incomplete abortion, the white blood cell count will be greater than 12,000/mm^3. The sedimentation rate will increase with abortion, anemia, or infection and therefore is not useful for diagnostic purposes.
- Endocrine. The human chorionic gonadotropin, estrogen, and progesterone titers can be minimal in abortions.

A detailed, accurate history focusing on the woman's recent health; menstrual, gynecologic, and obstetric history; contraceptive method used; and possible date of conception is necessary for a complete diagnostic evaluation. While obtaining the health history, gather all pertinent information related to the woman's physical state. To help refine the diagnosis, obtain complete information regarding the pain, including location, type, and duration. Assess the amount and consistency of blood to determine whether any products of conception have been passed.

Nursing diagnoses

After gathering assessment data, the nurse reviews it carefully to identify pertinent nursing diagnoses for the woman with antepartal complications. (See Appendix 1, NANDA taxonomy of nursing diagnoses.)

Planning and implementation

After assessing the woman with antepartal complications and formulating nursing diagnoses, the nurse develops and implements a plan of care centering on the following common nursing goals:

- promoting the physical well-being of the woman and her fetus
- preventing or controlling further complications
- preventing sequelae
- providing emotional support to the woman and her family.

A woman with suspected abortion should be referred to a doctor immediately because emergency medical intervention may be needed to decrease complications. The patient may have a nursing diagnosis of **denial related to impending loss of pregnancy**. To care for this woman, save all expelled tissues and clots; maintain a calm, confident, and sympathetic manner; alert the doctor to pertinent signs and history; and encourage bed rest. Administration of sedatives and analgesics may be needed based on each individual case and the doctor's orders. Rest will decrease bleeding, and the medications will ease the patient's anxiety. Try to stay with the woman, and provide comfort measures usually associated with labor. The woman may be sensitive to any suggestion that she has somehow caused the abortion. The nurse will need to be sensitive to this feeling of vulnerability and be cautious when caring for the family to avoid increasing anxiety and guilt. Prepare the woman physically and emotionally for dilatation and curettage (D&C), if indicated.

After an abortion, the woman may have a nursing diagnosis of *anticipatory grieving related to loss of pregnancy.* Current literature indicates that grief following abortion is often not recognized or supported by health professionals. Therefore, to care for this patient, the nurse must provide emotional support, answer all questions, or clarify any information for the woman and her family. Ask the patient and her family about their needs and coping mechanisms. Realize that these are directly influenced by religious beliefs. Care is enhanced by accommodating such needs within the facility's constraints. Notify clergy to visit and offer support as the woman wishes and as indicated.

Teach the woman to wear a comfortable support bra to reduce discomfort from breast engorgement, which may produce anxiety; intervene as appropriate, depending on the doctor's orders and the woman's preferences. Administer RhIg I.M. injection within 72 hours if the woman is Rh negative and has not formed Rh antibodies from a previous Rh-positive pregnancy (See "Rh Incompatibility," pages 140 to 144.).

Management of an abortion depends on its type and the extent of the woman's symptoms. An incomplete abortion may be followed by a D&C to remove the remaining tissues. The doctor uses dilators to open the cervix and then performs suction curettage. Analgesics or general or local anesthetics may be used. Intravenous oxytocin, in a dextrose 5% in water intravenous solution, may be required to induce uterine contractions. Because retained placental fragments can cause the uterus to remain relaxed following the abortion, the uterine muscles may not constrict uterine vessels, causing hemorrhage during or after the procedure. Additional oxytocin infusion may be required to prevent hemorrhage. Monitor I.V. infusion and vital signs before, during, and after the D&C. Assess the hemodynamics of the woman to maintain her optimal health.

Ergot products (such as methylergonovine) that cause uterine and cervical contractions are contraindicated until the uterus is empty. This reduces the chance of retaining placental fragments. After the procedure, however, the doctor may order three or four doses of ergonovine, orally or intramuscularly, if the woman's blood pressure is normal. Blood or antibiotics may be ordered in cases of extreme blood loss, anemia, or infection.

If the cause of the abortion can be determined and eliminated, the chance for a future normal pregnancy is excellent. If no complications, such as infection or hemorrhage, occur, the abortion probably will have no detrimental physical effects on the patient.

Evaluation

Examples of appropriate evaluation statements appear at the end of this chapter.

ECTOPIC PREGNANCY

Ectopic pregnancy results from fertilization of the ovum before it migrates through the fallopian tube, thereby delaying its transport. This delayed transport may leave the zygote in the fallopian tube at the time of implantation. The majority of extrauterine pregnancies result from impeded progress of the fertilized ovum through the fallopian tube. The primary causes of ectopic pregnancies are tubal obstruction and delayed tubal transport.

A previous episode of pelvic inflammatory disease with accompanying salpingitis is commonly implicated in cases of tubal obstruction. Salpingitis results in mucosal damage, tubal narrowing, and diverticula, and also may impair tubal motility.

Other conditions that predispose a woman to ectopic pregnancy include:

- presence of scar tissue from a previous therapeutic abortion or previous abdominal surgery that may affect tubal motility
- use of an intrauterine device (IUD) for more than 2 years, which can cause a low-grade inflammatory response within the fallopian tubes
- in vivo exposure to diethylstilbestrol, which can adversely affect tubal motility
- congenital anomalies that interfere with passage of the fertilized ovum or with implantation
- altered hormonal status that affects tubal motility.

Other predisposing factors include infertility, increased maternal age, and a previous ectopic pregnancy. A woman who has an ectopic pregnancy in one fallopian tube is at increased risk for developing an ectopic pregnancy in the opposite tube probably due to a previous salpingitis. Some studies have shown that women who have IUDs or take progestin-only birth control pills have a higher incidence of ectopic pregnancy. Furthermore, those with a history of tubal ligation have a 16% to 50% rate of ectopic pregnancy.

Classification

Ectopic pregnancies are classified by the site of implantation, such as tubal or ovarian. Abdominal pregnancies occur once in approximately 15,000 live births; however, the delivery of a live, term neonate from an abdominal pregnancy occurs only once in approximately 250,000 live births. Intra-abdominal pregnancies also are associated with increased maternal mortality caused by uncontrolled hemorrhage and sepsis.

Assessment

Gather and record such relevant history as occurrence of abdominal surgery, spontaneous or voluntary abortion, or ectopic pregnancy. Take note of the patient's religious preferences, should baptism be requested or administration of blood or blood products be necessary.

Observe for abdominal pain, amenorrhea, and abnormal vaginal bleeding. Abdominal pain is the most consistent finding, occurring in over 90% of cases. The quality of pain varies markedly but usually is described as cramplike. Nausea and vomiting also may occur, along with urinary frequency. Signs of ruptured ectopic pregnancy may occur, including pallor, tachycardia, hypotension, and temperature elevation. Adnexal tenderness occurs unilaterally in about 50% of women. (See *Unruptured and ruptured ectopic pregnancy: Comparing the signs and symptoms*.)

Complicating ectopic pregnancy diagnosis are the numerous disorders that share many of the same signs and symptoms. These disorders include appendicitis, salpingitis, abortion, ovarian cysts, and urinary tract infections. Because definitive diagnosis is difficult, the condition may become an obstetric emergency if the ectopic pregnancy is unrecognized until the tube ruptures. Many emergency departments admit women with a ruptured tubal pregnancy without previous signs or symptoms.

Tests such as the serum test for beta-subunit human chorionic gonadotropin (beta-hCG) aid in diagnosing ectopic pregnancy. Beta-hCG, a hormone produced by the trophoblastic cells of the developing placenta, can be detected in minute amounts by radioimmunoassay of the hormone in a blood sample 9 days after ovulation. It can also be detected quickly, accurately, and inexpensively by sensitive home urine tests for pregnancy.

Physical signs and laboratory tests other than those for beta-hCG have limited diagnostic value unless tubal rupture occurs. A missed period, adnexal tenderness, or a small adnexal mass, for example, may indicate ectopic pregnancy but also can indicate an ovarian or corpus luteum cyst.

Unruptured and ruptured ectopic pregnancy: Comparing the signs and symptoms

The nurse must be able to distinguish between the signs and symptoms of unruptured and ruptured ectopic pregnancy to act decisively and quickly.

If unruptured, patient experiences:
- unilateral abdominal cramps and tenderness
- menstrual changes, such as spotting or a missed period
- low-grade fever (99° to 100° F [37.2° to 37.7° C])
- normal pulse
- nausea and vomiting.

If ruptured (in addition to signs and symptoms described above), patient experiences:
- sudden onset of abdominal pain from blood accumulation in the peritoneal cavity or from tubal rupture
- shocklike state from ruptured tube or excessive blood loss
- shoulder pain resulting from diaphragmatic irritation caused by blood accumulation in the peritoneum
- rapid, thready pulse from blood loss and subsequent hypovolemia
- cold extremities from excessive blood loss and decreased blood pressure.

Once a positive pregnancy test has been obtained, an ultrasound can be performed. If a gestational sac is not visible 5 to 6 weeks after the last menstrual period, an ectopic or abnormal intrauterine pregnancy can be suspected. Although abdominal ultrasound can be helpful, it has been more effective in ruling out an intrauterine pregnancy than in confirming an ectopic one. First, a pseudogestational sac in the uterus occurs in 10% to 20% of patients with ectopic pregnancy. Rarely, intrauterine and ectopic pregnancies can coexist so that the identification of one does not automatically rule out the other. Finally, because of their relatively small size, ectopic pregnancies are difficult to detect with abdominal ultrasound.

However, with the more recent development of vaginal sonography, results have been reported to have a specificity and sensitivity for ectopic pregnancy of 96% to 99%. This is performed by placing a transducer at the external opening of the vagina and directing sound waves into the pelvic cavity. In the event that this is negative and pregnancy is suspected, the woman can be followed by serial sonography and serial beta-hCG levels.

A laparoscopy can also be performed to confirm a suspected ectopic pregnancy. Because blood is present in the abdominal cavity in about 65% of patients with unruptured ectopic pregnancies and other conditions not requiring laparotomy, laparoscopy is especially helpful in identifying the bleeding sites.

The most effective diagnosis of an ectopic pregnancy combines these three diagnostic tools. Serum hCG levels in conjunction with ultrasonography and laparoscopy provide accurate information without using an invasive procedure.

Culdocentesis—aspiration or incision through the posterior vaginal fornix—also can be performed to detect intraperitoneal bleeding. Retrieval of nonclotting blood is a positive indication of ectopic pregnancy or other peritoneal bleeding, but it does not definitively ensure the absence of a hemoperitoneum caused by an ectopic pregnancy.

Nursing diagnoses

After gathering assessment data, the nurse reviews it carefully to identify pertinent nursing diagnoses for the patient with antepartal complications. (See Appendix 1, NANDA taxonomy of nursing diagnoses.)

Planning and implementation

A woman who exhibits the signs and symptoms of ectopic pregnancy may have subsequent bleeding and a nursing diagnosis of **decreased cardiac output related to bleeding at the site of ectopic pregnancy rupture.** Contact the doctor immediately if signs and symptoms occur, and assess vital signs every 15 minutes or as prescribed. Gather appropriate laboratory data including blood type, complete blood count, Rh, crossmatch, and serum hCG. Take the following steps for emergency care:

- Prepare for I.V. fluids with port for medication and a large-bore needle to accommodate blood transfusions if needed.
- Have oxygen on hand to prevent hypoxia related to hypovolemia.
- Gather emergency medications and equipment in case of shock.
- Prepare the woman for surgery by explaining the procedure, checking to see if her consent has been obtained, administering prescribed preoperative medication, and completing the surgical checklist.
- Keep the woman and her family informed.
- Contact clergy to baptize the fetus if desired by the family and document their wishes.

After surgery, the woman may have a nursing diagnosis of **anticipatory grieving related to loss of pregnancy.** If the woman is Rh negative, check to determine if antibodies are present in her blood, and prepare to administer RhIg if she has not formed Rh antibodies from an earlier pregnancy with an Rh-positive fetus. Administer fluids, medications, and treatments as prescribed, based on the woman's preference and tolerance. Inform her and her family if the fetus was baptized. Clarify, if necessary, the doctor's explanation of cause, management, and recovery, including chances for future pregnancies.

Effective management of ectopic pregnancy is complex. Hemorrhage is the major problem; bleeding must be controlled quickly and effectively. Because extreme blood loss can lead to shock, ensure that sufficient blood is available for transfusions.

Immediately after an ectopic pregnancy is diagnosed, a laparotomy can be performed to remove the products of conception, control blood loss by evacuating blood and clots, and cauterize bleeding vessels. However, a laparoscopy is sometimes preferred to an incision because of decreased morbidity and lower cost.

An interstitial ectopic pregnancy—a pregnancy occurring within a segment of the fallopian tube closest to the uterus—presents a diagnostic and management challenge. This rare form of ectopic pregnancy occurs in about 2.5% of all cases. Because of its location and lack of specific signs and symptoms, interstitial ectopic pregnancy typically is diagnosed through laparoscopy after tubal rupture and hemorrhage. With advances in ultrasonography, however, an eccentric location of the gestational sac can be identified. Laparoscopic surgery can successfully remove the products of conception if interstitial pregnancy is identified early, before rupture. If identification occurs concurrently with or after rupture, salpingectomy usually is required. Because the location is adjacent to the uterus, damage may result that will require removal of the uterus.

Medical therapy of ectopic pregnancies using methotrexate to treat interstitial and ectopic pregnancies has been most effective with pregnancies of 6 weeks gestation or less. Use of methotrexate in this manner is still experimental as of this writing.

An ovarian pregnancy requires the removal of the affected ovary. An adherent fallopian tube also may require removal. An advanced ectopic pregnancy, which typically is abdominal, requires a laparotomy as soon as the woman is stable and able to withstand surgery. Generally, the fetus succumbs before it is viable. If the placenta in an abdominal pregnancy is attached to a vital organ such as the liver, no attempt is made to separate or remove the placenta. The umbilical cord is cut flush with the placenta and the placenta is left in situ. Degeneration and absorption of the placenta usually occurs without complications. However, placental degeneration can lead to disseminated intravascular coagulation in some individuals.

Evaluation

For examples of appropriate evaluation statements, see the end of this chapter.

GESTATIONAL TROPHOBLASTIC DISEASE

Gestational trophoblastic disease (GTD) may be benign (hydatidiform mole) or malignant (choriocarcinoma). In GTD, trophoblastic cells covering the chorionic villi proliferate, and the villi undergo cystic changes.

In benign GTD, a neoplasm forms on the chorion (the outer layer of the membrane containing amniotic fluid) when the chorionic villi degenerate and become transparent vesicles that hang in grapelike clusters. These vesicles contain a clear fluid and may involve all or part of the decidual lining of the uterus. Usually no embryo is present because it has been absorbed.

In malignant GTD—a serious, rapidly developing, but rare carcinoma—neoplastic trophoblasts proliferate without cystic villi and may metastasize.

Assessment

Ask the woman if she has experienced nausea, vomiting, and continuous or intermittent vaginal discharge. Also ask her about the size of her abdomen. Because GTD typically is accompanied by rapid uterine growth, she may tell you, "I've gotten so big so quickly!"

Assess her vaginal discharge, which usually is brownish red. Send a specimen to the laboratory to rule out other infectious causes of vaginal bleeding. Measure fundal height; usually the uterus is enlarged out of proportion to the weeks of gestation. A vaginal examination shows thinning and softness of the lower uterine segment. No fetal heart tones are heard and no fetal body parts can be palpated. Laboratory studies show a reduced hemoglobin level, hematocrit, and red blood cell count and an increased white blood cell count and sedimentation rate. Human chorionic gonadotropin (hCG) titers are extremely elevated. Urinalysis probably will show proteinuria. An ultrasound performed after the 3rd month will show grapelike clusters rather than a fetus.

Nursing diagnoses

After gathering assessment data, the nurse reviews it carefully to identify pertinent nursing diagnoses. (See Appendix 1, NANDA taxonomy of nursing diagnoses.)

Planning and implementation

Monitor the woman's vital signs, vaginal discharge, and urine for proteinuria. The patient may have a nursing diagnosis of ***anxiety related to the unknown,*** for which she, and probably her partner, will require support when they are given the diagnosis. If the woman has to wait for the uterine wall to become firmer before having a dilatation and curettage (D&C), she will be going home knowing that she is not carrying a fetus. Give her time to work this through and verbalize her feelings. Be sensitive to her ability to cope, and assess her family support. After the D&C, routine postoperative care is necessary. The patient may have a nursing diagnosis of ***knowledge deficit related to necessary follow-up care.*** GTD can be malignant, making follow-up care extremely important.

Management of GTD involves evacuation of the uterine contents. An induced abortion may be followed by D&C; however, a D&C cannot be performed until the uterine wall becomes firmer and less friable. Tissue obtained from curettage must be examined by a pathologist for residual trophoblastic cells.

Vacuum suction also may be used to evacuate the uterus. As with a D&C, vacuum suction requires dilatation of the cervix. Whatever the treatment, blood replacement may accompany it.

Because GTD can be malignant, follow-up care must continue for at least 1 year. Recommended care includes:

- monitoring hCG levels once a week until titers are negative for 3 consecutive weeks; then once monthly for 6 months; then every 2 months for 6 months
- taking a chest X-ray once a month until hCG titers are negative, then every 2 months for 1 year
- preventing pregnancy for at least 1 year after all titers and X-rays are negative; an oral contraceptive is indicated to prevent pregnancy.

Evaluation

Examples of appropriate evaluation statements appear at the end of this chapter.

INCOMPETENT CERVIX

Incompetent cervix or premature dilation of the cervix is characterized by painless dilation of the cervix in the second or third trimester, with prolapse and ballooning of membranes into the vagina, followed by rupture of membranes and expulsion of an immature fetus. De-

pending on the length of gestation, spontaneous abortion or premature delivery may result.

Up to 40% of all perinatal deaths occur in association with pregnancies that terminate between 20 and 28 weeks' gestation. Cervical
incompetence is a major contributor to those losses.

Assessment

The woman with this condition does not have uterine contractions
or other signs and symptoms of labor. A pelvic examination reveals
other signs and symptoms of a dilated cervix possibly accompanied by
a congenital problem such as a short cervix. A double uterus or a uterus
with an altered shape may be diagnosed most efficiently by sonogram.
The woman may report a previous traumatic delivery, incompetent
cervix, or dilatation and curettage.

Nursing diagnoses

After gathering assessment data, the nurse reviews it carefully to identify pertinent nursing diagnoses. (See Appendix 1, NANDA taxonomy of nursing diagnoses.)

Planning and implementation

Provide basic preoperative and postoperative care for the woman undergoing a cerclage of the cervix, paying special attention to vaginal
bleeding. Frequently assess for the presence and quality of fetal heart
tones. Cervical cerclage may lead to a nursing diagnosis of *pain from
abdominal cramping related to cerclage to repair an incompetent
cervix.* Decisions about the type of delivery the woman will have usually depend on the position of the suture when she begins labor. Many
doctors believe that if the suture is maintaining cervical closure, a cesarean delivery should be performed to preserve the suture, thereby
maintaining cervical closure in future pregnancies. However, others
believe that a cesarean delivery places the woman unnecessarily at
risk for maternal morbidity when the suture could easily be removed
transvaginally. A suture that has loosened or become displaced will
not maintain cervical closure in subsequent pregnancies. In that case,
the suture is clipped and removed when labor begins and vaginal delivery may proceed.

Because incompetent cervix usually is not diagnosed until after
one or more abortions, this probably is not the first time the woman
and her partner have had to face delivery complications or the loss of
a fetus. Therefore, she and her family will need much support. Applicable nursing diagnoses in this situation include *anticipatory grieving related to potential loss of a fetus through incompetent cervix,*

and *situational low self-esteem related to diagnosis of incompetent cervix.* Incompetent cervix, which has more muscle tissue than a normal cervix, can be corrected and the pregnancy maintained by wedge trachelorrhaphy (removal of a wedge of the extra muscle tissue from the anterior segment of the cervix with its closure) or by cervical cerclage. The procedure most frequently used is the transvaginal cervical cerclage (McDonald procedure), in which a band of nonabsorbable ribbon is placed around the cervix beneath the mucosa to constrict the opening. The suture works much like the string on a drawstring bag. The key to success for the procedure is placing the suture high enough on the cervix so that it will remain in place.

The doctor typically will wait until 14 to 16 weeks' gestation, if possible, before performing the procedure to avoid having to remove the suture for a spontaneous first trimester abortion. An ultrasound is usually done to rule out congenital anomalies before the procedure is performed.

The pregnancy usually is maintained after cerclage, provided the membranes remain intact and the cervix was not more than 3 cm dilated or more than 50% effaced at the time of the correction. The procedure also may be performed transabdominally if necessary.

Evaluation

For examples of appropriate evaluation statements, see the end of this chapter.

HYPEREMESIS GRAVIDARUM

Sometimes called "pernicious vomiting," this complication of pregnancy involves dehydration and malnutrition. This syndrome is defined as vomiting severely enough to cause weight loss, dehydration, starvation acidosis, and alkalosis and hypokalemia from vomiting that occurs after the 16th week of gestation. Because hyperemesis begins as simple nausea and vomiting, a definitive diagnosis can be difficult. The woman's tolerance for nausea and vomiting, the degree of hydration, her electrolyte balance, and her level of disability all affect the diagnosis. The nurse should realize that every case of nausea and vomiting during pregnancy can be serious.

Mild nausea and vomiting, commonly called "morning sickness," occurs in approximately 50% of all pregnant women during the first trimester. Its physiologic basis is not completely understood, but no one theory adequately explains the symptoms. Morning sickness is considered a minor, self-limiting problem that appears 4 to 6 weeks after a missed menses and disappears after about 14 to 16 weeks of gestation.

Assessment

Unremitting nausea and vomiting that persist beyond the first trimester are characteristic of hyperemesis gravidarum. Vomitus ranges from undigested food, mucus, and bile early in the disorder to a "coffee-grounds" appearance in later stages.

Continued vomiting leads to dehydration, ultimately causing hypovolemia. Laboratory studies may reveal hemoconcentration and, in severe cases, loss of hydrogen, sodium, potassium, and chloride. Signs of progressive dehydration and impending hypovolemia are ketonuria, weight loss, increased pulse rate, decreased blood pressure, changes in skin turgor, and dry mucous membranes. Dehydration also can lead to confusion and coma as well as hepatic and renal failure.

The loss of gastric juices from vomiting can lead to metabolic alkalosis. Simultaneously, the woman's altered nutritional state can cause metabolic acidosis. The acidosis may partially obscure the alkalosis and result in a mixed acid-base disorder.

Severe malnutrition also may cause hypoproteinemia and hypovitaminosis with resulting hypoprothrombinemia from severe malnutrition and possible hemorrhage.

In severe, long-term cases of hyperemesis gravidarum, the kidneys may cease concentrating urine effectively, causing increased serum levels of urea nitrogen and creatinine.

Nursing diagnoses

After gathering assessment data, the nurse reviews it carefully to identify pertinent nursing diagnoses. (See Appendix 1, NANDA taxonomy of nursing diagnoses.)

Planning and implementation

For the woman with a nursing diagnosis of *fluid volume deficit related to persistent vomiting and decreased fluid intake,* expect to administer parenteral fluids, electrolytes, vitamins, and proteins as prescribed to counteract dehydration and loss of nutrients. Also be prepared to administer antiemetics as prescribed to decrease vomiting and promote rest. Expect oral intake to be restricted for the first 48 hours followed by cautious resumption of small, dry meals and then by clear liquids. This allows the gastrointestinal system to rest from overstimulation. Monitor intake and output and levels of ketosuria.

For a woman with a nursing diagnosis of *pain related to persistent vomiting,* keep the room quiet, pleasant, and well-ventilated to promote rest and relaxation; maintain excellent daily hygiene, especially oral hygiene following vomiting episodes, to promote comfort; and limit visitors to promote rest.

A woman who appears clinically stable may be managed as an outpatient with close follow-up. Hydration with isotonic fluids is essential. In addition, teach the woman how to assist with her own treatment. For example, teach her that small, frequent meals containing easily digested, high-carbohydrate foods will help to reestablish adequate vitamin and protein levels. Drinking fluids after her meals will also help reduce nausea and vomiting. Heartburn and reflux esophagitis are common and typically are treated symptomatically.

Antiemetics, a mainstay in treating hyperemesis, also have a mildly sedating effect. (See *Drugs used to treat hyperemesis gravidarum*, pages 162 and 163.)

Many women report episodes of emesis in connection with a particularly stressful incident or aspect of their lives. If possible, a woman with hyperemesis should try to avoid or resolve situations that aggravate the condition or increase stress.

An essential aspect of outpatient care is reassurance and support. A debilitated woman who is worried about her pregnancy may experience a severe emotional crisis. Make a special effort to give the patient emotional support.

For a hospitalized woman with severe symptoms, treatment goals are to eliminate vomiting, restore hydration, reestablish electrolyte balance, and supplement vitamin intake. To achieve these goals, restrict oral intake, expect to begin parenteral administration of fluids with electrolytes and supplementary vitamins and minerals, and administer antiemetics. This treatment plan allows rest for the overstimulated gastrointestinal tract while providing necessary nutrients to the body.

Persistent weight loss, acidosis, and malnutrition require total parenteral nutrition to provide adequate protein intake for mother and fetus.

Before, during, and after hospitalization, the woman needs a quiet, aesthetically pleasing environment. A perceived lack of tolerance may indicate to the woman that the nurse feels the disorder is psychosomatic and that the woman does not need hospitalization. Therefore, maintain a calm, accepting attitude.

Evaluation

During this step of the nursing process, the nurse evaluates the effectiveness of the plan of care against subjective and objective criteria. Evaluation findings should be stated in terms of actions performed or outcomes achieved for each goal. The following examples illustrate appropriate evaluation statements for women with antepartal complications:

- The woman has verbalized understanding of the necessity for having a dilatation and curettage after a spontaneous abortion.

(*Text continues on page 164.*)

Drugs used to treat hyperemesis gravidarum

This chart summarizes the major antiemetic agents in current clinical use to treat hyperemesis gravidarum. Intravenous fluids should be given to initially reduce dehydration. Remember that, with persistent vomiting, the patient must be evaluated for diagnosis of other diseases. These include cholecystitis, pancreatitis, hepatitis, pyelonephritis, gastroenteritis, and fatty liver of pregnancy.

DRUG AND MECHANISM OF ACTION	USUAL DOSAGE	NURSING IMPLICATIONS
promethazine (Phenergan)		
Depresses central nervous system and inhibits acetylcholine	I.M. or P.R.:12.5 to 25 mg every 4 to 6 hours p.r.n. Also available in oral form if the patient can tolerate it.	• May cause drowsiness, dizziness, increased or decreased blood pressure, mouth dryness. May impair platelet aggregation in the newborn. • Safety during pregnancy has not been established. Should only be used if potential benefits outweigh the hazards.
prochlorperazine (Compazine)		
Blocks dopamine receptors in medullary chemoreceptor trigger zone	Oral: 5 to 10 mg t.i.d. or q.i.d. I.M.: 5 to 10 mg every 3 to 4 hours, injected deeply into buttocks. No doses should exceed 40 mg daily.	• May cause glycosuria, dry mouth, nasal congestion, restlessness, insomnia, anorexia, dizziness, postural hypotension, blurred vision. Reported cases of prolonged jaundice, extrapyramidal symptoms, hyperreflexia or hyporeflexia in newborn infants.

Drugs used to treat hyperemesis gravidarum *(continued)*

DRUG AND MECHANISM OF ACTION	USUAL DOSAGE	NURSING IMPLICATIONS
prochlorperazine (Compazine) *(continued)*		
		• Safety during pregnancy has not been established; therefore, should only be used when potential benefits outweigh the hazards.
metoclopramide (Reglan)		
Blocks dopamine receptors in medullary chemoreceptor trigger zone	Oral: 10 mg q.i.d. I.M. or I.V.: 10 mg q.i.d.	• May cause restlessness, anxiety, drowsiness, lassitude, extrapyramidal symptoms, tardive dyskinesia. • Safety and efficacy have not been established for therapy that continues longer than 12 weeks. • Safety during pregnancy has not been established in humans; should only be used when absolutely necessary. • Patient should not operate machinery while taking; drug impairs judgment and motor skills.

- The woman's vital signs are stable after cervical cerclage.
- The woman's ectopic pregnancy rupture site pain has been controlled with an analgesic agent.
- The woman has listed the necessary follow-up for monitoring of gestational trophoblastic disease.
- The woman has responded to small, frequent feedings by a reduced emesis.

NURSING CARE DURING THE INTRAPARTAL PERIOD

PHYSIOLOGY OF LABOR AND CHILDBIRTH

8

Impending labor and childbirth typically trigger both excitement and apprehension in a pregnant patient. Whether the patient is a primipara about to give birth for the first time, or a multiparous woman experienced from previous childbirth, she will have many physical and psychological needs. To meet these needs, the nurse must understand the labor process and how it affects the woman and fetus.

THEORIES OF LABOR ONSET

Although several theories of labor onset have been proposed, the exact mechanism has eluded researchers. Instead of a single initiating factor, several maternal, fetal, and placental factors probably interact to initiate labor. These include oxytocin stimulation, progesterone reduction, estrogen stimulation, fetal cortisol production, and the effects of fetal membrane phospholipids, arachidonic acid, and prostaglandins.

FACTORS AFFECTING LABOR

Successful labor and childbirth require coordination of five essential factors, sometimes termed the "five P's":

- passenger
- passageway
- powers
- placental position and function
- psychological response.

For the fetus to move successfully through the pelvis, the contractions and bearing-down efforts must be of adequate intensity and frequency, the placenta must be properly positioned and provide adequate oxygen to the fetus, and the woman must be psychologically prepared. Problems involving any of these essential factors may jeopardize safe labor and childbirth and require medical or surgical intervention.

Fetus (passenger)

Fetal factors affecting labor and childbirth include size and shape of the head, lie, attitude, presentation, position, and station.

Head

The skull is composed of several small, thin, incompletely developed bones, including two frontal bones, two parietal bones, two temporal bones, and one occipital bone. The largest part of the fetus, the skull, is also the least compressible part. However, the skull bones are connected by flexible, membrane-occupied spaces called sutures, which allow alterations in skull shape called molding. During labor, the skull bones are pressed together and may overlap, reducing the size of the head and facilitating passage through the more rigid maternal pelvis. These bones eventually fuse after birth to form the rigid cranial cavity characteristic of the adult.

Besides allowing for molding, the sutures separating these bones aid in identifying fetal position during labor. The sagittal suture, which runs in an anteroposterior direction, separates the two parietal bones. The frontal suture, an extension of the saggital suture, separates the two frontal bones. The coronal suture separates the parietal bones from the frontal bones. The lambdoidal suture separates the parietal bones from the occipital bone.

Sutures intersect at membranous spaces called fontanels. The anterior fontanel is located at the junction of the sagittal, coronal, and frontal sutures. The diamond-shaped, anterior fontanel measures 3 to 4 cm long and 2 to 3 cm wide. By remaining open until the infant is about 18 months old, this fontanel gives the brain space to grow. The posterior fontanel is located at the junction of the sagittal and lambdoidal sutures. This triangular-shaped fontanel, approximately 2 cm wide, normally closes within 6 to 8 weeks after birth.

During labor, the head usually moves so that its smallest diameter, the occipito-bregmatic, enters the pelvis. The head can flex or extend about 45 degrees and can rotate about 180 degrees. This ability to flex, extend, and rotate allows its smallest diameters to move down the birth canal and pass through the maternal bony pelvis.

Lie

Fetal lie refers to the position of the fetal spine in relation to the maternal spine. When the two spines are parallel, the fetus is in a longitudinal lie. When the spines are perpendicular, the fetus is in a transverse lie. When the fetal spine is at an angle between the parallel and perpendicular position, the fetus is in an oblique lie. Typically, a fetus in an oblique lie will convert either to a longitudinal or a transverse lie before birth.

Unless the fetus is positioned in a longitudinal lie, a vaginal birth is impossible, and surgical intervention becomes necessary.

Attitude

Fetal attitude refers to overall body flexion or extension, which determines the relationship of fetal parts to one another. The usual fetal attitude in the uterus is vertex, with the head flexed so that the chin rests against the chest, the legs and arms folded in front of the body, and the back curved slightly forward.

The fetus normally exhibits varying degrees of flexion and extension throughout pregnancy with no ill effects. However, fetal attitude becomes significant during labor and childbirth. With the fetus in a cephalic presentation, a fully flexed attitude enables the occiput to enter the pelvis. As the degree of extension increases, the diameter of the head entering the pelvis also increases, making labor and childbirth more difficult.

Position

Fetal position refers to the relationship of the presenting part to the front, back, or side of the maternal pelvis. The nurse establishes fetal position by determining three factors: a landmark on the fetal presenting part, whether this landmark faces the right or left side of the maternal pelvis, and whether the landmark faces the front, back, or side of the maternal pelvis. (See *Determining fetal position.*)

Presentation

Fetal presentation refers to the manner in which the fetus enters the pelvic passageway. The portion of the fetus that enters the pelvic passageway first determines how presentation is classified:

- cephalic (head first)
- breech (buttocks or feet first)
- shoulder
- compound.

Approximately 95% of all births occur with the fetus assuming a cephalic presentation. A shoulder presentation occurs when the fetal spine is perpendicular to the maternal spine. Unless the fetus in this presentation moves to a longitudinal lie, cesarean delivery is necessary. Predisposing factors in a shoulder presentation include placenta previa, neoplasms, fetal anomalies, hydramnios, preterm labor, uterine atony, multiple gestation, and premature rupture of membranes.

Before the 28th week of gestation, approximately 25% of fetuses are in a breech presentation. By the 34th week of gestation, however, most fetuses move to a cephalic presentation. Nevertheless, 3% to 4% of all term pregnancies involve breech presentation.

Determining fetal position

Fetal position is determined by the relationship of a specific presenting part to the front, back, or side of the maternal pelvis. A notation system identifies three features: a landmark on the presenting part (O for occiput, M for mentum, S for sacrum, A for acromion process, and D for dorsal); whether this landmark faces the right (R) or left (L) side of the pelvis; and whether the landmark faces the front (A for anterior), the back (P for posterior), or a side (T for transverse) of the pelvis. Thus, for a fetus with the occiput (O) as the presenting landmark, positioned facing the right side (R) and front (A) of the maternal pelvis, the nurse would identify the position as ROA.

In a vertex presentation, the fetus may assume one of the six positions illustrated below: LOP, LOT, LOA, ROP, ROT, or ROA.

LEFT OCCIPUT POSTERIOR (LOP)

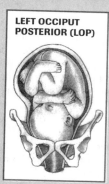

LEFT OCCIPUT TRANSVERSE (LOT)

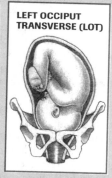

LEFT OCCIPUT ANTERIOR (LOA)

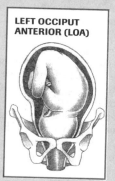

RIGHT OCCIPUT POSTERIOR (ROP)

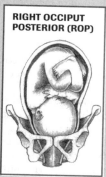

RIGHT OCCIPUT TRANSVERSE (ROT)

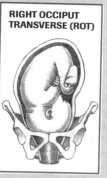

RIGHT OCCIPUT ANTERIOR (ROA)

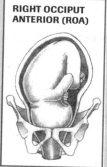

In most cases, the cause of breech presentation cannot be pinpointed; however, numerous maternal, placental, and fetal predisposing factors have been identified. Maternal factors associated with breech presentation include uterine anomalies, uterine relaxation resulting from previous childbirth, myometrial neoplasm, contracted pelvis, oligohydramnios, and hydramnios. Placental factors include the implantation of the placenta in either cornual-fundal region. Also reported to cause a higher incidence of breech presentations is placenta previa, a condition in which the placenta partially or totally covers the cervical os and blocks the fetus from leaving the uterus. Fetal factors include prematurity, multiple gestation, anencephaly, hydrocephaly, intrauterine fetal death, and other fetal anomalies.

Station
Fetal station refers to the relationship of the presenting part to the maternal ischial spines. The ischial spines, located at midpelvis, form the narrowest portion of the pelvis through which the fetus must pass. When the largest diameter of the presenting part (usually the biparietal diameter of the head) is level with the ischial spines, the fetus is at station 0. Numbers from 1 to 3 indicate how many centimeters the presenting part is above or below the ischial spines. Thus, a presenting part above the ischial spines is designated as −1, −2, or −3; a presenting part below this point, +1, +2, or +3. When the presenting part is classified as being at greater than +3 station, it is at the pelvic outlet and visible on the perineum.

Successful vaginal birth requires progressive fetal descent from a minus station to 0 and then to a plus station during labor. Lack of this progressive descent with effective uterine contractions may indicate cephalopelvic disproportion or an inappropriately short or tangled umbilical cord. In such cases, cesarean delivery may be necessary.

Pelvis (passageway)
The passageway through which the fetus must travel during labor consists of the pelvis and soft tissues. Pelvic types and diameters affect labor and childbirth.

The pelvis is partly ligamentous and partly bony. Although there are four basic pelvic types—gynecoid, android, anthropoid, and platypelloid—a woman usually has features of two or more types.

The true pelvis contains three levels, or planes: the pelvic inlet, the midpelvis, and the pelvic outlet. Diameters measured in these three planes indicate the amount of space available for the fetus during birth.

The pelvic inlet has four diameters: the anteroposterior diameter, the bi-ischial (or transverse) diameter, and two oblique diameters. The pelvic inlet's anteroposterior diameter is further divided into the obstetric conjugate, the true conjugate, and the diagonal conjugate diameters. The diagonal conjugate can be measured during a pelvic examination; the other two diameters are estimated from this measurement.

The pelvic diameters can be affected by the woman's position during labor, by the hormone relaxin in the system, and by the amount of fat or soft tissue surrounding the pelvis. Relaxin helps to relax the pelvis and increase the pelvic diameters. Therefore, assuming a squatting or lateral Sims' position may help increase the pelvic diameters.

Uterine contractions (powers)

Rhythmic tightening of the upper uterine segment musculature, uterine contractions serve several purposes during labor and childbirth. (See *Palpating uterine contractions*, page 172.) Coordinated and effective uterine contractions promote fetal descent and rotation, cervical effacement and dilation, separation and expulsion of the placenta, and constriction of the uterine vasculature to prevent postpartal hemorrhage.

A uterine contraction begins as a series of biochemical interactions in response to a change in electrical activity. This change, referred to as a wave of excitation, originates in pacemakers located near the uterotubal junctions. The downward movement of the electrical charge from the upper segment of the uterus to the cervix is known as fundal dominance. Contraction intensity and duration are both greater in the upper uterine segment than in the lower uterine segment.

These three characteristics—fundal dominance, intensity, and duration—help create a coordinated uterine contraction that produces maximum expulsive force. The muscular structure of the uterus (the myometrium) is unique because the fibers remain shortened even after the contraction is over, instead of reverting to their precontraction size; that is, the fibers shorten progressively during labor. This is known as retraction or brachystasis. As labor continues, this progressive shortening of fibers results in a thickening of the upper uterine segment and a decrease in uterine size, which impels fetal descent.

For uterine contractions to propel the fetus through the birth canal effectively, several biochemical interactions must occur. A uterine contraction occurs in three phases: increment, acme, and decrement. (See *Phases of a uterine contraction*, page 173.) During the increment and acme phases, waves of excitation, initiated in the pacemakers, induce contractions. As the waves subside, contractions decrease in intensity and duration and conclude in the decrement phase.

During labor, the nurse evaluates the duration, frequency, and intensity of contractions. The duration of a contraction refers to the

PSYCHOMOTOR SKILLS

Palpating uterine contractions

Assessing uterine contractions by palpation requires no special equipment, but it does require nursing skill and sensitivity to touch. To palpate uterine contractions effectively, the nurse should follow these steps:

1 Place the palmar surface of the fingers on the patient's uterine fundus and palpate lightly. Note the uterine tightening and abdominal lifting that occur with contractions. Keep in mind that each contraction has three phases: the increment (building up) phase, the acme (peak) phase, and the decrement (letting down) phase.

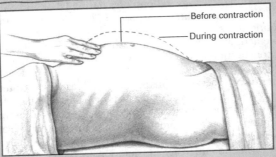

Before contraction

During contraction

2 Palpate during several contractions, determining their frequency, duration, and intensity. To assess frequency, time the period between the beginning of one contraction and the beginning of the next. To evaluate duration, time the period from the onset of uterine tightening to its relaxation. While the uterus is tightened, determine the intensity of the contraction by pressing the fingertips into the fundus. During mild contractions, the fundus indents easily and feels like a chin. In moderate contractions, the fundus indents less easily and feels more rigid, like the tip of a nose. With strong contractions, the fundus is firm, resists indenting, and feels like a forehead.

time between the beginning and end of the contraction. Duration usually ranges from 15 to 30 seconds in early labor to 45 to 90 seconds in later stages. The frequency of contractions is measured from the beginning of one contraction to the beginning of the next. In early labor, frequency ranges from 20 to 30 minutes; in the later stages, it ranges from 2 to 3 minutes.

Phases of a uterine contraction

As shown in the diagram below, a uterine contraction occurs in three phases: increment (building up), acme (peak), and decrement (letting down). Between contractions is a period of relaxation. The two most important features of contractions are frequency and duration. Frequency refers to the elapsed time from the start of one contraction to the start of the next contraction. Duration is the elapsed time from the start to the end of one contraction.

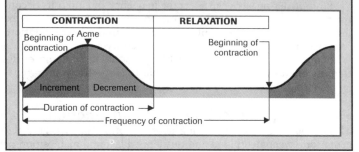

The duration and frequency of contractions affect both the patient and the fetus. Duration greater than 90 seconds and frequency less than 2 minutes increase the risk of uterine rupture and also put the fetus at high risk for hypoxia from uterine vasoconstriction. Excessively long and overly frequent contractions also sap the woman's energy and strength during labor, hindering her voluntary bearing-down efforts.

The intensity of a contraction refers to its strength during the acme phase. Intensity can be measured fairly directly with an intrauterine catheter and indirectly by palpation or external monitoring. The normal resting pressure of the uterus between contractions measured via intrauterine catheter is 10 mm Hg; this pressure can increase to 50 mm Hg during acme. When the pressure reaches 15 to 20 mm Hg, blood supply to the uterus and placenta is compromised, and the woman usually begins to feel pain.

Bearing-down efforts

Once uterine contractions have fully effaced and dilated the cervix, the second stage of labor begins and the woman's voluntary bearing-down efforts become effective. In these efforts, she contracts the diaphragm and abdominal muscles to increase intra-abdominal pressure. This action, which applies pressure to the uterine walls, adds to the pressures from uterine contractions and aids fetal descent and expulsion. The woman also experiences a great involuntary urge to push as the head of the fetus descends and pushes against the sacral and obturator nerves.

Positions for labor

Throughout most of the world today, labor and childbirth most often occur with the woman in an upright position. In contrast, the recumbent position remains a Western tradition.

Position during labor can affect the frequency and intensity of contractions. For a woman in the supine position, contractions may be less intense but more frequent. For a woman in the lateral position, contractions tend to be more intense but less frequent.

Some women prefer being upright, as in walking, standing, or sitting. Inconclusive evidence suggests that these positions may shorten labor.

Placenta (placental position and function)

Throughout pregnancy and during labor, the fetus depends on the placenta for oxygenated blood and nutrients. Placental malposition or malfunction can hinder labor and childbirth and may compromise the well-being of the fetus. In most cases, the placenta is attached to the upper uterine segment. However, 1 in every 200 to 300 pregnancies involves placenta previa—implantation of the placenta in the lower uterine segment, where it partially or totally covers the cervical os. Besides blocking the os, placenta previa causes the placenta to separate from the uterine wall partially or totally as the cervix dilates, typically causing hemorrhage.

Other conditions can cause placental malfunction. For example, in abruptio placentae, which occurs in about 1 in 250 pregnancies, the placenta prematurely separates from the uterine wall. Another condition, uteroplacental insufficiency, impairs the ability of the fetus to withstand the rigors of labor.

Psychological response

The role that a pregnant woman's mental and emotional state plays in labor and childbirth has received increasing attention over the last several decades. Research has identified a relationship between a woman's perception of her health state during pregnancy and her behavior during labor. Women who adopted a "sick role" during pregnancy had a higher incidence of prolonged, difficult labor. More recent studies point to a relationship between anxiety and the length and difficulty of labor. In particular, high epinephrine levels triggered by maternal anxiety can lead to diminished uterine activity and longer labors. Also, women who experienced severe pain or distress-related thoughts may be more likely to experience an inefficient labor.

These and other studies indicate the importance of an appropriate psychological response to the physiologic and emotional demands of labor. Factors that may influence a woman's psychological response include preparation for labor, support systems, and coping mechanisms.

MECHANISMS OF LABOR

For most women, labor follows a consistent pattern. As uterine contractions intensify, the cervix effaces and dilates. Propelled by uterine contractions and the woman's bearing-down efforts, the fetus descends through the birth canal via its cardinal movements.

Cervical effacement and dilation

Myometrial activity at the onset of labor leads to full cervical effacement and dilation. Effacement refers to a progressive shortening of the vaginal portion of the cervix and thinning of its walls. Effacement is described in percentages, ranging from 0% (noneffaced and thick) to 100% (fully effaced and paper thin). With the cervix fully effaced, its constrictive uterine neck is obliterated, and the cervix becomes continuous with the lower uterine segment.

Cervical dilation refers to progressive enlargement of the cervical os, from less than 1 cm to about 10 cm (full dilation), to allow passage of the fetus from the uterus into the vagina. Because uterine muscle fibers remain shortened even after a contraction ceases, the uterus elongates and the uterine cavity decreases in size. These actions force the fetus downward toward the cervix. Cervical dilation results from the pressure plus the upward pulling of longitudinal muscle fibers over the fetus. Typically, effacement and dilation occur more quickly in multiparous women than in primiparous women. (See *Comparing the average length of labor*, page 176.)

Cardinal movements

Cardinal movements refer to the typical sequence of positions assumed by the fetus during labor and childbirth. (See *Cardinal movements of labor*, pages 177 and 178.)

Descent

Descent refers to the downward movement of the fetus into the pelvic passageway. In a primiparous woman, this process may begin several weeks before labor, but further descent usually does not occur until the second stage of labor. In a multiparous woman, descent usually

Comparing the average length of labor

The four phases of labor often occur within somewhat predictable time frames. The chart below compares the average length of the phases of labor for the primigravida and multipara.

	PRIMIGRAVIDA	MULTIPARA
Latent phase	8.6 hrs	5.8 hrs
Active phase	5.8 hrs	2.5 hrs
First stage of labor	13.3 hrs	8.3 hrs
Second stage of labor	60 min	24 min

begins with engagement. This downward motion results from one or more forces: contraction of the abdominal muscles, pressure from the amniotic fluid, direct fundal pressure upon the fetus, and the extension and straightening of the fetus. The progression of this downward movement is described as follows:

- Floating. The presenting part, the portion of the fetus that enters the pelvic passageway first, moves freely above the pelvic inlet.
- Fixed. The presenting part has entered the pelvic inlet and no longer moves but is not yet engaged.
- Engaged. The widest part of the presenting part has reached the level of the ischial spines.
- Midpelvis. The presenting part has descended halfway to the pelvic floor.
- On the pelvic floor. The presenting part has descended to the perineum.

One other consideration involved in fetal descent is synclitism or asynclitism. When the diameter of the fetal parietal bones is parallel to the plane of the pelvic passageway, it is said to be synclitic. Some deviation from the plane, asynclitism, is normal but marked asynclitism can interfere with the normal progress of labor.

Flexion

Resistance from the cervix, pelvic walls, or pelvic floor normally flexes the head of the fetus. When the head flexes downward so that the chin rests against the chest, the smallest diameter of the head, the occipito bregmatic diameter, will pass through the woman's pelvis.

Cardinal movements of labor

For a fetus in the vertex (crown or top of head) presentation, labor follows a typical sequence. Illustrations on the right show the relationship of the fetal skull to the maternal pelvis.

1 Engagement, descent, flexion. The widest diameter of the head passes the level of the pelvic inlet; as the fetus moves downward toward the ischial spines, the head flexes on the chest.

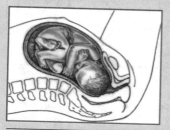
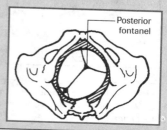

Posterior fontanel

2 Internal rotation. The anteroposterior diameter of the head comes into line with the anteroposterior diameter of the pelvic outlet.

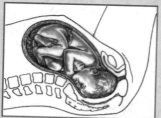
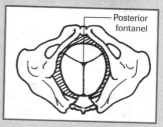

Posterior fontanel

3 Extension. The head extends from the perineum after passing under the symphysis pubis.

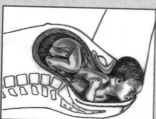
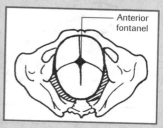

Anterior fontanel

(continued)

Cardinal movements of labor (continued)

4 External rotation (restitution). The head rotates 45 degrees back to its original position.

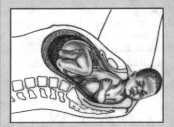
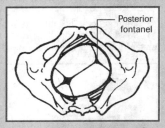

Posterior fontanel

5 External rotation (shoulder rotation). The head rotates an additional 45 degrees to a transverse position; the anterior shoulder passes the perineum.

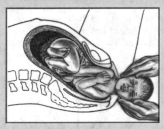
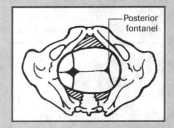

Posterior fontanel

6 Expulsion. The rest of the body is easily delivered by lateral flexion.

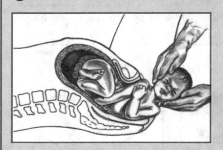

Internal rotation

In most cases, internal rotation occurs during the second stage of labor, sometimes during one contraction. During internal rotation, the anteroposterior diameter of the head comes in line with the anteroposterior diameter of the pelvic outlet. When the head meets resistance from the pelvic floor, it rotates under the symphysis pubis approximately 45 degrees left of the midline of the anterior abdominal wall. Internal rotation does not involve movement of the shoulders, which remain oblique. Although most fetuses assume an occiput anterior position following internal rotation, some rotate instead to an occiput posterior or occiput transverse position. These positions occur primarily in women with abnormal pelvic configurations, such as android or anthropoid pelves. Approximately 70% of fetuses in either position rotate spontaneously to the anterior position. However, failure of the fetus to assume an anterior position can lead to prolonged labor caused by the inability of the fetal occiput to fill the pelvic cavity adequately or to exert equal pressure around the cervical os.

Extension

The head of the fetus remains in a flexed position until it passes under the symphisis pubis and reaches the perineum. The head then extends as it is born. As the head extends, it passes over the anterior margin of the perineum; then the head drops down and the chin lies over the woman's perineum.

External rotation

Once the head passes over the perineum, it rotates 45 degrees, returning to the position it originally assumed during engagement. This is called restitution. Next, the fetus rotates an additional 45 degrees to assume a transverse position as the delivery proceeds. This movement positions the shoulders in line with the anteroposterior diameter of the woman's pelvis. The anterior shoulder usually appears first, under the symphysis pubis; the posterior shoulder follows.

Expulsion

Once the shoulders are born, the remainder of the body is easily pulled upward and away from the perineum, following the natural curve of the pelvic passageway.

SIGNS AND SYMPTOMS OF LABOR

Although the exact mechanism that triggers labor remains unclear, certain physiologic signs and symptoms typically predict the onset of true labor. Some of these signs and symptoms may occur up to 3 weeks before labor onset; others coincide with the beginning of labor.

Lightening

Lightening occurs as the fetal presenting part settles lower in the pelvis, leaving more space in the upper abdomen. In primiparous women, lightening normally occurs 2 to 3 weeks before labor begins; in multiparous women, it may not occur until labor actually begins. This downward fetal movement decreases pressure on the diaphragm, easing respiratory effort and allowing the woman to breathe more deeply. It also reduces compression of the stomach, allowing the woman to eat more at each meal. Accompanying these sensations are a change in abdominal shape and a visible decrease in fundal height, at which time the fetus is commonly said to have "dropped."

Lightening also may cause discomfort. In some patients, the frequent urge to urinate experienced early in pregnancy returns because the uterus and fetal presenting part can push against the bladder. The patient may feel fetal movements much lower in the abdomen, producing a sensation of pressure.

Also, downward pressure on deep leg veins from the enlarged uterus may cause pelvic pressure and edema of the legs. Increased pelvic pressure can lead to or aggravate hemorrhoids or varicose veins; this pressure may cause leg cramps or pain when it impinges on nerves.

Braxton Hicks contractions

Throughout pregnancy, the uterus undergoes a series of painless, irregular contractions known as Braxton Hicks contractions. These help prepare for labor by causing cervical changes late in pregnancy.

Braxton Hicks contractions have been described as pulling or tightening sensations in the uterine fundus. Although these contractions may occur every 5 to 20 minutes throughout pregnancy, they typically become most noticeable during the last 6 weeks of gestation in primiparous women and the last 3 to 4 months in multiparous women. They are the primary cause of false alarms that bring pregnant patients to the hospital thinking that labor has begun. The nurse should assure the patient that these contractions are normal and that they may become stronger during and after intercourse or strenuous physical activity. Advise her about rest and relaxation techniques if they produce discomfort. Assure the woman that unless these contractions become longer, stronger, closer together, and persistent, regardless of activity level, they are not labor contractions. However, offer encouragement by teaching her that Braxton Hicks contractions assist the cervix in effacement and occasionally in dilation before the onset of labor.

Cervical changes

Late in pregnancy, the cervix begins to change in preparation for dilation and onset of labor. Braxton Hicks contractions move the cervix upward as the lower uterine segment is formed. As a result, the fibrous connective tissue of the cervix loosens, causing the cervix to become softer, thinner, shorter, and more pliable—a process known as effacement. Prostaglandin release may also contribute to cervical effacement.

As the cervix undergoes its prelabor changes, the mucus plug—which blocks the cervix throughout pregnancy—becomes dislodged. At the same time, some of the cervical capillaries rupture; blood mixes with the mucus, producing what is known as "bloody show." The woman may detect a blood-tinged mucus discharge anytime from several days before labor to the onset of labor. Normally, only a few drops of blood mix with the mucus plug. The nurse should advise the woman to notify the doctor or nurse-midwife if she passes a larger amount of blood.

Rupture of membranes

Approximately 12% of all pregnant women experience a spontaneous rupture of membranes (SROM) before labor begins. Within 24 hours, labor will spontaneously begin in about 80% of these women. The time between SROM and labor initiation depends on the length of gestation. A woman who does not deliver within 24 hours after SROM is considered to have prolonged rupture of membranes, a condition that puts her and the fetus at increased risk for infection. (See "Premature Rupture of the Membranes," pages 121 to 125.)

When the rupture occurs, the amniotic fluid may flow profusely or it may dribble. A woman may confuse rupture of membranes with urinary incontinence caused by uterine pressure on the bladder. Testing of vaginal discharge with nitrazine paper allows the examiner to distinguish between the two conditions. Normal vaginal discharge and urine are both acidic, but amniotic fluid is alkaline (pH 7.2), which turns yellow nitrazine paper a deep blue on contact.

Another simple test performs the same function. When allowed to dry on a microscopic slide, amniotic fluid assumes a characteristic fernlike pattern. This is called ferning. Neither urine nor vaginal secretions assume this same pattern.

Another way to identify amniotic fluid is by directly observing pooled fluid in the vagina. The examiner inserts a sterile speculum and then asks the woman to cough or bear down. If the membranes have ruptured, the examiner will observe fluid leaking into the vagina.

Other signs and symptoms

Women have reported other signs and symptoms shortly before labor onset. A weight loss of 1 to 3 pounds, representing water loss, may result from changes in electrolyte concentrations of body fluids, which are linked to altered estrogen and progesterone levels. Relaxin, a hormone secreted only during pregnancy, seems to soften the sacroiliac, sacrococcygeal, and pubic joints, and increase their mobility. The effect of relaxin on pelvic joints may cause or increase sacroiliac discomfort. Increased vaginal secretions may also occur, resulting from blood vessel congestion of vaginal mucous membranes.

In the last few days before labor onset, the woman may experience a burst of energy known as the "nesting instinct." She may feel compelled to clean house and otherwise ensure that everything is ready for the neonate's arrival. The nurse should caution each woman against overexertion and encourage her to rest and build up energy reserves for labor and childbirth if this occurs.

STAGES OF LABOR

Labor consists of four distinct stages. Understanding what occurs during each stage will help the nurse anticipate and meet the woman's needs in labor. The average length of labor for a primigravida is 14.5 hours and for a multigravida, 7.75 hours. True labor is characterized by progressive cervical dilation and fetal descent.

First stage of labor

The first stage is divided into latent and active phases. (See *Charting the progression of labor using the Friedman graph.*)

Latent phase

First described by Friedman, the latent phase precedes active labor. In primiparous women, this phase averages 8.6 hours; in multiparous women, 5.8 hours. During this time, irregular, short, and mild contractions occur; and the cervix dilates to 3 to 4 cm. The woman may remain at home during the early part of the latent phase. When she enters the health care facility or birthing center, she may complain of abdominal cramping and lower back discomfort. Her behavior typically displays various degrees of excitement and apprehension. If she has not yet passed the mucus plug, she commonly will do so during this phase.

Active phase

Moving from the latent to the active phase occurs when the cervix dilates faster than 1.2 cm/hour in a primiparous woman and 1.5 cm/hour in multiparous women. In about 90% of women, labor has progressed

Charting the progression of labor using the Friedman graph

The Friedman graph represents the progression of labor of a primiparous woman. An "O" indicates cervical dilation and an "X" represents station.

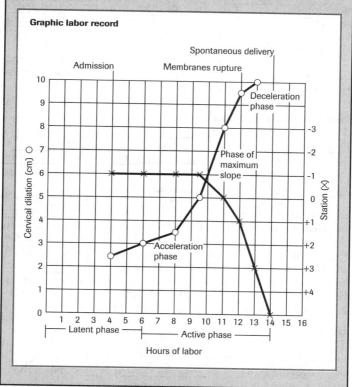

Graphic labor record

to the active phase by the time cervical dilation reaches 5 cm. During the active phase, the cervix dilates to 10 cm. Contractions occur every 2 to 5 minutes, last 40 to 50 seconds, and are moderately intense. In primiparous women, this phase averages 5.8 hours; in multiparous women, 2.5 hours. Fetal descent continues throughout the active phase. The rate of descent is at least 1 cm/hour in primiparas and 2 cm/hour in multiparas. It is referred to in relationship to the station, or the relationship of the lowest portion of the presenting part to the ischial spines of the woman's pelvis.

Transition

Transition is the shortest phase, occurring when the cervix is dilated between 8 and 10 cm. It averages less than 3 hours in primiparas and less than 1 hour in multigravidas. However, this phase is the most difficult for the woman. Intense contractions lasting between 45 and 60 seconds occur every $1^{1}/_{2}$ to 2 minutes. The woman may thrash about, become irritable, lose control of breathing techniques, and experience nausea and vomiting.

Using the Friedman graph, the nurse can follow the rate of cervical dilation and fetal descent. By plotting these, the nurse can identify normal and abnormal labor patterns.

Second stage of labor

The second stage begins with complete cervical dilation and ends with birth. Intense contractions occur every 2 to 3 minutes and last 60 to 90 seconds. For primiparous women, this stage averages 1 hour; for multiparous women, 24 minutes. In either case, a second stage lasting longer than 2 hours is considered abnormal.

The beginning of this stage is characterized by an increase in bloody show, rupture of membranes (if this has not already occurred), severe rectal pressure, and a maternal reflex bearing-down with each contraction. As the fetus approaches the perineal floor, the perineum bulges and flattens. As the labia spread, the head appears at the vaginal opening. At this time, the woman should assume an active role and push with each contraction. Research has shown that labor progress and outcome can be enhanced if the nurse encourages pushing that reinforces involuntary bearing-down instead of sustained breath-holding.

Head

To prevent maternal lacerations and damage to the fetal intracranium, the birth attendant must control the speed at which the head passes over the perineum. When necessary, the birth attendant should apply pressure over the perineum to maintain flexion of the head and decrease the occurrence of perineal lacerations. Once the head emerges, the oral and nasal pharynx are suctioned with a bulb syringe to remove any secretions blocking the airway. Then the doctor or nurse-midwife must check for the presence of the umbilical cord around the infant's neck. While this is happening, the nurse should encourage the woman to breathe easily and not push. If the cord is loose around the neck, it will be slipped over the infant's head. If the cord is very tight, fetal hypoxia may occur; therefore, the birth attendant must clamp and cut the cord and unwrap it from around the infant's neck before the birth of the shoulders.

Shoulders

Following external rotation of the head, the shoulders pass through the pelvic inlet. Holding the head, the birth attendant applies slight downward traction to deliver the anterior shoulder. After it emerges, gentle upward traction is applied to the head to allow the birth of the posterior shoulder.

Body and extremities

Once the shoulders emerge, the rest of the body, which is narrower than the shoulders, slides out with little or no traction needed.

Third stage of labor

The third stage begins immediately after birth and ends with the separation and expulsion of the placenta. Strong but generally less painful contractions continue during this stage. Their frequency may decrease to every 5 minutes. Normally, the placenta emerges approximately 5 minutes after the neonate's delivery.

Placental separation

As labor nears completion and birth becomes imminent, the uterus begins to contract forcefully. By the time the neonate is delivered, the uterus consists of an almost solid mass of muscle with walls several centimeters thick above the lower segment. This differs greatly from the large cavity that previously housed the fetus. The fundus now lies just below the umbilicus. Signs indicating placental separation include lengthening of the umbilical cord, a sudden gush of dark blood from the vagina, maternal report of vaginal fullness, and a change in uterine shape from disklike to globular. The nurse can palpate or see this above the symphysis.

Placental delivery

The placenta is expelled through one of two mechanisms. In the Schultze mechanism, the central portion of the placenta separates from the uterine wall before the outside edges do. Then the central portion folds or buckles outward, away from the retroplacental hematoma. When the placenta is expelled, the shiny, fetal side is visible; thus the name "shiny Schultze." In the Duncan mechanism, the placental edges separate first, followed by the central portion. The central portion then rolls up and is expelled sideways so that the cotyledons of the maternal side are visible; thus the name "dirty Duncan." In the Duncan mechanism, separation may be incomplete, leaving placental fragments in the uterus that could lead to hemorrhage or infection. In both cases, careful evaluation must be done of the placenta for completeness and of the woman for bleeding. (See Chapters 17 and 18 for more information.)

Fourth stage of labor

Beginning with delivery of the placenta and extending through the first 4 postpartal hours, the fourth stage is the time the woman's body adjusts to the postpartal period. She should be assessed for uterine atony, postpartal hemorrhage, abnormal vital signs, and urine retention. Ideally, the woman and her partner should hold and examine their infant and begin parent-infant bonding.

MATERNAL SYSTEMIC RESPONSE TO LABOR

Labor produces significant changes in many body systems. Understanding these changes will help the nurse provide better care for the woman during labor.

Cardiovascular system

In the first and second stages of labor, cardiovascular system changes primarily affect blood pressure. Cardiac output increases dramatically between contractions as labor progresses, rising 10% to 15% in the first stage of labor and 30% to 50% in the second stage. Contractions during the first stage of labor raise systolic blood pressure readings about 10 mm Hg and diastolic readings from 5 to 10 mm Hg. Because of this fluctuating increase, blood pressure readings between contractions will be the most reliable ones. Contractions in the second stage raise systolic and diastolic readings an average of 30 mm Hg and 25 mm Hg, respectively. Between contractions, blood pressure may remain elevated by 10 mm Hg systolic and 5 to 10 mm Hg diastolic. This persistent elevation puts a woman who already has hypertension at increased risk for complications such as cerebral hemorrhage.

The woman's position during labor also can affect blood pressure. In a supine woman, the inferior vena cava and other vessels are compressed from the weight of the uterus and its contents. This causes a reduction in the blood return to the maternal heart, which in turn has decreased cardiac output. Therefore, the woman experiences a hypotensive episode. Factors that may increase a woman's risk of supine hypotensive syndrome include dehydration, hypovolemia, obesity, multiple gestation, hydramnios, and a supine position. This can be remedied by turning the woman on her side or sitting her up, which moves the uterus and its contents off the inferior vena cava.

A strong contraction reduces blood flow through the uterine artery into the intervillous spaces. Consequently, blood flow is redirected into the peripheral circulation, leading to increased peripheral resistance. This leads to increased blood pressure and decreased pulse rate.

The woman's voluntary bearing-down efforts in the second stage of labor greatly alter intrathoracic pressure. As the woman performs Valsalva's maneuver, intrathoracic pressure increases, venous return decreases, and venous pressure increases. As blood from the lungs is forced into the left atrium, cardiac output, blood pressure, and pulse pressure all increase, and bradycardia temporarily occurs. These processes reverse when Valsalva's maneuver ceases; however, the nurse must be aware of the long-term effect on the woman with a history of cardiac disease. Also, the fetus may experience hypoxia during this time.

Other factors that may alter blood pressure during labor include anxiety, pain, and certain medications. For example, hypotension may result from administration of a narcotic such as meperidine because of its vasodilating effects or from a regional anesthetic because of its sympathetic blocking effects.

A slow, progressive rise in pulse rate typically occurs during labor. Factors that may exacerbate this rise include pain, anxiety, hemorrhage, infection, certain medications (such as tocolytics), dehydration, increased cardiac output, and decreased plasma volume.

Gastrointestinal system

During labor, gastric motility and absorption decrease and gastric emptying time increases. As a result, a woman in labor may vomit food she consumed as long as 24 hours before labor began. These normal physiologic responses are enhanced by narcotic administration, which also slows labor.

Solid foods usually are withheld during labor to prevent the risk of aspiration if an emergency arises and general anesthesia is needed. For similar reasons, some doctors advocate giving the woman antacids to neutralize gastric acid either during labor or immediately before anesthetic administration. Because gastrointestinal absorption of fluids is not altered, sipping water or chewing ice chips is allowed during labor.

Respiratory system

Oxygen consumption increases dramatically during labor, from a normal rate of about 250 ml/minute to approximately 750 ml/minute during contractions. Both during and between contractions, oxygen consumption increases progressively throughout labor. By the second stage of labor, a woman's oxygen consumption may be twice that of her consumption before the onset of labor. This dramatic increase is especially likely in an unmedicated woman experiencing extreme anxiety. Resulting hyperventilation can lead to respiratory alkalosis, hypoxia, or hypocapnia. Signs and symptoms include nausea, vomiting, dizziness, disorientation, and tingling of fingers. The nurse must monitor the woman for signs of such problems and intervene promptly to avoid endangering the fetus.

Hematopoietic system

The normal leukocyte count of 5,000 to 11,000/mm³ may increase to about 25,000/mm³ during labor. This rise occurs particularly during prolonged labor, showing a possible link to strenuous muscle activity or increased stress. Other significant hematologic changes include increased plasma fibrinogen levels and decreased plasma glucose levels and blood coagulation times.

Renal and urologic system

During labor, decreased sensory perceptions may impair the woman's ability to feel bladder fullness and the urge to void. Also, compression of the ureters by the uterus may impede urine flow. Either of these factors can lead to urinary stasis and, if bladder fullness is profound, possibly impede fetal descent. For this reason, the nurse should encourage the woman to empty her bladder every 2 hours during labor.

When engagement occurs and the presenting part of the fetus enters or passes the pelvic inlet, the base of the bladder is pushed upward and forward. Pressure from the presenting part may interfere with blood and lymph drainage from the base of the bladder, leading to tissue edema.

During labor, trace amounts of protein in urine commonly occur because of muscle breakdown. However, levels above trace amounts should alert the nurse to the possibility of pregnancy-induced hypertension.

Fluid and electrolyte balance

Labor can have several effects on the woman's fluid and electrolyte balance. Increased muscular activity increases body temperature, which causes fluid and electrolyte loss through diaphoresis. Increased respiratory rate and resultant hyperventilation increase fluid loss through evaporation. Vomiting, which may occur during transition in the active phase of labor, also can cause fluid and electrolyte loss. For these reasons, careful monitoring of fluid intake and output is essential during prolonged labor to prevent dehydration and related problems.

FETAL SYSTEMIC RESPONSE TO LABOR

Understanding the normal fetal response to labor helps the nurse quickly identify variations from normal and intervene promptly to prevent further complications.

Cardiovascular system

The normal fetal heart rate ranges from 120 to 160 beats/minute. A rate greater than 160 beats/minute for more than 10 minutes is considered tachycardia; a rate of 100 to 119 beats/minute is considered bradycardia. Normal rhythm is fairly constant, with the baseline reflecting a fluctuation of ±5 to 10 beats over a selected time interval. (See Chapter 9, Fetal assessment.)

Fetal blood pressure is one of several factors responsible for ensuring an adequate exchange of gases and nutrients to and from the fetal capillaries and the intervillous space. Adequate placental and fetal reserve ensures that the fetus can withstand the stresses of anoxia brought on by uterine contractions.

Respiratory system

The fetus's breathing activity decreases sharply during labor. Through ultrasonography, an examiner can study these breathing movements and distinguish true preterm labor from false labor.

Acid–base status

During pregnancy, the fetus is at risk for both respiratory and metabolic acidosis. Because a major role of the placenta is to function as a fetal lung, any conditions interrupting normal blood flow to or from the placenta will increase fetal partial pressure of arterial carbon dioxide and decrease fetal pH.

Since the technique of monitoring fetal scalp capillary blood pH was introduced in the early 1960s, it has gained widespread clinical acceptance because it indicates how adequately tissues are being supplied with oxygen. Measuring partial pressure of arterial oxygen (PaO_2) indicates the status of the fetus at the time of sampling; however, compared to the pH, PaO_2 may be difficult to measure correctly and may fluctuate rapidly. Because the blood pH is influenced by respiratory and metabolic factors, both rapid (respiratory) and prolonged (metabolic) changes can be detected.

During the first stage of labor, the fetal scalp capillary blood pH is approximately 7.35; during the second stage, approximately 7.25. Values below 7.2 indicate fetal distress. This decrease results from uterine contractions, which inhibit placental exchange, and from de-

creased maternal pH. Decreased values become more evident during
the second stage of labor because the hypoxia associated with pushing leads to metabolic acidosis.

Fetal activity

The term fetus moves between 20 and 50 times per hour. These movements remain largely unchanged during labor until the membranes
have ruptured; then the movements decrease.

Using ultrasound to study movement during labor, researchers found
that fetal behavioral states present during pregnancy continue during
labor. The fetus periodically changes from quiet to active sleep states,
in spite of ruptured membranes and uterine contractions that progressively increase in frequency, duration, and intensity.

Vital signs

During the fetus's quiet sleep state, which normally lasts about 40 minutes, the heart rate variability may decrease. A decrease lasting more
than 40 minutes, however, may indicate fetal hypoxia and requires
further investigation.

A low maternal temperature has been shown to lead to fetal bradycardia; however, the fetal heart rate returns to normal as maternal
temperature rises. The temperature of amniotic fluid and the fetus
parallels the woman's temperature. The fetus responds to lower tem-
peratures with decreased metabolic requirements and a decreased pulse
rate.

9

FETAL ASSESSMENT

Early and informed nursing judgments about fetal heart rate (FHR) data can be crucial to performing timely and appropriate nursing interventions.

PHYSIOLOGIC BASIS OF FETAL MONITORING

Fetal monitoring provides data about fetal status during the intrapartal period. Hypoxic or nonhypoxic stress on the fetus produces characteristic FHR patterns detectable through electronic monitoring techniques. To detect such patterns accurately, the nurse must understand basic physiologic principles of uteroplacental-fetal circulation and FHR regulation.

Uteroplacental–fetal circulation

During labor, fetal well-being depends on effective oxygen exchange from the maternal circulation through the placenta to the fetus. Any condition or factor that disrupts this circulatory route can compromise fetal well-being.

Factors affecting uteroplacental-fetal circulation

Any condition that decreases maternal cardiac output reduces placental blood flow. During labor, uteroplacental-fetal circulation can be affected by maternal position, uterine contractions, placental surface area and diffusion distance, anesthetics, maternal hypertension or hypotension, and cord compression. The nurse's primary goal is to maintain adequate maternal circulation and perfusion to the placenta so that the fetus can receive the needed oxygen and nutrients.

Fetal heart rate regulation

The FHR is regulated by the sympathetic and parasympathetic divisions of the autonomic nervous system and chemoreceptors and baroreceptors. The normal range of the FHR is 120 to 160 beats/minute.

Through the vagal reflex, the parasympathetic nervous system controls the FHR and is responsible for its beat-to-beat changes. When the vagal reflex is stimulated, the FHR decreases. Conversely, stimulation of the sympathetic nervous system increases the FHR.

The autonomic nervous system receives information on blood pressure and oxygen status from chemoreceptors and baroreceptors, which help the autonomic nervous system stabilize blood pressure.

Chemoreceptors detect even minute changes in tissue oxygen levels and trigger the sympathetic nervous system to increase the FHR so that more blood will circulate to the affected area, increasing tissue oxygenation. As a result, fetal blood pressure increases.

Baroreceptors are extremely sensitive to any elevation in blood pressure. An increase in blood pressure provokes baroreceptors to signal the parasympathetic nervous system to rapidly decrease the FHR. As the FHR decreases, so does fetal cardiac output and blood pressure.

FETAL AND UTERINE MONITORING

Careful monitoring of fetal and uterine functions during labor helps the nurse identify problems before they cause serious complications. Monitoring methods include manual techniques and internally and externally applied devices for electronic fetal monitoring (EFM).

Fetal monitoring

The nurse can monitor the FHR through auscultation, using a fetoscope or an ultrasound stethoscope (Doppler blood flow detector), or through EFM. Each method carries distinct advantages and disadvantages.

Fetoscope and ultrasound stethoscope

Historically, auscultating the FHR during labor has been considered sufficient monitoring for the low-risk patient and fetus. The fetoscope is a special stethoscope that enhances the nurse's ability to hear the fetal heartbeat. Each type uses an enlarged bell with a small plate attached to it and the nurse's forehead is pressed against this plate. This allows the sound of the FHR to be conducted through the nurse's skull, thus making it easier to hear.

In contrast, the ultrasound stethoscope uses ultra-high-frequency sound waves to detect fetal heartbeats. The ultrasound stethoscope can be used as early as the 10th week of gestation to listen to the FHR.

According to guidelines originally developed by the Nurses' Association of the American College of Obstetricians and Gynecologists (now called the Association of Women's Health, Obstetric, and Neonatal Nurses), the nurse should perform auscultation for the low-risk patient every 60 minutes during the latent phase and every 30 minutes during the active phase of the first stage of labor and every 15 minutes during the second stage; for the high-risk patient, every 30 minutes during the latent phase and every 15 minutes during the active phase of the first stage and every 5 minutes during the second stage.

A disadvantage of auscultation is that it cannot be used to assess the most important sign of fetal well-being: beat-to-beat variability of the FHR. (See *Auscultating for fetal heart tones*, page 194.)

Electronic fetal monitoring

EFM can be used externally or internally to establish a continuous record of the FHR and its relationship to uterine contractions. A heart rate pattern that is normal or otherwise within EFM guidelines is a reliable indicator of fetal well-being. At times, abnormal patterns may occur without indicating fetal distress; however, fetal hypoxia reliably produces changes in the FHR pattern.

External EFM. This technique allows safe, ongoing assessment of the FHR. One widely used method of external EFM is the ultrasound transducer. A transducer is guided over the patient's abdomen to determine the area closest to the fetal heart. After placement, the transducer emits low-energy, high-frequency ultrasound waves and directs them through the abdominal wall toward the fetal heart. These ultrasound waves strike the heart wall and are deflected back through the abdominal wall, where the transducer receives them. The transducer then relays the waves to the fetal monitor, which translates them two ways: into a signal that sounds like a heartbeat and into waveform lines on the monitor strip.

Besides being noninvasive, ultrasound poses no apparent risk for the fetus or mother. This method allows the nurse to monitor short-term (but not beat-to-beat) variability, long-term variability, and periodic accelerations and decelerations of the FHR. (See the section "Fetal heart rate patterns.")

Unfortunately, the monitor can make errors in counting when the FHR falls below 60 beats/minute. It may count both motions of the cardiac cycle, which falsely doubles the heart rate, a condition known as doubling. Conversely, with an accelerated FHR of 200 beats/minute or above, the monitor counts only half the beats, a situation known as halving. These problems demonstrate the hazards of relying solely on technology. A nurse who has any question about the accuracy of external EFM should auscultate for the FHR to verify the rate.

PSYCHOMOTOR SKILLS

Auscultating for fetal heart tones

The nurse auscultates for fetal heart tones to assess the fetal heart rate (FHR), which provides information about fetal viability and stress. To auscultate for fetal heart tones, follow these guidelines.

1 Place the earpieces of an ultrasound stethoscope in your ears and press the bell gently on the patient's abdomen. Start listening at the midline about midway between the umbilicus and the symphysis pubis. As an alternate auscultation method, listen with a fetoscope on your head with the bell extending from the center of your forehead. Then press the bell about 1/2" (1 cm) into the patient's abdomen. Remove your hands. With either method, move the bell slightly from side to side, if needed, to the point where the heart tones are loudest.

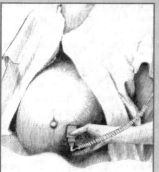

ULTRASOUND STETHOSCOPE

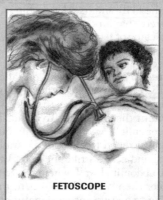

FETOSCOPE

2 Listen throughout several contractions and for at least 60 seconds after to establish the well-being of the fetus. The normal FHR is 120 to 160 beats/minute. Check the FHR every 30 to 60 minutes during early labor, every 15 minutes during active labor, and every 5 minutes during the second stage of labor. Remember that heart rate accelerations and decelerations occur periodically during contractions and fetal movements.

Internal EFM. Nurses may wonder why internal EFM is used when external EFM is noninvasive and easier to use. With external EFM, extraneous noises from pulsating maternal vessels and from maternal and fetal movement may interfere with an accurate, clear tracing. The trans-

Auscultating for fetal heart tones (continued)

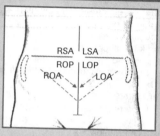

3 If fetal heart tones are difficult to hear, perform Leopold's maneuvers to determine the fetal position and find the site where the heart tones are likely to be heard best. This illustration divides the abdomen into quadrants; start listening at the point indicated by the position of the fetus. If the fetal heart tones are still not clear, move in the direction indicated by the arrows. The fetus is likely to be in one of the following positions: left sacral anterior (LSA), left occiput anterior (LOA), left occiput posterior (LOP), right sacral anterior (RSA), right occiput anterior (ROA), or right occiput posterior (ROP). For example, with the fetus in a cephalic presentation, fetal heart tones are loudest midway between the patient's umbilicus and the anterior superior spine of the ilium; in a breech presentation, tones are loudest at or above the level of the umbilicus.

ducer must be repositioned frequently to maintain a clear signal. In contrast, the waveforms produced by internal EFM are not affected by maternal or fetal movement and can produce an accurate tracing of the fetal heartbeat with beat-to-beat variability and uterine contractions.

Internal EFM is performed by attaching a small, corkscrew-type spiral electrode to the fetal presenting part during a pelvic examination. The electrode penetrates the presenting part about 1.5 mm and must be attached securely to ensure a good signal. Internal EFM can be used only when the patient's membranes are ruptured, when the cervix is dilated at least 2 cm, and when the presenting part is at least at the −1 station. In many health care facilities, nurses with special preparation are allowed to attach these electrodes. (See *Applying an internal EFM*, page 196.) A plate is attached to the patient's leg to hold the wires from the electrode in place. Most women consider the leg plate less distracting than the belts used with the ultrasound unit.

The spiral electrode picks up the fetal heartbeat and transmits it to the monitor. The monitor transforms the impulse into a fetal electrocardiogram waveform on an oscilloscope screen and a waveform on the printout. These data are more accurate than those provided by external EFM and allow the nurse to track and calculate beat-to-beat variability in the FHR.

PSYCHOMOTOR SKILLS

Applying an internal EFM

Internal electronic fetal monitoring (EFM) provides the most accurate information for assessing fetal status in utero. The fetal heart rate is monitored via an electrode. The uterine contractions are monitored via an internal catheter connected to a pressure gauge. Use sterile technique when placing internal monitors.

The spiral electrode (at left) is inserted during a vaginal examination. The electrode is attached to the presenting fetal part, usually the scalp or buttocks.

The internal catheter (at right) is inserted up to the black mark during a vaginal examination and connected to a monitor that interprets uterine contraction pressures.

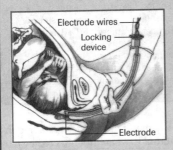
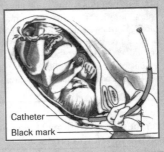

Uterine activity monitoring

Like any muscle, the uterus can contract and relax. Its normal resting tone is 5 to 15 mm Hg. In the first stage of labor, when the uterus contracts, the tone rises to 50 to 75 mm Hg. During the second stage of labor, when the patient does not push, it may rise to 75 to 100 mm Hg with contractions.

Increased uterine activity can result from factors other than normal contractions during labor, including incautious use of oxytocin and abruptio placentae.

Contractions that occur at 3-minute intervals dilate the cervix most effectively and allow sufficient time for the fetus and uterine muscle to reoxygenate.

Contractions that occur less than 2 minutes apart or last longer than 90 seconds reflect increased uterine activity, which can indicate hyperstimulation. This reduces perfusion to the placenta and can lead to fetal distress. In response to hyperstimulation, the fetus typically displays a prolonged deceleration or late decelerations of the heart rate.

Therefore, the nurse must monitor uterine activity as closely as FHR. Uterine activity can be monitored externally by using palpat. or a tocodynamometer or internally with an intrauterine pressu. catheter. Telemetry also can be used to monitor the patient in labor.

Manual palpation

The manual method of monitoring uterine contractions, palpation, requires no special equipment. It does, however, require skill and sensitivity to touch. To palpate uterine contractions, the nurse places the palmar surfaces of the fingers on the top of the uterine fundus where it contracts.

During mild contractions, the fundus indents easily and feels like a chin. In moderate contractions, the fundus indents less easily and feels more rigid, like the tip of the nose. With strong contractions, the fundus is firm, resists indenting, and feels like a forehead. The nurse must remember to palpate a set of at least three contractions to obtain sufficient data to evaluate a uterine contraction pattern.

External tocodynamometer

The tocodynamometer, a pressure-sensitive disk, is attached to an elastic belt strapped on the patient's abdomen so that the disk lies directly over the fundus. The pressure exerted by uterine contractions is then amplified and relayed to the FHR monitor, which records the frequency and duration of the contractions. It does not record the intensity of contractions.

If the tocodynamometer is not placed properly on the fundus, contractions may not be recorded. Also, the tighter the belt is strapped, the stronger the contractions appear on the graph, and vice versa.

Internal intrauterine pressure catheter

When oxytocin is used to stimulate labor, or when labor fails to progress normally, an internal intrauterine pressure catheter is used. When properly inserted, this device accurately and continuously records uterine tone and the frequency, duration, and intensity of uterine contractions. It can be inserted after the cervix has dilated 2 to 3 cm and the membranes have ruptured.

In this sterile procedure, the nurse assists the doctor or nurse-midwife by filling and irrigating the end of a pliable plastic catheter with sterile water. Then the doctor or nurse-midwife inserts the catheter through the vagina and into the cervix, alongside the fetus. The catheter is advanced approximately 18" (46 cm) until its black mark is visible at the introitus. (See *Applying an internal EFM.*) After insertion is completed, the catheter is irrigated again to clear any bubbles or vernix that may interfere with transmission, and then it's taped to the woman's leg; the syringe and catheter are attached to their proper outlets on the strain gauge.

Each uterine contraction compresses the water in the catheter. This pressure is relayed through the plastic tubing to an external pressure-sensitive device, which relays the pressure to an attached monitor that records the pressure as mm Hg on the monitor strip. The contraction appears on the graph as an inverted "U."

The intrauterine pressure catheter can use various pressure-sensitive devices. One device, the strain gauge, has a plastic dome filled with sterile water that exerts pressure on a membrane within the unit. A disposable unit does not require water or a strain gauge. This unit eliminates the time-consuming set-up, irrigation, and calibration required by other types. However, the disposable unit is more expensive and may have to be replaced if the unit is disconnected when the patient arises to use the bathroom.

The nurse can speed intrauterine catheter insertion by preparing the equipment in advance and explaining the procedure to the woman. This gives the nurse time for any necessary troubleshooting.

Telemetry

By using remote monitoring, or telemetry, the nurse can monitor the woman in labor as she moves about. External and internal methods are available. For the woman with external EFM equipment, a battery-powered, two-way radio transmitter on a shoulder strap allows remote monitoring of the FHR and uterine contractions. Internal EFM equipment requires insertion of a transmitter into the vaginal vault after the pressure catheter is placed in the uterus and a scalp electrode is applied to the fetal presenting part. Both telemetry methods provide close assessment of the woman's labor and allow her to move freely within a specified area and not be confined to bed earlier than desired.

A fetus coping well with the stress of labor will typically exhibit a reassuring FHR pattern; a fetus in distress will demonstrate an abnormal pattern. Fetal distress may reveal itself in various combinations of symptoms: An increasing baseline FHR may indicate the fetus is trying to compensate for decreased oxygen reserves; late decelerations indicate placental insufficiency and the need for prompt intervention.

FETAL HEART RATE PATTERNS

Labor and delivery put stress on even the healthiest fetus. Accurate interpretation of a monitor strip of fetal heart patterns can help the nurse determine when a fetus has crossed the line from normal stress to distress. (See *Reading a fetal monitor strip*.)

Baseline fetal heart rate

The starting point for all fetal assessment is the baseline FHR. Accurate baseline FHR determination serves as a reference for all subsequent FHR readings taken during labor.

Reading a fetal monitor strip

The monitor strip is divided into two sections. The top section shows the fetal heart rate (FHR) measured in beats/minute (bpm). The nurse reads both sections of the strip horizontally and vertically. Reading horizontally, each small square represents 10 seconds. Between each vertical dark line are six squares, which represent 1 minute. Reading vertically, each square represents an amplitude of 10 bpm.

The bottom section shows uterine activity (UA), measured in mm Hg. Reading horizontally, each small square represents 10 seconds; the space between each vertical black line represents 1 minute. Reading vertically, each square represents 5 mm Hg of pressure.

The baseline FHR, or "resting" heart rate, is assessed between uterine contractions and when no fetal movement is occurring. The baseline FHR—normally 120 to 160 bpm with a variability of ±10 bpm—serves as a reference for subsequent heart rate readings taken during contractions.

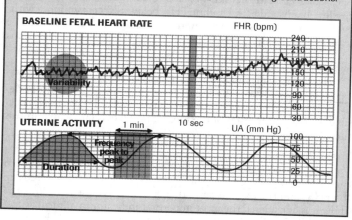

Establish the baseline FHR between uterine contractions and when there is no fetal movement. In a full-term fetus, baseline FHR normally ranges between 120 and 160 beats/minute. Initially, the nurse establishes the baseline FHR by examining approximately 5 to 10 minutes of the FHR on the monitor strip; the baseline FHR is the average rate between contractions during that 5- to 10-minute period. Once a baseline FHR is established, it does not change unless a new rate is present for 15 minutes. Deviations from the normal baseline FHR include tachycardia, bradycardia, and increased or decreased variability. (See *Variations of baseline fetal heart rate,* pages 201 and 202.)

Baseline tachycardia

A baseline FHR exceeding 160 beats/minute and lasting for more than 10 minutes indicates baseline tachycardia. Several factors can produce tachycardia in the fetus. The most common cause is maternal fever, which raises the fetal metabolic rate and, consequently, the baseline FHR. Baseline tachycardia also may be the first sign of intrauterine infection with prolonged rupture of membranes. Another possible cause is maternal anxiety, which releases epinephrine that crosses the placenta and increases the baseline FHR. Drugs that can cause fetal baseline tachycardia when used by the mother include parasympathetic blocking agents, such as atropine and scopolamine, and beta sympathomimetics, such as ritodrine and terbutaline. Baseline tachycardia also may be a response to hypoxia.

Baseline bradycardia

A baseline FHR in the range of 100 to 119 beats/minute is termed baseline bradycardia. A baseline FHR below 120 beats/minute without late decelerations but with normal beat-to-beat variability can be reassuring. Baseline bradycardia accompanied by late decelerations and little or no variability is an ominous sign of advanced fetal distress from hypoxia and acidosis.

The rare case of congenital heart block produces a baseline bradycardia of 60 to 80 beats/minute. A fetus with heart block must be delivered in a facility where cardiac surgery is available. Whenever possible, intrapartal transfer of the mother and fetus is indicated in this situation.

Variability

Variability refers to the beat-to-beat changes in FHR that result from the interaction of the sympathetic nervous system, which speeds up the FHR, and the parasympathetic nervous system, which slows the FHR. It is considered the most important indicator in clinical assessment of fetal well-being. Beat-to-beat variability can only be evaluated while using an internal scalp electrode.

Variability has two components—long-term and short-term. Long-term variability refers to the larger periodic and rhythmic deviations above and below the baseline FHR. Normal long-term variability ranges from 5 to 20 beats/minute in rhythmic fluctuations, three to five times per minute.

Short-term variability describes the differences in successive heartbeats, as measured by the R-R wave interval of the QRS cardiac cycle. It represents actual beat-to-beat fluctuations in the FHR and the balance between the sympathetic and parasympathetic nervous systems. Short-term variability is classified as present or absent. Normal

Variations of baseline fetal heart rate

By properly interpreting baseline fetal heart rate (FHR), the nurse can determine fetal well-being. This chart presents possible causes, clinical significance, and nursing interventions associated with baseline tachycardia and baseline bradycardia as well. The strips below show representative baseline FHR and various baseline variations.

Baseline tachycardia: FHR > 160 bpm for more than 15 minutes

POSSIBLE CAUSES	CLINICAL SIGNIFICANCE	NURSING INTERVENTIONS
• Early fetal hypoxia • Maternal fever or infection • Parasympathetic agents, such as atropine and scopolamine • Beta-sympathomimetic agents, such as ritodrine and terbutaline • Amnionitis • Maternal hyperthyroidism • Fetal anemia • Fetal heart failure • Fetal cardiac arrhythmias	Persistent tachycardia without periodic changes usually does not adversely affect fetal well-being—especially when associated with maternal fever. However, tachycardia is an ominous sign when associated with late decelerations, severe variable decelerations, or absence of variability (See chart below.)	Intervene to alleviate the cause of fetal distress and provide supplemental oxygen (7 to 8 L/minute), as prescribed. Also administer I.V. fluids, as prescribed. Patient should be on her left side for best circulation to the fetus.

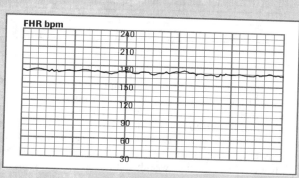

FHR bpm

(continued)

Variations of baseline fetal heart rate *(continued)*

Baseline bradycardia: FHR < 120 bpm for more than 15 minutes

POSSIBLE CAUSES	CLINICAL SIGNIFICANCE	NURSING INTERVENTIONS
• Late fetal hypoxia • Beta-adrenergic blocking agents, such as propranolol, and anesthetics • Maternal hypotension • Prolonged umbilical cord compression • Fetal congenital heart block	Bradycardia with good variability and without periodic changes is not a sign of fetal distress if the FHR remains above 80 bpm. Bradycardia caused by hypoxia is ominous when associated with loss of variability and late decelerations. (See chart below.)	Intervene to alleviate the cause of fetal distress. Administer supplemental oxygen (7 to 8 L/minute), start an I.V. line, and administer fluids, as prescribed. Patient should be positioned on her left side for the best circulation to the fetus.

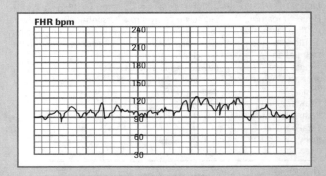

short-term variability—2 to 3 beats per amplitude—is considered the most reliable single indicator of fetal well-being. Variability is described as normal, increased, decreased, or absent.

Factors increasing variability. In the healthy fetus, movement accelerates the heart rate and increases long-term variability. This concept serves as the basis for assessing fetal well-being with the nonstress test. This test can be performed weekly as indicated, usually after week 32 of pregnancy.

The nonstress test (NST) indicates fetal well-being if the fetus can accelerate its heart rate two or more times in 15 minutes in response to a stimulus from contractions or fetal movement. If each acceleration increases 15 beats/minute above the baseline and lasts 15 seconds or more, the NST is considered within normal limits.

Variability also increases during the second stage of labor, which begins when the cervix is fully dilated and ends with birth. This increase may be related to a mild hypoxia caused by the increased intensity, duration, and frequency of uterine contractions. As the fetus descends the birth canal, a prolonged deceleration or bradycardia typically results.

Commonly, short- and long-term variability increase when the fetus assumes the occiput posterior position.

When hypoxemia occurs, the fetus responds initially by increasing short- and long-term variability. If this hypoxemia is untreated, it can lead to fetal heart rate decelerations. For example, if a woman is on an oxytocin drip to induce or augment labor and uterine contractions occur closer than every 2 minutes or last longer than 90 seconds (a condition known as uterine tachysystole), contractions occur too quickly, preventing complete fetal oxygenation. The fetal stress liberates epinephrine, and variability increases. In this situation, the nurse should reduce the frequency of contractions by decreasing the oxytocin as prescribed and by having the woman turn to her left side, which decreases the frequency of contractions.

Factors decreasing variability. Although decreased variability can endanger the fetus, the nurse never should presume fetal distress based solely on a decrease in variability.

A benign cause of decreased variability is quiet fetal sleep. The fetus normally has sleep-awake cycles lasting 20 to 30 minutes. After a period of normal variability, short- and long-term variability suddenly decrease. This sudden onset, and the absence of other signs of fetal distress such as late decelerations, should reassure the nurse that this is a sleep state, not a sudden catastrophe. When the fetus awakens, the variability reappears just as suddenly.

Drugs that depress the fetal central nervous system (CNS), such as narcotics, or block the action of the fetal parasympathetic nervous system, such as atropine, can decrease variability. When these drugs are administered to the mother, the nurse should expect a decrease in variability and be reassured if no other signs of fetal distress, such as late decelerations, are present.

Fetal arrhythmias, such as paroxysmal atrial tachycardia and complete heart block, will decrease variability. The sympathetic nervous system becomes dominant and increases the FHR. The nurse should be aware that the higher the FHR, the lower the variability.

Hypoxia and acidosis develop gradually and are two of the more dangerous causes of decreased variability. Initially, the fetus may react to hypoxemia with increased heart rate variability. As a continued decrease in oxygen progresses to hypoxia, the heart rate accelerates as the fetus attempts to increase oxygenation. The result is baseline tachycardia and decreased or absent variability. Over time, the lack of oxygen harms the fetal CNS. If this cycle of deterioration continues, acidosis develops and direct myocardial depression of the FHR occurs. At this stage, the fetus will be near death and may display baseline bradycardia.

Periodic changes

Transient accelerations or decelerations from the baseline FHR are called periodic changes and are caused by uterine contractions and fetal movements. They represent the normal rhythmic fluctuations from the fetal resting pulse.

Accelerations

Transient accelerations in the FHR normally are caused by fetal movements and uterine contractions. This type of acceleration typically indicates fetal well-being and adequate oxygen reserve. Accelerations also may be caused by partial umbilical cord compression.

Decelerations

Periodic decelerations from the normal baseline FHR are classified as early, late, or variable, depending on when they occur and their waveform shape. (See *Common decelerations*.)

Early decelerations. Decelerations that begin early in the contraction are associated with normal FHR variability and are well tolerated by the fetus. They are unaffected by maternal oxygen administration or position changes and require no nursing intervention.

Early decelerations exhibit a uniform waveform shape on the monitor strip, typically mirroring that of the uterine contractions. They arise from pressure on the fontanels produced by uterine contractions when the cervix is dilated 4 to 7 cm. This pressure produces localized hypoxemia that stimulates the chemoreceptors. As the baroreceptors are stimulated, the vagal system decreases the FHR in response. The onset, the lowest point of descent, and the recovery from early decelerations occur exactly in sequence with the contraction.

Late decelerations. These decelerations start after the beginning of a contraction. The lowest point of a late deceleration occurs after the contraction ends; descent and return are gradual and smooth. The FHR rarely falls more than 30 to 40 beats/minute below the baseline FHR. Late decelerations typically produce U-shaped waveforms.

(*Text continues on page 208.*)

Common decelerations

Decelerations—periodic decreases in fetal heart rate (FHR)—are caused by uterine contractions, fetal movements, or fetal distress. This chart illustrates early, late, and variable decelerations, and then lists their possible causes, clinical significance, and appropriate nursing interventions.

Early deceleration

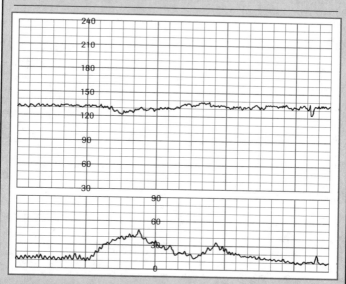

Possible causes
• Compression of the fetus's head

Characteristics
• Descent, peak, and recovery of deceleration waveform mirrors the contraction.

Clinical significance
• Is benign
• Indicates head compression at 4 to 7 cm dilation

Nursing interventions
• Reassure the patient that the fetus is not at risk.

(continued)

Common decelerations (continued)

Late deceleration

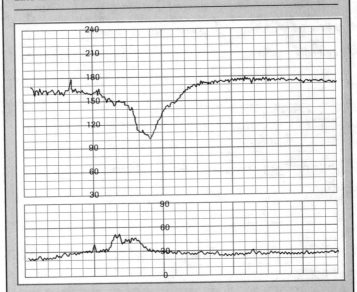

Possible causes
- Uteroplacental circulatory insufficiency (placental hypoperfusion) caused by decreased intervillous blood flow during contractions or structural defect in placenta, such as abruptio placentae
- Uterine hyperactivity caused by excessive oxytocin infusion
- Maternal hypotension or maternal supine hypotension syndrome

Characteristics
- Deceleration waveform begins about 30 seconds after the contraction begins.
- Lowest point of deceleration waveform occurs after the peak of the contraction.
- Recovery occurs after the contraction ends.

Clinical significance
- Indicates uteroplacental insufficiency
- May lead to fetal hypoxia and acidosis if underlying cause is not corrected

Common decelerations *(continued)*

Late deceleration *(continued)*

Nursing interventions
- Turn the patient on her left side to increase placental perfusion and decrease contraction frequency.
- Increase the I.V. fluid rate to increase intravascular volume and placental perfusion, as prescribed.
- Administer oxygen by mask at 7 L/minute to increase fetal oxygenation, as prescribed.
- Notify doctor or nurse-midwife.
- Assess for signs of the underlying cause, such as hypotension and uterine tachysystole.
- Take other measures, such as discontinuing oxytocin, as prescribed.
- Explain rationales for interventions to the patient and support person.

Variable deceleration

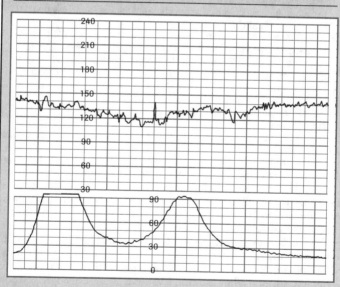

Possible causes
- Umbilical cord compression causing decreased fetal oxygen perfusion

(continued)

Common deceleration *(continued)*

Variable deceleration *(continued)*

Characteristics
- Deceleration waveform shows abrupt onset and recovery.
- Waveform shape varies and may resemble the letter U, V, or W.
- FHR commonly decreases to 60 beats/minute.

Clinical significance
- Is most common deceleration pattern in labor because of contractions and fetal movement
- May indicate cord compression
- Is well tolerated if the fetus has sufficient time to recover between contractions and if the deceleration does not last more than 50 seconds

Nursing interventions
- Help the patient change positions. No other intervention is necessary unless fetal distress is evident.
- Assure the patient that the fetus tolerates cord compression well. Explain that cord compression affects the fetus the same way that breath-holding affects the patient.
- Assess deceleration pattern for reassuring signs: baseline FHR not increasing, short-term variability not decreasing, abrupt beginning and ending of decelerations, and deceleration lasting less than 50 seconds.
- If assessment does not reveal reassuring signs, notify the doctor or nurse-midwife; then start I.V. fluids and administer oxygen by mask at 7 L/minute, as prescribed.
- Explain the rationales for nursing interventions to the patient and her support person.

Usually repetitive, late decelerations occur with each contraction, although in some cases they will occur only with stronger contractions.

Late decelerations are nonreassuring, or an ominous sign, because they indicate uteroplacental insufficiency, which comes from decreased intervillous blood flow. This decreased blood flow leads to inadequate oxygen exchange.

The nurse may counter the underlying cause of uteroplacental insufficiency and may reverse its course by removing it. Maternal hypotension usually can be remedied by changing the patient's position to her left side and administering I.V. fluids as prescribed. If oxytocin is overstimulating the uterus, it should be discontinued. Then contractions should occur less frequently, giving the fetus more time to reoxygenate, and the late decelerations may disappear.

However, intrinsic causes of uteroplacental insufficiency usually cannot be reversed. Such conditions as diabetes, pregnancy-induced hypertension, and pregnancy of 42 weeks or more may foster a placenta that is structurally incapable of meeting fetal oxygen needs, particularly during labor.

The nurse who recognizes a late deceleration pattern and intervenes appropriately may help prevent fetal hypoxia and asphyxia. If a second late deceleration occurs, the nurse should notify the doctor or nurse-midwife and intervene to decrease uterine activity by discontinuing oxytocin, maximize uterine perfusion by turning the woman on her left side, administer oxygen by mask at a rate of 7 L/minute, and increase I.V. fluids as prescribed.

If decelerations persist for more than 30 minutes and birth is not imminent, the nurse should alert the doctor or nurse-midwife again and notify other appropriate personnel. A cesarean delivery may be necessary. The need for cesarean delivery depends on the woman's parity and degree of cervical dilation. For example, a primiparous woman at 2 cm dilation with uncorrectable late decelerations is not a candidate for a vaginal delivery, but a multiparous woman at 9 cm dilation possibly could deliver vaginally without jeopardizing the fetus.

Variable decelerations. When fetal movements or contractions compress the umbilical cord, variable decelerations occur. Dramatic and unpredictable, they vary in shape, duration, depth, and timing. To the woman and support person, a variable deceleration may seem to indicate that the fetus's heart has stopped. The nurse should reassure them that these decelerations are the most common patterns during labor and usually are no cause for alarm. The nurse should explain that the decrease in FHR is analogous to the fetus holding its breath during a contraction and then resuming breathing.

Variable decelerations seem dramatic and they can resemble early and late deceleration patterns. Cord compression stimulates the chemoreceptors and baroreceptors, causing the FHR to drop rapidly. A deceleration to 60 beats/minute or below is common.

The deceleration in the FHR produces shapes like the letters V, U, or W on the monitor strip. To tolerate these episodes well, the fetus must have sufficient time between contractions to reoxygenate.

In many cases, variable decelerations are preceded and followed by slight accelerations called shoulders. The FHR accelerates slightly, then decelerates suddenly and sharply; the deceleration ends just as suddenly as it begins. Finally, a small acceleration (the other shoulder) occurs before the baseline FHR is reestablished. These shoulders occur because the contraction occludes only the umbilical vein at first. When the umbilical arteries also are occluded, the deceleration occurs. Shoulders are a reassuring sign.

Variable decelerations can be mild, moderate, or severe. The nurse should know the differences but also should realize that certain fetuses can tolerate severe variable decelerations, while other fetuses have difficulties even with mild ones. Therefore, the nurse must assess the monitor strip according to reassuring and nonreassuring criteria.

A reassuring variable pattern has an abrupt onset and end, the baseline FHR does not increase, and short-term variability does not decrease. A nonreassuring pattern includes signs of hypoxemia. At first, variability increases, but the baseline FHR remains within normal limits. Eventually, the FHR accelerates to a baseline tachycardia as the fetus tries to compensate for the growing oxygen deficit. Hypoxia becomes more evident as variability decreases. The shape of the variables may become more rounded, and the onset and end smoother, indicating that the CNS is adversely affected.

To help correct variable decelerations, the nurse should try to alleviate cord compression by changing the woman's position, using the knee-chest, Trendelenburg, or other positions as needed. In most cases, maternal repositioning alleviates cord compression, allowing resumption of oxygen flow and fetal reoxygenation. Amnio-infusion, administration of fluid directly into the amniotic sac by the doctor or certified nurse-midwife, is also used to alleviate cord compression. As always, the nurse monitors the patient carefully.

If maternal repositioning is unsuccessful, the nurse should observe for reassuring and nonreassuring signs. If reassuring signs disappear, the nurse should administer oxygen. If variable decelerations persist, other interventions are necessary.

Prolonged decelerations. Prolonged decelerations, also known as a reflex bradycardia, are defined as FHR decelerations lasting 60 to 90 seconds. These occur in response to sudden stimulation of the vagal system by a vaginal examination, electrode application, or similar occurrence, and may persist for several minutes or more. During deceleration, the FHR exhibits normal or increased variabililty.

Although the nurse must notify the doctor or nurse-midwife as soon as a prolonged deceleration occurs, it does not automatically indicate uncorrectable fetal distress or cord prolapse. The vagal reflex itself may be caused by sudden hypoxemia with or without accompanying carbon dioxide retention and acidosis.

Other common factors also may trigger the vagal reflex that causes prolonged decelerations. When contractions occur closer than every 2 minutes or the uterus develops hypertonus, the sustained pressure on the fetus triggers the vagal reflex and decelerates the FHR. Variability also may increase. While the stimulus is operating, the FHR remains decelerated.

Prolonged decelerations also can be caused by such drugs as bupivacaine and lidocaine when used for regional and paracervical blocks. These drugs temporarily increase uterine tone and contraction frequency, which can decrease the FHR. Also, maternal supine hypotension syndrome may cause prolonged decelerations.

Maternal pushing in the second stage of labor puts pressure on the fetus's body. This pressure can trigger a vagal reaction, particularly in the last few minutes before birth. This is one way labor personnel know delivery is imminent.

When prolonged decelerations occur, the nurse first must assess for cord prolapse or imminent delivery. If the woman is receiving oxytocin, the nurse should discontinue the drug as prescribed and perform or assist with a vaginal examination. If the examination reveals a pulsating cord, the nurse should intervene using traditional techniques. (See *Umbilical cord prolapse*, page 353.)

If the vaginal examination rules out cord prolapse and imminent delivery, the nurse should assess the woman and monitor strip.

If the deceleration is the result of uterine hypertonus, drugs, or maternal pushing, the nurse should stay with the patient and ask another nurse to call the doctor or nurse-midwife, then stop the oxytocin, turn the woman on her left side, tell her to stop pushing, administer oxygen by mask, and increase the I.V. fluid rate as prescribed.

In most cases, the deceleration corrects itself in 10 minutes, and the fetus resuscitates itself in 30 to 60 minutes after the deceleration ends. During the recovery, the FHR shows a baseline tachycardia and a few late decelerations. Because tachycardia is a compensatory mechanism that aids fetal reoxygenation, it is a reassuring sign after a prolonged deceleration. The late decelerations verify that the fetus has just experienced hypoxia; they disappear as the fetus recovers.

OTHER FETAL ASSESSMENT TECHNIQUES

Although a normal FHR pattern during labor is a reliable indicator of fetal well-being, an abnormal pattern does not always signal distress. Several tests exist to distinguish the fetus that is in danger from the fetus that exhibits an abnormal pattern requiring no intervention. These tests are performed by the doctor or nurse-midwife.

Fetal scalp blood sampling test

At times, fetal hypoxia is suggested by a confusing FHR pattern, such as a sustained flat heart rate without late decelerations. In this case, fetal scalp blood sampling—a process for evaluating the fetus's acid-base status—can be used with fetal monitoring to assess fetal status. When vaginal delivery is anticipated within 30 to 60 minutes but the FHR shows uncorrectable late decelerations with normal variability, fetal scalp sampling can indicate that a cesarean delivery may not be necessary. The nurse can assist the health practitioner by setting up the equipment for the test and explaining it to the patient.

Fetal scalp stimulation test

Some researchers have suggested that more widespread use of the fetal scalp stimulation test could reduce by half the need for fetal scalp blood sampling. A positive (or reactive) response to stimulating the fetal scalp, either with gentle digital pressure or by applying an Allis clamp, is considered a reliable indicator of fetal well-being. A positive response is marked by an acceleration of the FHR by 15 beats/minute for at least 15 seconds.

Fetal acoustic stimulation test

The fetal acoustic stimulation (FAS) test, also called the vibratory acoustic stimulation test, may be a promising alternative to fetal scalp blood sampling. A positive test for FAS eliminates the need for the more invasive and difficult-to-perform scalp sampling procedure.

In FAS, an electrolarynx vibratory device used at 80 decibels is applied to the patient's abdomen for 3 seconds. The sound and vibrations cause an accelerated FHR. A positive result is indicated by an FHR acceleration of at least 15 beats/minute above the baseline FHR for at least 15 seconds occurring two or more times within 10 minutes, and indicates fetal well-being. A study has shown that no fetus with a positive test result had a pH less than 7.25, which is considered within the normal range.

NURSING RESPONSIBILITIES

According to nursing practice standards, the nurse using EFM when caring for a patient in labor is held legally responsible for any procedures performed. This means that the nurse is responsible for recognizing abnormal fetal heart patterns and uterine activity, intervening appropriately, and notifying the doctor or nurse-midwife whenever necessary. To meet this responsibility, the nurse must have received the special preparation to perform EFM procedures and interpret results.

The monitor strip is considered a vital part of the medical record. Therefore, the nurse must document all assessments, procedures, and interventions on the monitor strip as well as on the chart. If time is short, the nurse should make the monitor strip the primary place to document because it provides a chronological record of events. (See *Documentation checklist for fetal monitoring.*)

The nurse can be held liable for preparing a woman for a procedure to which she did not consent. Therefore, once the doctor or

Documentation checklist for fetal monitoring

The nurse should ask the following questions when assessing the fetal monitor strip and documenting findings:
- What is the frequency of contractions?
- How long do the contractions last?
- What is their intensity?
- What is the baseline fetal heart rate (FHR)?
- Is the baseline FHR within the normal range?
- If not, is baseline tachycardia or bradycardia present?
- Is long- or short-term baseline FHR variability present?
- Are accelerations present?
- Are decelerations present? If so, are they early, late, variable, or prolonged?
- Based on monitor readings, have appropriate nursing interventions been performed and documented?
- What was the outcome of the interventions?

nurse-midwife has explained the procedure and obtains informed consent, the nurse must make sure that the woman fully understands the procedure that will be performed.

If a nonreassuring pattern occurs, standards of care dictate that the nurse notify the doctor or nurse-midwife and then intervene appropriately to prevent further deterioration of fetal status. If they do not respond in a timely fashion, the nurse must follow the policy established by the health care facility. In most cases, this means informing the nurse-manager, who can intervene as necessary.

Patient teaching and support

The nurse should ask the woman what she knows about fetal monitoring. The greatest resistance to EFM typically comes from patients who do not understand its purpose. As simply as possible, the nurse should emphasize that a normal FHR is a highly reliable indicator of fetal well-being. The nurse should explain how evaluating FHR and uterine contractions can identify possible sources of danger to the fetus.

Also, the nurse should describe how EFM can assist the patient during labor and delivery by helping her time the frequency and duration of contractions.

The nurse should explain that EFM allows constant tracking of the FHR. Even the nurse who is not in the room can view the tracing on the central display at the nursing station and evaluate the data.

Maternal teaching should include all the possible situations that may cause undue anxiety. The woman should hear the fetal heartbeat and understand that the normal heart rate varies. Therefore, the nurse should demonstrate how moving the belt or changing maternal position can cause a false FHR reading. Turning off the microphone on the monitor will eliminate distracting noises.

Applying a fetal scalp electrode and an intrauterine pressure catheter also may cause anxiety about fetal injury. To allay these fears, the nurse should demonstrate the insertion of the scalp electrode so that the woman can see that only the tip of the wire slips under the fetal scalp, and explain that the procedure is no more painful than sticking a pin into a thick or calloused area of the finger. The nurse should explain that if the heart rate transmission stops suddenly after the electrode is in place, the electrode has probably fallen off and that this is no cause for alarm.

Before the intrauterine catheter is inserted, the nurse should use an unsterile sample to demonstrate how soft and pliable it is and show the woman an illustration of where the catheter is placed in the uterus. The nurse should explain the function of the catheter and the need for data on the strength of contractions, particularly if the woman is receiving oxytocin.

Despite the advantages of EFM, the nurse should remember that the woman is the focus of the care. She needs to feel that the nurse is monitoring and concerned about her, not a machine.

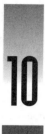

COMFORT AND SUPPORT DURING LABOR AND CHILDBIRTH

Few women experience painless labor. In fact, many describe it as intolerable, crushing, grueling, and searing. An international study of primiparous and multiparous women reported that 15% experienced little or no pain, 35% moderate pain, 30% severe pain, and 20% very severe pain.

Pain experienced during normal labor follows a predictable cycle of peaks and valleys. Despite its predictable course, however, each woman perceives labor pain as a unique, personal experience based on her physical condition, pain tolerance, and psychological background. The nurse must collaborate with other health care providers to assess the woman's perception of pain and the degree of comfort achieved through therapy. Because childbirth is a stressful experience for the woman, her partner, and other family members, steadfast support by the nurse can help ease emotional stress and physical discomfort during this time. The nurse not only gives direct support to the woman and her family, but also plays a key role in helping the woman's primary support person function effectively.

PAIN DURING LABOR

Even though each woman responds to pain uniquely, nursing interventions can help reduce pain perception and alter pain response for most women. To intervene properly, the nurse should understand the type of pain typically experienced during labor, physical and psychological factors that influence pain perception, and how observation of behavior patterns can clarify a woman's response to pain.

During the first stage of labor, pain results primarily from cervical effacement and dilation. At 0 to 3 cm of cervical dilation, the woman may describe the pain as an ache or discomfort; at 4 to 7 cm, as moderately sharp; at 7 to 10 cm, as severe, sharp, and cramping.

During the second stage of labor, pain results from friction between the fetus and birth canal and from pressure on the perineum, bladder, bowel, and uterine ligaments.

During the third stage of labor, pain results from ischemia caused by contraction of uterine blood vessels. The pain will continue until the placenta has been expelled.

Factors that influence labor pain

Many factors affect a woman's perception of and ability to cope with pain. These factors may be physiologic, social, or psychological; they include parity, fetal size and position, certain medical procedures, anxiety, fatigue, education level, cultural influence, and coping mechanisms. Knowledge of these influences can help the nurse anticipate, assess, and meet a woman's needs. (See *Response to pain*.)

Behavioral responses to labor pain

During the latent phase, the patient typically can respond to teaching and interventions because contractions have not become intensely painful. Moving to active labor typically marks the point when pain alters the woman's behavioral responses. She may lose the ability to focus attention, have difficulty following instructions, and forget proper breathing techniques. She also may withdraw from social interaction, yet fear being abandoned or left alone even for brief periods.

CULTURAL CONSIDERATIONS

Response to pain

Although each woman has her personal beliefs and values, her cultural background may influence her behavior.

Studies have shown that the response to pain varies among women and among cultures. One study of 75 Lamaze-trained women found that, among ethnic groups, response to labor pains differed significantly—even when anxiety was minimal. Patients from some groups, such as Italians and Hispanics, tend to use body language and expressions freely; those from other groups, such as Vietnamese, Irish, and Native Americans, tend to respond passively and do not openly display discomfort.

To help a woman from a different cultural background cope with her pain effectively, be aware of your personal and cultural views and take a nonjudgmental approach. During the health history, identify the woman's cultural background and determine how it may affect her response to pain.

By monitoring for reactions common to women in labor, the nurse can gauge the comfort promotion needs of each patient. Such reactions include:

- facial grimacing or groaning
- muscle tension and grunting (with bearing-down efforts)
- increased blood pressure, pulse rate, and respirations
- desire for personal contact and touch in early active labor
- withdrawal, irritability, and resistance to touch during the transition to active labor.

NURSING CARE

To provide care for the woman in labor, the nurse must be familiar with various nonpharmacologic and pharmacologic pain-relief methods.

Assessment

Assessment of a woman experiencing labor pain includes three parts. First is the health history, which investigates any medical factor that could affect the safety or efficacy of pain-reducing pharmacologic agents, plus ongoing questions about the woman's pain perception. Second is physical assessment of the woman, the fetus, and labor progress. Third is follow-up assessment, performed after implementing pain-relief measures to determine their effectiveness.

Health history

Review the woman's medical history, asking specifically about medication allergies and any obstetric problems that could affect the choice of pain-relief methods. Determine how much the woman knows about childbirth and pain-relief measures, ask about previous experiences with pain and pain-relieving agents, and assess the woman's current pain level and psychological reaction to it.

Consider the patient's obstetric history when assessing the need for pain-relief measures. Pertinent assessment topics include the length of previous labors, the woman's perception of previous labor pain, pain-relief measures used in previous labors, and her perception of their effectiveness. Also assess the woman for a drug use history. Chronic drug use can lower pain thresholds and decrease coping abilities, thereby increasing the perceptions of pain severity.

Check carefully for chronic and acute illnesses that could affect labor progress or place the patient at risk, including hypertensiive disorders, diabetes mellitus, bleeding disorders, complications of pregnancy, chronic respiratory disease, and severe dehydration. The nurse will determine the need for and level of ongoing intervention and assessment, based on her findings.

If the patient has pregnancy-induced hypertension (PIH), utero-placental perfusion may be inadequate and gas exchange may be poor. In mild cases of PIH, most analgesic and anesthetic options remain available as long as fetal assessment reveals no signs of compromise. However, regional anesthesia increases the risk of hypotension, which may cause hypoxia in the woman and fetus. Also note renal or liver disease that can accompany PIH, which may affect the metabolism of some agents, possibly resulting in toxicity.

If the patient has diabetes mellitus with no evidence of fetal distress, small doses of narcotic analgesics or an epidural block may be used for pain relief. The patient will require continuous fetal monitoring, glucose surveillance, and vital sign assessment.

The patient with placenta previa or abruptio placentae usually requires cesarean delivery. The anesthesia used for a cesarean section depends on the presence or absence of active bleeding and fetal distress. Assess for a history of any chronic respiratory disease, which could cause respiratory depression in the anesthetized patient.

Some obstetric problems may recur in successive pregnancies, resulting in longer, more painful labor or possibly necessitating surgical intervention. These include persistent posterior fetal position and cephalopelvic disproportion.

Assess the patient's knowledge of relaxation techniques, positioning, and pharmacologic options for pain relief. Assess her reaction to her partner. Is the partner helpful and supportive? Is the partner's anxiety level disturbing to her?

Cultural beliefs

Assess the woman's and family's birth culture for any beliefs and practices that could influence labor and delivery. Birth culture refers to a set of beliefs, values, and norms surrounding the birth process and shared to various degrees by members of a cultural or ethnic group. It informs members of the group about the nature of conception, the proper conditions for procreation and childbearing, the mechanism of pregnancy and labor, and the rules and rationales of antepartal and postpartal behavior. The birth culture may influence the woman's diet, her response to labor, preferred positions for childbirth, activity restrictions, and family members' roles during childbirth.

Physical assessment

When evaluating possible implementation of comfort promotion or pain-relief measures, consider maternal status, fetal status, and labor progress.

Maternal status. Observe the patient's spontaneous verbal and nonverbal expressions to assess discomfort. Keep in mind that excessive anxiety may impede cervical dilation; a small dose of an analgesic agent may relax an anxious patient sufficiently to allow cervical dilation and shorten labor.

Fetal status. Carefully consider fetal age and development before administering prescribed pain-relief agents. An immature fetus has a diminished ability to metabolize analgesic or anesthetic agents used to reduce labor pain; the doctor or nurse-midwife must carefully consider fetal status before drug administration. (See *Fetal factors that affect drug choice*.)

Heart rate offers the primary indicator of fetal well-being. Obtain and document baseline fetal heart rate and pattern before pharmacologic measures are instituted.

Labor progress. Before implementing prescribed pain-relief measures, consider labor progress. Narcotics and epidural anesthesia may slow labor further when given to a patient experiencing slow labor progress or infrequent contractions. Also consider intensity, frequency, and duration of contractions to help determine the need for pain relief.

Assess cervical dilation to ensure that pharmacologic agents are given at the safest times during labor. Systemic narcotics may be given for analgesia during the first stage of labor, but may prolong labor if administered too early in the latent phase and may depress the neonate if given too close to delivery. Antianxiety agents also may be used in the latent phase to decrease anxiety and fear. Timing is essential to achieve appropriate pain relief without adversely affecting the fetus.

FETAL STATUS

Fetal factors that affect drug choice

Certain fetal body systems mature more slowly than others. Rates of development and fetal physiology must be evaluated before the doctor or nurse-midwife selects pain-relief agents for the woman. The following development factors affect drug choice:

- A fetus with an immature blood-brain barrier has increased risk for high drug concentrations in the central nervous system.
- An immature fetus will have less plasma protein available to bind with analgesic and anesthetic agents. As a result, the plasma concentration of free (active) drug is increased.
- A fetus with an immature liver has insufficient enzymes to metabolize such agents.
- A fetus with an immature renal system cannot excrete analgesic and anesthetic agents.

Follow-up assessment

To determine the effectiveness and safety of comfort promotion and pain-relief measures, continue to assess the patient and fetus throughout labor. Observe maternal and fetal vital signs frequently, assess the patient's cardiovascular response, and watch for such adverse drug reactions as vomiting, itching, and drowsiness.

Pain relief. Assess pain relief continually during nonpharmacologic measures and at 30-minute intervals after analgesic administration. Pain should abate soon after administration of an anesthetic. Assess the duration and degree of pain relief to help anticipate additional pain-relief measures if necessary.

Effects on patient and fetus. Assess the patient's level of consciousness, respiratory rate, blood pressure, and pulse rate frequently. Narcotic analgesics may produce respiratory depression and hypotension. Narcotic analgesics can cause drowsiness that may interfere with effective bearing-down efforts in the second stage of labor.

To prevent maternal injury, assess for adverse drug reactions and allergic reactions. Watch for aspiration if a patient, made drowsy by narcotic analgesics, begins to vomit.

After administering pharmacologic agents, assess fetal heart rate according to health care facility protocol. After birth, the neonate's muscle tone, color, and respirations can reflect the effects of pharmacologic agents used on the patient.

Nursing diagnosis

After assessing the patient and fetus, review the findings and formulate nursing diagnoses related to comfort promotion and pain relief. (See Appendix 1, NANDA taxonomy of nursing diagnoses.)

Planning and implementation

The nurse provides or assists with comfort promotion and pain-reduction measures when caring for a woman in labor.

Comfort measures

Intervene to decrease anxiety, promote hygiene, and help the woman find comfortable positions that reduce labor pain and facilitate childbirth. Some women find these actions adequate to maintain comfort throughout labor.

Decrease anxiety

As contractions grow more frequent and intense, anxiety may increase. The patient may fear withdrawal of support, abandonment, the unknown, or loss of control. Increased epinephrine and norepinephrine levels raise blood pressure and pulse, diminish myometrial activity, exhaust glucose reserves, and decrease adenosine triphosphate synthesis necessary for uterine contractions.

Anxiety also leads to tension, which may cause additional pain. Nursing interventions should seek to reduce anxiety, thus decreasing blood pressure and heart rate, allowing greater energy production for effective uterine contractions, and reducing muscle tension and the heightened pain perception caused by tension.

The nurse's presence, confidence, attention, and concern help control the patient's anxiety. As labor progresses, keep her informed, teach and reinforce coping strategies, and assure her that labor is progressing normally. If assessment reveals that labor is not progressing normally, notify the doctor immediately. If she becomes discouraged or frustrated, reassure her and help her to choose an alternate method of comfort promotion.

A support person provides comfort, reassurance, and assistance with such pain-control techniques as breathing exercises, imagery, and distraction.

Helping the patient's partner also helps reduce her anxiety. Support the partner's efforts to comfort the patient. Offer instructions and assistance as appropriate.

Examples include giving the patient ice chips, rubbing her back, and bringing her items she may want. Verbal support could include coaching breathing or other pain-coping techniques and praising her for her progress. Nonverbal support could include holding her hand and stroking her face.

Promote hygiene

Nursing interventions to maintain hygiene can increase the patient's comfort level by boosting self-esteem, providing distraction, removing an additional source of discomfort, and blocking pain perception. For a patient with a nursing diagnosis of self-esteem disturbance related to inability to cope with labor pain or negative perception of behavior, the nurse may implement the following hygiene measures.

Showers and bathing. Many labor and delivery areas have showers. A warm water massage directed at the patient's back promotes relaxation and counter stimulates pain transmission. Provide a stool in the shower and a supportive bar for the patient to grasp or press against during contractions. Assist the patient or ask her partner to assist her in the shower, as needed.

Perineal care. Clean the vulva after the patient has a vaginal examination, urinates, or defecates. Provide a sanitary pad and belt to help her feel secure while walking. Change the disposable underpad as needed.

Oral hygiene. Provide frequent mouth care, as necessary. For a dry mouth, offer the patient ice chips, mouthwash, or a toothbrush or apply a cool, moistened cloth to her lips. For dry lips, suggest petroleum jelly or lip balm.

Linens and clothing. Change soiled or damp linens and gowns frequently. Offer extra pillows for comfort and socks and additional clothing to prevent chilling. If the patient grows warm during active labor, help her remove extra clothing.

Position the patient for comfort. For a patient with a nursing diagnosis of pain related to the frequency and intensity of uterine contractions, suggest that she change position to enhance comfort. During the latent and early active stages, encourage her to move about. A patient in an upright position will have stronger, more regular, and more frequent contractions because gravity helps align the fetus with the pelvic angle as the uterus tilts forward with each contraction. Maintaining this position may shorten labor and reduce pain and medication requirements.

As labor progresses and an upright position becomes uncomfortable, the patient might alternate walking with sitting, side-lying, or kneeling to provide rest and vary the intensity and frequency of contractions. If she must remain in bed during labor because of obstetric or fetal conditions, advise her to assume a side-lying position as often as possible to minimize fetal stress and enhance circulation.

Posterior fetal positions typically prolong labor and cause severe sacral pain known as back labor. To encourage rotation of the presenting part to an anterior position, therefore making the patient more comfortable, take the following steps:

- Using Leopold's maneuvers, determine the position of the fetus's back. Direct the patient to lie on the same side as the fetus's back with her upper leg propped on pillows.
- Suggest that the patient straddle a chair or lean on her partner during contractions.
- During the second stage of labor, encourage her to use a squatting or side-lying position for pushing. Many birthing beds have squatting bars that allow her to assume more comfortable, efficient positions for childbirth. After a contraction, the patient can lean back on a supportive wedge or pillow until her next contraction begins. Squatting increases the pelvic angle by approximately 30% and enhances pushing efforts as the vagina widens and shortens. A side-lying position may slow descent in the second stage of labor, but it provides more effective relief for back pain than squatting.
- Advise the patient to assume an all-fours position and to rock her pelvis to encourage fetal rotation and decrease pain. Kneeling or squatting also may be combined with pelvic rocking, but these positions can be uncomfortable and tiring for a patient not accustomed to them.

Relaxation techniques

The goal of relaxation techniques is to reduce anxiety and muscle tension, thus quieting or calming the mind and muscles. Studies indicate that relaxation decreases oxygen consumption, heart rate, respiratory rate, arterial blood lactate concentration, and sympathetic nervous system activity.

Typically, relaxation techniques distract the patient from pain, increase her sense of control over the pain, and aid sleep and rest. However, not all techniques succeed with all women; a patient may have to try several before finding relief. Even when a relaxation method succeeds, relief from fatigue may last only 5 to 20 minutes. Although these methods may reduce distress, they may not relieve pain. Assess whether and when the patient needs analgesia or an anesthetic for pain reduction. If and when this becomes necessary, relaxation techniques may increase effectiveness.

Techniques used to promote relaxation include distraction, progressive muscle relaxation, yawning, controlled breathing, imagery, touch, and music therapy. Ensure that the environment is conducive to relaxation. Remove the telephone, dim glaring lights, and maintain the room temperature at 68° to 70° F (20° to 21° C). Minimize unnecessary interruptions.

Interventions for the unprepared patient

A patient with no childbirth education presents a special challenge to the nurse, who must provide information and guide her through comfort promotion and pain reduction. Use all of the previous ideas, but keep in mind several issues.

If the patient has no support person, remain with her and assume the support role. Because the patient's anxiety and stress level may be high, teach simple relaxation techniques, including controlled breathing. Inform her of what will happen during labor, why it will happen, and how long labor may last.

If the patient has a support person, focus on that person's supporting role. Demonstrate touch, massage, and simple breathing patterns. Describe normal labor stages, expected behaviors, and typical interventions, including comfort measures and pain-relieving agents.

If an unprepared patient feels out of control, it may be difficult to shift her focus from pain to relaxation techniques. To get her attention, try such simple techniques as establishing direct eye contact, calling her by name, asking questions, and whispering into her ear. Coach the patient through relaxation techniques during a contraction; then have her practice the techniques immediately so that she knows how to use them before the next contraction.

Nonpharmacologic pain control

Comfort measures typically fall short of pain relief, which becomes important for many women as labor progresses. Methods to accomplish this goal using nonpharmacologic agents include hypnosis, transcutaneous electric nerve stimulation, and acupressure or acupuncture. These techniques require special preparation and education of the practitioner.

Pharmacologic pain control

Analgesic and anesthetic agents are the two types of pharmacologic pain relief used during labor. (For a summary, see *Drugs used to relieve labor pain*.)

Analgesia refers to pain reduction without loss of consciousness. Although the patient may continue to perceive pain, an analgesic agent can make it more tolerable.

Anesthesia refers to partial or complete loss of sensation, sometimes with loss of consciousness. Affecting the entire body or only a region of the body, an anesthetic agent blocks conduction of impulses along pain pathways to the brain.

Regional anesthetic agents are injected into areas surrounding nerves. Types used for labor pain include pudendal block, epidural block, spinal block, saddle block, or paracervical block.

General anesthetic agents render the patient unconscious and thus unable to feel pain. These agents may be inhaled or administered I.V. Typically, they are used only for emergency cesarean delivery or other surgical interventions because they greatly increase the risk of aspiration, the leading cause of anesthesia-related maternal death.

Ideally, the patient should receive information and make choices about pharmacologic options before labor begins. Childbirth education classes typically include this information. The patient's health care practitioner and anesthesiologist must describe obstetric analgesia and anesthesia and obtain written consent to administer these therapies. Provide additional information as needed, including the route of administration, degree and timing of pain relief, impact on labor and the fetus, potential adverse drug reactions, and the effectiveness of the technique selected. In addition, explain how analgesia and anesthesia may interfere with the patient's active participation in labor. Describe the immediate and prolonged effects of pharmacologic agents on the neonate. Take steps to ensure that the patient's support group will support her decision for or against pharmacologic intervention. If a patient who planned a "natural" childbirth requires pharmacologic pain relief during labor, help her work through any feelings of guilt or failure, and provide reassurance about her decision.

(Text continues on page 230.)

Drugs used to relieve labor pain

The drugs listed here are commonly used for analgesia or anesthesia in the first and second stages of labor.

DRUG, INDICATION, AND USUAL DOSE	POSSIBLE ADVERSE EFFECTS	NURSING CONSIDERATIONS
Narcotic agonists		
meperidine, morphine *Indication:* Alter pain perception; used for pain relief and mild sedation. *Dose:* meperidine 50 mg I.M., 12.5 to 25 mg I.V.; morphine 10 to 15 mg I.M. or I.V.	*Maternal:* decreased respirations, orthostatic hypotension, nausea and vomiting, itching, drowsiness *Fetal:* moderate central nervous system (CNS) depression, decreased beat-to-beat variability *Neonatal:* moderate CNS depression, mild behavioral depression	• Give meperidine during active labor; administer morphine during prodromal labor or prolonged latent phase or with hypertonic uterine dysfunction. • Review maternal history for drug allergy, substance abuse, chronic respiratory disease, and renal and liver disease. • Frequently assess maternal vital signs, respirations, and level of consciousness. • Assess labor stage and progress. • Use continuous electronic fetal heart rate (FHR) monitoring, if possible. • A degree of neonatal respiratory depression can be anticipated if administered 1 to 2 hours prior to birth. Administer naloxone as ordered.
Narcotic antagonists		
naloxone *Indication:* Reverse systemic narcotic depression, including respiratory depression caused by	*Maternal:* may reverse analgesia if given 5 to 10 minutes before delivery, increasing pain perception *Fetal:* none	• May be administered when acute opioid overdosage is suspected. • Keep resuscitation equipment nearby during administration. • Do not administer to patient with known drug dependency. • Develop a plan for alternative pain relief.

(continued)

Drugs used to relieve labor pain *(continued)*

DRUG, INDICATION, AND USUAL DOSE	POSSIBLE ADVERSE EFFECTS	NURSING CONSIDERATIONS
Narcotic antagonists *(continued)*		
narcotic toxicity in mother or neonate. *Dose:* 0.4 to 2 mg I.V. for adult; 0.01 mg/kg body weight for infant (I.V., I.M., or S.C.)	*Neonatal:* may induce withdrawal symptoms in a narcotic-depressed neonate	• Narcotic antagonists will not reverse respiratory depression caused by sedatives, hypnotics, anesthetics, or nonnarcotic CNS depressants.
Narcotic agonist-antagonists		
butorphanol tartrate, nalbuphine *Indication:* Alter pain perception; for pain relief and mild (nalbuphine) to moderate (butorphanol) sedation. *Dose:* butorphanol 1 to 2 mg I.M. or I.V.; nalbuphine 1 to 2 mg S.C., I.M., or I.V.	*Maternal:* withdrawal symptoms in a narcotic-dependent patient; decreased respirations, orthostatic hypotension, nausea and vomiting, itching, drowsiness *Fetal:* moderate CNS depression, decreased beat-to-beat variability *Neonatal:* moderate CNS depression, mild behavioral depression	• Give during active labor. • Review the patient's history for drug allergy, substance abuse, chronic respiratory disease, and renal and liver disease. • Frequently assess maternal vital signs, respirations, and level of consciousness. • Assess labor stage and progress. • Use continuous electronic FHR monitoring, if possible.
Sedative-hypnotics (tranquilizers)		
phenothiazines (promethazine, propiomazine), piperazine (hydroxyzine)	*Maternal:* may cause dizziness, lassitude, incoordination, fatigue, euphoria, or excitation	• Administer in early or active labor. • Review the patient's history for drug allergies before administration.

Drugs used to relieve labor pain *(continued)*

DRUG, INDICATION, AND USUAL DOSE	POSSIBLE ADVERSE EFFECTS	NURSING CONSIDERATIONS

Sedative-hypnotics (tranquilizers) *(continued)*

Indication: Phenothiazines and piperazine provide moderate sedation, decrease nausea and vomiting, may reduce narcotic requirements; piperazine may decrease apprehension. *Dose:* phenothiazines 50 mg I.M. or I.V.; hydroxine 25 to 100 mg I.M.	*Fetal:* decreased beat-to-beat variability; moderate CNS depression, especially with larger doses *Neonatal:* possible hypotonia, decreased feeding, lethargy, and hypothermia	• Usually given only during the early first stage of labor.
barbiturates (secobarbital, nembutal) *Indication:* Decrease anxiety and apprehension during the prodromal or early latent phase of labor; provide mild sedation. *Dose:* secobarbital 100 mg P.O.; nembutal 100 mg I.M.	*Maternal:* possible paradoxically increased pain and excitability *Fetal:* none *Neonatal:* possible CNS depression that can persist for several days	• Nembutal may be given during early labor; secobarbital may be given during false labor. • Barbiturates are administered less commonly than other tranquilizers because of their prolonged depressant effect on the neonate. • Barbiturates should be administered only if delivery is not expected for 12 to 24 hours.

(continued)

Drugs used to relieve labor pain *(continued)*

DRUG, INDICATION, AND USUAL DOSE	POSSIBLE ADVERSE EFFECTS	NURSING CONSIDERATIONS

Regional anesthetic agents

bupivacaine, lidocaine, chloroprocaine, mepivacaine
Indication: Preferred regional method for analgesia and anesthesia during first and second stage of labor; provide anesthesia for vaginal or cesarean delivery; relieve uterine pain; pudendal block relieves perineal pain.
Dose: varies

Maternal: hypotension (epidural and spinal); delayed analgesia (10 to 20 minutes); one-sided block or ineffective pain relief (spinal); prolonged labor if epidural block given too early; urine retention (epidural and spinal); increased toxicity from vascularity of region (pudendal); hematoma (pudendal); diminished bearing-down efforts (epidural)
Fetal: transient decreased beat-to-beat variability with lidocaine and mepivacaine; late decelerations; fetal distress secondary to maternal hypotension; about 30% incidence of bradycardia (paracervical)

- Determine baseline maternal vital signs and FHR; assess throughout labor as needed.
- Explain procedure and expected feelings as anesthesia is initiated.
- *Pudendal:* Assess for diminished bearing-down reflex and fetal symptoms associated with accidental scalp injection.
- *Epidural:* Ensure adequate patient hydration by administering 500 to 1,000 ml I.V. fluid before injection. Take vital signs every 5 minutes for 30 minutes after injection and report hypotension. Monitor vital signs every 15 minutes throughout continuous epidural infusion. Catheterize if patient retains urine. Labor may be augmented with oxytocin if uterine contractions diminish. Assist with positioning and maintain safety (put up side rails).
- *Spinal:* Ensure adequate hydration by administering 500 to 1,000 ml I.V. fluid before injection. Take vital signs every 5 minutes until delivery. Report hypotension, and treat as prescribed with increased fluids, left-lying position, lowering the head of the bed, and other treatments per facility protocol. Observe for signs of total spinal block (apnea, unconsciousness,

Drugs used to relieve labor pain *(continued)*

DRUG, INDICATION, AND USUAL DOSE	POSSIBLE ADVERSE EFFECTS	NURSING CONSIDERATIONS

Regional anesthetic agents *(continued)*

| | *Neonatal:* CNS depression in presence of severe hypotension; neonatal bradycardia, hypotonia, and decreased responsiveness with accidental fetal intracranial injection (pudendal block) | absent blood pressure, absent pulse, or pupil dilation). Encourage the patient to lie flat for 8 to 10 hours after administration. |

General anesthetic agents

| halothane, enflurane, thiopental sodium *Indication:* Anesthesia for cesarean delivery; surgical intervention for obstetric complications, version, extraction, or uterine manipulation. *Dose:* varies | *Maternal:* increased risk of regurgitation and aspiration; increased risk of uterine atony; decreased risk of hypovolemia compared to regional anesthesia *Fetal:* increased risk of fetal CNS depression | • Assess for risk of aspiration. Maintain nothing by mouth status.
• Administer antacid or H_2-blocking agent, as prescribed.
• Continuously monitor FHR, especially during induction of anesthesia and in response to anesthesia.
• Maintain respiratory support, I.V. fluids, and uterine fundal massage, as necessary, during recovery from anesthesia.
• Drowsiness may persist after recovery. Assist with positioning and maintain safety by putting up side rails. |

Analgesia. The patient may receive an analgesic agent when active labor is established. Administration usually takes place via an intravenous or intramuscular injection.

Analgesic agents may cause drowsiness, euphoria, orthostatic hypotension, and dizziness. Use side rails on the bed to ensure the patient's safety if a member of the health care team or a support person cannot be in constant attendance. Caution the patient and support person that she should not get out of bed without a nurse's help.

Categories of systemic analgesic agents used during labor include sedatives, narcotic agonists, mixed narcotic agonist-antagonists, antianxiety agents, and inhalation analgesics.

Regional anesthesia. By blocking pain transmission without altering consciousness, regional anesthesia allows the patient to participate in labor and childbirth while decreasing pain perception and the amount of drug that crosses to the fetus. Many doctors advocate regional anesthesia. Its disadvantages include potential central nervous system toxicity, hypotension, diminished bearing-down efforts, pruritus, urine retention, nausea, and vomiting.

The doctor, anesthesiologist, or nurse-midwife administers the anesthetic depending on the site. Drugs used most commonly include ester-type agents (chloroprocaine hydrochloride, procaine hydrochloride, and tetracaine hydrochloride) and amide-type agents (bupivacaine hydrochloride, etidocaine hydrochloride, lidocaine hydrochloride, and mepivacaine hydrochloride). The choice of agent will differ with the type of anesthetic block used.

Regional anesthesia techniques include local infiltration, such as pudendal and paracervical blocks, epidural block, and spinal block. Epidural and spinal blocks carry the risk of hypotension caused by sympathetic blockage.

Local infiltration. The doctor or nurse-midwife may use local infiltration before delivery to perform an episiotomy or after delivery to repair perineal lacerations. This simple method of anesthesia, commonly chosen by prepared patients or those seeking a more "natural" birth, produces few complications for the patient or neonate. The agent is injected directly into perineal tissue with a 22G needle. The patient may report a brief burning sensation after injection.

Pudendal block. Another form of local infiltration, this block is used during the second stage of labor to numb the perineum and vagina for delivery, episiotomy repair, or forceps delivery. The pudendal block is especially effective for difficult episiotomies or repairing lacerations after delivery. It does not block pain perceived from uterine contractions, but it may decrease bearing-down efforts.

During a vaginal examination, the needle is inserted across the sacrosciatic notch and passes the tip of the ischial spine. The doctor or nurse-midwife injects 3 to 5 ml of the drug into the pudendal nerve on each side of the sacrum. Complications include accidental injection into a blood vessel, hematoma, and perforation. If the needle enters the fetus's scalp or cranium, neonatal brachycardia, apnea, and diminished responsiveness may be present after birth.

Paracervical block. Also a type of local infiltration, this technique blocks nerves on either side of the cervix, thereby anesthetizing the uterus and cervix during the active phase of labor. This technique involves insertion of an Iowa trumpet (or needle guide) into the lateral fornix of the vagina and injecting 5 to 10 ml of anesthesia. Duration of action is approximately 1 hour, which generally provides relief through the second stage of labor.

Use of the paracervical block is infrequent today; 20 to 30 percent of fetuses develop bradycardia and subsequently may develop fetal acidosis. Also, a risk exists for inadvertent intracranial injection into the fetus.

Epidural block. The most commonly used method of pain relief during labor, the epidural block can provide continuous anesthesia to the lower half of the body during the first and second stages of labor. This type of anesthesia is commonly used during cesarean deliveries. The anesthesiologist or nurse anesthetist inserts an 18G needle into lumbar interspace 3, 4, or 5. The needle tip is advanced into the epidural space to administer the anesthetic. Although the patient's pelvis and legs feel heavy, she retains some ability to move and bear down.

Continuous epidural infusion is a variation on the epidural block. The patient receives continuous infusion of dilute anesthetic agents through an indwelling epidural catheter, a method that maintains continuous drug levels, reduces the amount of drug needed, and decreases the risk of hypotensive crisis. The same precautions should be exercised with the indwelling epidural catheter as with the standard method.

Contraindications for epidural anesthesia include coagulopathy problems, allergic reactions, placental insufficiency, and infection at the puncture site. If a virus such as herpes is present on the skin at the site of epidural injection, further dissemination of the virus may occur. An epidural block should be used with caution if the patient has high or low blood pressure. (See *Hypotensive crisis*, page 232.)

Disadvantages of epidural anesthesia include the need to have skilled anesthesia personnel or a doctor on hand to monitor the patient and fetus. Further, it may prolong labor, cause difficulty in voiding, increase oxygen use, and increase the risk of forceps delivery because of the patient's diminished bearing-down efforts.

Administering epidural anesthesia requires much skill. Areas of unanesthetized tissue, ineffective anesthesia, or inadvertent spinal anesthesia may result from improper injection. Maternal hypotension may

---

EMERGENCY ALERT

Hypotensive crisis

Hypotensive crisis may occur after spinal or epidural anesthesia as the anesthetic agent spreads through the spinal canal. A sympathetic blockade produces marked hypotension from loss of peripheral resistance, decreased venous return, and decreased cardiac output. Decreased placental perfusion occurs with maternal hypotension, resulting in fetal bradycardia.

Signs and symptoms of hypotensive crisis
- Fetal bradycardia
- Decreased beat-to-beat variability
- Maternal hypotension (20% or greater drop from baseline blood pressure or less than 100 mm Hg systolic)

Treatment and nursing considerations
- Turn patient to left lateral position to increase uterine perfusion.
- Infuse I.V. fluid rapidly, as prescribed.
- Administer oxygen by mask at 8 to 10 L/minute, as prescribed.
- Elevate the patient's legs.
- Notify the anesthesiologist.
- Administer vasopressor I.V. or I.M., as prescribed.
- Stay with the patient and monitor blood pressure and fetal heart rate frequently.

---

occur from sympathetic blockade, which causes vasodilation, loss of peripheral resistance, and central nervous system toxicity. The patient may feel chilled from peripheral temperature changes and may experience postpartal urine retention, necessitating catheterization. To help prevent hypotension, the nurse should place a blanket roll under the patient's right hip. This takes uterine pressure off major vessels and increases cardiac return.

Spinal block. This technique resembles the epidural block except that the needle penetrates the meninges and enters the subarachnoid space. The anesthesiologist mixes a single injection of anesthesia with a sample of the patient's cerebrospinal fluid and injects it into the third, fourth, or fifth lumbar inner space. The patient loses feeling and motor ability in the lower portion of her body. Numbness extends from the umbilicus to the toes (T10 level) for vaginal delivery and from the xiphoid process to the toes (T8 level) for cesarean delivery. A low spinal block, or saddle block, may be used during the second stage of labor if placental extraction or instrumental delivery becomes necessary.

As with an epidural, a spinal block may lead to vasodilation that can cause hypotension and fetal hypoxia. The anesthetic agent could spread, causing a total spinal block, apnea, reduced blood pressure and pulse, and unresponsiveness. Contraindications for spinal block are similar to those for epidural block. Adverse reactions include post-spinal headache, shivering, and urine retention.

Because epidural and spinal anesthesia cause hypotension, I.V. fluids (preferably lactated Ringer's solution) are necessary. Expect to infuse 500 to 1,000 ml of fluid before administration of epidural or spinal anesthesia and to maintain an I.V. infusion for fluid and possible emergency drug administration should hypotension occur. Monitor vital signs every 5 minutes for the first 30 minutes after initiation of epidural anesthesia and every 15 minutes throughout epidural infusion. Monitor vital signs according to facility protocol after administration of spinal anesthesia until delivery, and monitor as prescribed for up to 24 hours after delivery.

Signs and symptoms of anesthesia overdose include circumoral numbness, dizziness, and slurred speech. Maternal and fetal hypoxia may result, causing tachycardia. Be alert for these signs and symptoms, and notify the doctor or anesthesiologist if they occur. Treatment of toxicity includes administering oxygen and I.V. fluids.

Administration of epidural or spinal anesthesia requires that the patient be placed in a sitting or side-lying position, with shoulders parallel and legs slightly flexed to reduce hypotension. Epidural anesthesia does not affect motor pathways but, because the legs are numb, they seem heavy and are difficult to move. A spinal block produces motor paralysis. Ensure the patient's safety by using side rails and assisting with position changes.

General anesthesia

Because it requires intubation and increases the risk of aspiration, general anesthesia usually is used only when the patient undergoes emergency cesarean delivery, intrauterine manipulation, or other surgical intervention. General anesthesia may be attained through inhalation or I.V. drug administration. Inhalation involves high concentrations of the same agents used for inhalant analgesia (nitrous oxide, halothane, and enflurane). The I.V. agent thiopental sodium (Pentothal) produces deep anesthesia and may cause depression in the neonate.

Once the tube is in place, avoid compressing the vena cava by moving the patient from the supine position before anesthesia administration begins. Many obstetric operating room tables provide left lateral tilt capability to displace the gravid uterus off the vena cava. If the table cannot be tilted, insert a wedge beneath the patient's right hip. After positioning her, administer oxygen and fluids as prescribed just before anesthesia administration.

Administer a clear antacid—such as sodium citrate—a few hours before surgery to reduce the patient's risk of aspiration of acidic stomach contents while anesthetized. If she requires emergency surgery, the antacid may be administered 30 minutes or less before the procedure. Turning the patient from side to side enhances antacid effectiveness and promotes mixing of the antacid with gastric contents. In addition, many anesthesiologists now routinely decrease gastric acidity by administering an H_2 antagonist such as cimetidine (Tagamet) before surgery.

Because of delayed gastric emptying during pregnancy, the patient who requires emergency surgery may be at increased risk for regurgitation, which can cause chemical pneumonitis and death. To reduce gastric volume, some obstetricians forbid all women from drinking anything while in labor in case an emergency should arise.

Because inhalation agents may cause cardiac arrhythmias, monitor maternal electrocardiogram continuously throughout anesthesia administration and during recovery. Uterine atony, also produced by inhalants, may lead to uterine hemorrhage. Fetal and neonatal hypoxia also may occur with deep induction anesthesia, which reaches the fetus in about 2 minutes. If the patient received an I.V. anesthetic agent, monitor the neonate closely for depression.

Evaluation

Evaluation findings should be stated in terms of actions performed or outcomes achieved for each goal. The following examples illustrate appropriate evaluation statements for the woman experiencing labor pain.

- The patient controlled breathing and progressive muscle relaxation.
- The patient expressed understanding of pain-relief measures available to her.
- The patient reported relief from pain after administration of regional anesthesia.
- Fetal heart rate remained stable after anesthesia administration.

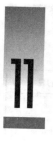

THE FIRST STAGE OF LABOR

The first stage of labor begins with the onset of regular, rhythmic uterine contractions that cause progressive cervical changes. It ends with complete cervical dilation of 10 cm. Labor, however, is much more than a physiologic process that allows the fetus to enter the world. It is also the dramatic culmination of the gestational period—a significant life event that represents a pivotal point in the lives of the mother, father, neonate, and other family members. It is a psychological and developmental task that demands rigorous adaptation. During the first stage of labor, nursing care must meet the patient's physical, psychosocial, and cultural needs.

NURSING CARE BEFORE ADMISSION

Before any patient can be admitted for care in the labor and delivery area, she should be in true labor, defined as progressive cervical dilatation and fetal descent, or show signs of a medical complication such as hypertension that could affect her or the fetus during labor and delivery. To make this determination, the nurse performs an initial assessment that focuses on the imminence of the birth and on fetal stability. This assessment, which includes a brief history and physical examination, should provide sufficient data to distinguish true labor from other conditions that mimic it, such as false labor, urinary tract infection (UTI), "terminal pregnancy blues" (generalized physical discomfort and emotional distress near the end of pregnancy), and abruptio placentae. However, if delivery appears imminent, omit the preadmission assessment and admit the patient immediately. (See *Characteristics of true and false labor*, page 236.)

Initial assessment

Set the tone for the initial assessment by making appropriate introductions. Briefly describe nursing activities during this assessment and

Characteristics of true and false labor

Compare the characteristics listed here to help determine whether a patient is in true or false labor.

CHARACTERISTIC	TRUE LABOR	FALSE LABOR
Contractions	Regular and rhythmic	Irregular
Pain	Discomfort moves from the back to the front of the abdomen	Mild discomfort or pressure in the abdomen and groin; may be relieved by walking
Fetal movement	Unchanged	May intensify
Fetal descent	Progressive	Unchanged
Show	Pinkish mucus, possibly with the mucus plug from the cervix	None
Cervix	Progressive effacement and dilation	Unchanged after 1 to 2 hours

maintain the patient's privacy and confidentiality to gain her trust and ease anxiety.

During the introductory period, observe the patient closely to identify clues to her labor status. Postures, facial expressions, or gestures that connote tension, anxiety, or pain may accurately reflect a patient's labor progress. Perspiration, varying breathing patterns, lack of concentration, and frequent position changes can indicate discomfort or stress during and between contractions. Involuntary grunting or breath holding may signal the onset of the second stage of labor. To help form an accurate initial impression, relate the patient's behavior to her cultural background.

If the patient is in active labor, shorten the initial assessment and prioritize the questions. Focus on collecting data about her current labor status. Refer to prenatal records, if available, and use the previously documented information.

Perform a brief physical examination to determine labor progress and fetal well-being. Be sure to help the patient find a comfortable position for the assessment. Calmly and efficiently conduct the history and physical assessment between contractions.

Health history

During the initial health history and review of the prenatal record, gather biographical data and investigate the woman's health status, health promotion and protection behaviors, and roles and relationships as they relate to her pregnancy, labor, and forthcoming delivery.

To help prioritize this information, obtain health history information in this order:

- biographical data
- expected delivery date
- previous pregnancies and outcomes
- previous labors and deliveries
- contractions
- rupture of amniotic membranes
- bloody show or vaginal bleeding
- pregnancy-related health problems
- other health problems
- fetal movements
- prenatal care
- primary caregiver
- support person
- family members or friends.

Also obtain and document any other information required by the health care facility.

Physical assessment

The initial physical assessment includes evaluation of:

- vital signs
- fetal heart tones
- uterine contractions
- fetal lie
- fetal presentation
- fetal position
- engagement
- estimated fetal weight
- edema and deep tendon reflexes
- amniotic membranes
- cervical changes, fetal descent, and other factors determined by vaginal examination.

Vital signs. For a woman in labor, vital signs provide necessary information about maternal and fetal health. They also provide baseline data for future comparisons.

First, check the patient's blood pressure, which should normally range from 90 to 138/60 to 88 mm Hg. A rise of 30 mm Hg systolic and 15 mm Hg diastolic above the patient's usual blood pressure may signal pregnancy-induced hypertension (PIH), anxiety, or fear. Blood pressure will increase during contractions.

The patient's temperature should range from 98° to 99.6° F (36.2° to 37.6° C). A temperature elevation may signal dehydration, a serious obstetric infection such as chorioamnionitis, or another type of infection such as a UTI.

Pulse rate should typically range from 60 to 90 beats/minute. An elevated pulse rate may be caused by anxiety, pain, infection, dehydration, or drug use.

Respirations should normally range from 16 to 24 breaths/minute. Increased respirations may indicate hyperventilation, anxiety, pain, or infection. Decreased temperature, pulse, and respirations do not commonly occur during labor.

Fetal heart tones. Assess the fetal heart tones for fetal well-being. If the health care facility requires, use a fetal heart monitor for this part of the assessment. (See Chapter 9, Fetal assessment.) Otherwise, assess the heart tones via auscultation. A variation above or below the normal fetal heart rate of 120 to 160 beats/minute may indicate fetal distress.

Uterine contractions. Use an external fetal monitor or palpate the patient's abdomen. Note the frequency, duration, and intensity of the uterine contractions. Also observe the patient during and between contractions to evaluate her level of discomfort. Ask the patient's support person to record the contraction pattern, if appropriate.

Fetal lie, presentation, and position. Perform Leopold's maneuvers to determine the fetal lie, presentation, and position. (See *Performing Leopold's maneuvers.*)

Leopold's maneuvers help detect potential problems, such as breech presentation or transverse lie, that require evaluation by the doctor or nurse-midwife. In diagnosing these problems, the course of labor may be determined.

Engagement. Palpate the abdomen to verify engagement. After engagement, labor may progress more quickly. In any patient, an unengaged fetus during labor increases the risk of umbilical cord prolapse with ruptured membranes and warrants close supervision. If the nurse is able to palpate and move the presenting part freely, engagement has not occurred.

Estimated fetal weight. Assess the fetal weight by measuring the fundal height and performing Leopold's maneuvers. Then correlate the estimated weight with the gestational age to identify a fetus that may be large or small for gestational age.

PSYCHOMOTOR SKILLS

Performing Leopold's maneuvers

Leopold's maneuvers allow the nurse to systematically evaluate the patient's abdomen to determine fetal position. This technique is generally reliable except in women who are obese or who have hydramnios.

Before performing Leopold's maneuvers, have the patient void and lie supine with her abdomen uncovered. To reduce abdominal muscle tension, place a pillow under her shoulders and ask her to draw her knees up slightly. Warm your hands before touching the patient's abdomen to avoid startling her or causing discomfort.

1 Use the first maneuver to determine which part of the fetus lies in the upper uterus. Facing the patient, lightly palpate her upper abdomen with both hands. The head feels round and firm. The buttocks feel softer and have a bony prominence.

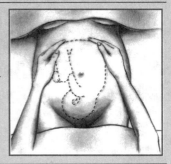

2 Perform the second maneuver to locate the back. Using gentle pressure, palpate the left side of the patient's abdomen with the palm of your right hand, while steadying the opposite side with your left hand. Repeat the maneuver with your right hand steadying and your left hand palpating. On one side of the patient's abdomen, the back of the fetus should feel firm and smooth; on the opposite side, the extremities should feel like small irregularities or protrusions.

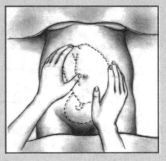

(continued)

Performing Leopold's maneuvers (continued)

3 Carry out the third maneuver to identify the presenting part (the part of the fetus above the pelvic inlet). Using the thumb and fingers of your dominant hand, grasp the patient's abdomen just above her symphysis pubis. The fetal part found here should be the opposite of the one found in the upper abdomen. If the head is palpated and can be moved gently back and forth, it is not yet engaged.

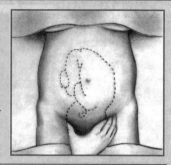

4 Perform the fourth maneuver to determine the descent of the presenting part. Stand facing the patient's feet. Then gently move your hands down the sides of her abdomen toward the symphysis pubis, noting which side has greater resistance. This resistance is caused by normal bony prominence of the fetus's head, either the brow or the occiput. If the head is flexed, the brow will palpated on the side opposite where the back was identified. If the head is extended, the occiput will be palpated on the same side as the back.

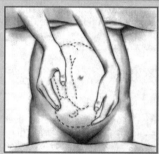

Edema and deep tendon reflexes. Inspect and palpate the patient's extremities for edema. Slight localized edema of the feet and ankles is normal late in pregnancy. However, edema of the face, hands, or pretibial area may signal generalized edema and PIH, especially if accompanied by brisk deep tendon reflexes or clonus and elevated blood pressure. If these signs are present, notify the doctor or nurse-midwife immediately.

Amniotic membranes. Whether or not the woman reported a sudden gush of fluid or a slow, continuous trickle of fluid during the health history, check the amniotic membranes. Inspect the vaginal opening for obvious fluid leakage. If fluid is present, test it with nitrazine paper. A positive test result—where the paper turns blue—may confirm rupture of the amniotic membranes or indicate nitrazine paper contamination with sterile lubricant, semen, or bloody show.

If the membrane status is in doubt, expect the doctor or nurse-midwife to confirm or rule out ruptured membranes by inspecting the cervical os through a speculum and examining the fluid through a microscope.

Vaginal examination. The vaginal examination determines the patient's labor progress by assessing cervical changes, confirming amniotic membrane status, and evaluating fetal position and descent. If specially educated in this skill, the nurse may conduct the vaginal examination. Otherwise, the nurse assists a doctor or nurse-midwife.

To prepare for a vaginal examination, gather the appropriate equipment based on the health care facility's procedures and the maternal and fetal status. For example, if the fetus shows signs of distress, obtain electronic fetal monitoring equipment with an internal catheter or electrode for insertion during the examination. Then help the patient into a comfortable lithotomy position, and drape her to maintain dignity.

During the examination, support the patient appropriately. Help her relax her vaginal muscles by suggesting conscious relaxation techniques. After the examination, clean the patient's perineum and change the disposable pad under her buttocks, as needed. Cover the patient with her bed sheet. Reaffirm and reexplain the examiner's findings, as appropriate, and answer any questions.

Immediately document vaginal examination findings. Include the date, time, findings, the examiner's name, and any procedures that were performed, such as an amniotomy or placement of fetal scalp electrode or intrauterine pressure catheter.

In some facilities, a properly trained nurse may conduct a vaginal examination to assess cervical position, dilation, effacement, and station.

Before labor begins, the cervix typically lies in the posterior part of the vagina. During labor, it rotates forward to midposition. A tight muscular band in the vagina may be mistaken for cervical dilation when the cervix actually is closed and posterior. To locate cervical position accurately, palpate the vaginal fornices thoroughly with the fingertips.

Dilation, effacement, and station vary as labor progresses. The initial assessment findings will provide a baseline for later evaluations of labor progress and will help in planning the patient's care.

If dilation is present without fetal descent, use caution during later vaginal examinations to prevent membrane rupture and umbilical cord prolapse.

Preparation for admission or discharge

Review all of the health history and physical assessment findings to develop a complete clinical picture of the patient. Consider the health care facility's policy for admission. If the patient is in true labor or meets the standards for admission, continue to prepare her for delivery. If she is in false labor and she and the fetus are in stable condition, call the doctor or nurse-midwife for discharge orders and instructions for the patient's return.

For a patient who must be discharged for false or prodromal labor, suggest comfort measures and explain medical orders. Keep the patient's safety in mind when providing instructions. Suggest that a warm tub bath or shower assisted by a family member can ease discomfort. Propose drinking warm milk or herbal tea and reclining semi-upright with pillows under her knees to promote rest. Encourage hydration with clear liquids and nourishment with light meals rich in carbohydrates. Suggest a massage by the patient's support person to promote comfort.

Instruct the patient to return to the health care facility if her membranes rupture, if she develops bleeding, if her contractions become more intense, or if she shows signs of infection, such as fever. Advise her to return if normal fetal movements change dramatically. Document the patient's discharge. Record the initial assessment findings and recommendations that the patient received for follow-up with the health care provider.

The patient may base her decision to leave the facility on such factors as her distance from the health care facility, access to transportation, ability to cope with her current status, or her family's concerns and ability to assist her at home. Remind her that active labor will occur and encourage her to go to her next prenatal visit if she hasn't delivered by that time.

NURSING CARE AFTER ADMISSION

Patients and their support people enter the labor and delivery unit in widely varying emotional states and degrees of preparedness. Regardless of the family's emotional state or preparation on admission, the nurse should make every effort to create a calm, welcoming environment. This will help decrease their apprehension and stress and promote a more positive childbirth experience.

Orientation

After the patient has been officially admitted, acquaint her and her support person with their physical environment. Initiate introductions among the patient, her support people, and the staff in order to establish an environment of mutual respect. Orient the patient and her support person to the call light, bed adjustment control, equipment to be used, and to the location of the bathroom, lounge, and telephone. A thorough orientation will help reduce their anxiety and convey openness to their needs, encouraging them to participate fully.

Informed consent is obtained before any procedure is performed on a patient in labor. The doctor or nurse-midwife should inform her of each procedure's benefits, risks, and alternatives, and obtain the consent. Then the nurse should allow time to answer the patient's questions and discuss her concerns. If medications or the stress of labor compromises the patient's ability to make rational decisions, include her support person or a family member in discussions about care and procedures. Document the patient's—or her family's—consent in her records.

Ongoing assessment

After the patient is admitted, complete her health history, perform a detailed physical assessment, and collect laboratory data. The assessment data will serve as the basis for developing a plan of care for the patient and her family.

Health history

This interview supplements the initial health history, which emphasized the patient's current labor status, with questions that review all body systems and assess her psychosocial status. If the patient's prenatal record includes this information, do not collect it again. If her record is unavailable or if she does not have frequent contractions or severe pain, assess the following areas in this order:

- family history
- medical and surgical history
- activities of daily living
- psychosocial status.

Vary the length of the ongoing health history based on the woman's condition. If the labor is progressing rapidly, prioritize the interview to collect the most important information to manage the birth and immediate postpartum period.

Physical assessment

Focus the physical assessment on findings that could affect labor, delivery, and maternal or fetal well-being. The following health history findings require detailed physical assessment:

- Dysuria (burning or pain on urination). This symptom suggests a UTI, which could increase the patient's discomfort during labor and delivery.

- Edema. A patient with generalized or excessive edema may have PIH or a kidney disorder that may cause labor complications.
- Visual difficulties. These symptoms may result from elevated blood pressure, which occurs in PIH.
- Headaches, dizziness, or syncope. These symptoms also may be linked to PIH.
- Vulvar varicosities or hemorrhoids. A patient with these swollen, tortuous veins should be monitored for pain or thrombosis during labor.
- Varicosities in legs. A patient with this condition may develop thrombosis and reduced blood flow to the legs during contractions.
- Calf pain. This symptom may indicate that thrombosis has occurred.
- Indigestion, nausea, vomiting, or diarrhea. These gastrointestinal problems can lead to dehydration, which depletes the energy needed for labor.
- Signs and symptoms of dehydration, such as thirst or dry mucous membranes. A dehydrated patient will need fluids to maintain her blood volume and prevent further problems.
- Signs and symptoms of upper respiratory tract infections, such as congestion or rhinorrhea (nasal discharge). Such effects may cause problems if the patient receives general anesthesia or undergoes intubation. They also may indicate cocaine use or allergies.
- Vaginal pruritus. This symptom may signal a vaginal infection that could be transmitted to the fetus.
- Skin rash or lesions, especially on the genitals. These signs may indicate a sexually transmitted disease, such as herpes, that could be transmitted to the fetus.
- Problems with back, pelvis, or abduction of legs that involve stiffness, difficulty in moving, or pain. Any of these problems may make the patient uncomfortable when in the lithotomy position. Back problems may worsen during labor.
- Jaundice. This sign may signal liver disease, which could reduce the patient's ability to clear anesthetics and medications from her body.

Laboratory studies

Review all of the patient's laboratory data. Consider the results of routine antepartal studies, special antepartal tests, and the routine studies performed on admission to the labor and delivery area. (See *Determining the significance of routine admission tests.*)

Determining the significance of routine admission tests

These studies are commonly ordered for pregnant patients. Their significance is described below.

Hemoglobin and hematocrit
Track levels of these blood components because many patients develop anemia, especially late in pregnancy.

Venereal disease research laboratory test or rapid plasma reagin test
Detects infection with syphilis.

ABO blood typing and Rh typing
Identifies blood type and Rh factor—vital information if the patient needs a blood transfusion; determines potential Rh incompatibility with the fetus if the patient is Rh-negative. Most health care facilities require these tests when admitting a patient who has not had a prenatal workup or whose results are not available.

Urinalysis
Assesses for changes in urine composition, which may occur as pregnancy stresses the kidneys.

Nursing diagnosis
The nurse reviews all health history, physical assessment, and laboratory test findings. Based on these, the nurse formulates nursing diagnoses for the patient, fetus, support person, or other family members, as needed. (See Appendix 1, NANDA taxonomy of nursing diagnoses.)

Initial planning and implementation
After assessing the patient and fetus, the nurse plans and implements routine admission procedures according to facility protocols. The nurse should prioritize these procedures based on the labor progress, the ease of implementation, and the patient's comfort, safety, preference, and need to move about. Each facility has different standard procedures, but most include I.V. fluid infusion and skin preparation.

I.V. fluid infusion
Some doctors are likely to limit the patient's intake to minimum oral fluids and ice chips because anesthetics delay gastric emptying and re-

lax the swallowing reflex, which may cause subsequent aspiration. Other providers encourage intake of clear fluids by mouth to avoid excessive acidity of gastric contents and provide nutrition during labor. If fluids are restricted or oral intake is inadequate or there is potential for fetal distress or complicated labor, continuous I.V. fluid will most likely be ordered.

Expect to administer I.V. fluids to a patient with a nursing diagnosis of **risk for fluid volume deficit related to restricted oral intake and increased fluid output.** Also plan to use this intervention under the following circumstances: maternal exhaustion and dehydration; fetal distress; oxytocin induction or augmentation; grand multiparity; history of postpartal hemorrhage; history of prenatal anemia in this pregnancy; potential for uterine atony secondary to uterine overdistention caused by such factors as multiple gestation, macrosomia, or hydramnios; a life-threatening obstetric or medical condition, such as abruptio placentae, PIH, or diabetes; or potential need for surgery or regional anesthesia.

If an I.V. is ordered, prepare the specified I.V. fluid and begin the I.V. in the cephalic vein just above the wrist to minimize dislodging it with maternal movement with labor. If blood samples have not yet been obtained for laboratory studies, gather the appropriate vials and take samples before starting the I.V. Then infuse the fluid at the prescribed rate.

During the infusion, watch for signs of fluid overload, infiltration, and phlebitis. Also, watch for restlessness or agitation, which can dislodge the catheter.

Perineal skin preparation

In most health care facilities, complete skin preparation has been omitted. If any type of preparation is ordered, perform the procedure according to health care facility policy.

Ongoing planning and implementation

During the first stage of labor, continually monitor the status of the patient, fetus, and labor progress. Also provide comfort and support to the patient, and plan and implement care for her family.

Do not let any activities interfere with the patient's ability to work with her body or with her support person's assistance during labor. Instead, encourage the support person's active involvement, use gentle touch and calm verbal assurance to show respect for their efforts and, when appropriate, communicate that all is going well.

Monitor vital signs

To help provide safe care, evaluate the patient's vital signs as often as indicated by the patient's condition and as required by the health care facility policy.

During the latent phase (0 to 3 cm of cervical dilation), assess the patient's blood pressure, pulse, and respirations hourly, if no problems are anticipated or discovered. Monitor her temperature every 2 to 4 hours throughout labor as indicated.

During the active phase of labor (4 to 10 cm of cervical dilation), check blood pressure, pulse, and respirations every hour. When the woman reaches transition, the final part of the active phase of labor, evaluate at least every 30 minutes.

Monitor uterine contractions

The policy of the health care facility—and the doctor's or nurse-midwife's orders—will determine exactly how often uterine contractions must be monitored. However, most facilities provide similar guidelines. Unless a deviation occurs, the nurse must assess contractions every hour during the early phase and every 30 minutes during the active phase of the first stage of labor.

The facility's policy and doctor's or nurse-midwife's orders also will determine whether uterine contractions are monitored by abdominal palpation or electronic fetal monitoring. Regardless of the method used, monitor the intensity, frequency, and duration of the contractions. Uterine activity can be affected by maternal exhaustion or dehydration, rupture of membranes, medication, position changes, and increased anxiety.

When monitoring contractions, pay careful attention to the relaxation period between them. Resting uterine tonus can become abnormally elevated, making the intensity of the contractions difficult to assess. If palpation reveals that the uterus is not relaxing adequately between contractions, the patient may have dysfunctional labor or, rarely, abruptio placentae. This uterine hypertonicity can decrease placental perfusion, causing severe fetal hypoxia and distress.

Monitor fetal response to labor

Frequently evaluate the fetus to maintain well-being. (See *Fetal evaluations during labor,* page 248.)

Depending on the health care facility's policies, assess the fetus by auscultating for fetal heart tones or using an electronic fetal monitor. Note the application of internal scalp electrodes or an intrauterine pressure catheter.

FETAL STATUS

Fetal evaluations during labor

During labor, the nurse must frequently monitor the fetus—as well as the patient—to help maintain their health. To assess the fetal status accurately, the nurse follows these steps:
- Auscultate for the fetal heart rate, rhythm, and response to contractions with a fetoscope or an electronic monitor at least every 30 minutes in the early phase of labor, every 15 minutes during active labor, and every 5 minutes in the second stage of labor.
- Note the amniotic fluid color, amount, and odor when the membranes rupture.
- Evaluate the results of fetal scalp sampling and pH testing, if prescribed.

Monitor labor progress

Perform or assist with vaginal examinations, as needed, to monitor cervical dilation, effacement, station, and other indicators of labor progress.

The frequency of vaginal examinations generally depends on the patient's condition and the nurse's ability to observe the contraction pattern, bloody show, patient's behavior, level and location of discomfort, and fetal heart tones.

Vaginal examination frequency also depends on the risk of introducing infection. A vaginal examination must be done on admission, before the patient receives any medication, and after spontaneous rupture of membranes. It may also be done whenever it is necessary to evaluate progress, such as when the patient enters into second stage of labor, when there is a change in fetal status, or when the patient wants to get out of bed. Document the administration of medications, oxygen, I.V. fluids, and epidural anesthesia as well as the patient's response to treatments received and any changes in the patient's or fetus's status.

Monitor urinary function

Evaluate the patient's urine output and assess for proteinuria and ketonuria. The patient should urinate at least every 2 hours and the urine should be checked for protein or ketones.

During active labor, the patient may develop bladder distention with decreased urine output. This increases her discomfort, impedes labor progress by preventing fetal descent, and can lead to postpartal hemorrhage and UTIs. To detect bladder distention, check for an irregularity in the lower abdomen or a distinct bulge over the symphysis pubis while monitoring uterine contractions and fetal heart tones. If she cannot urinate and shows signs of increasing distention, inform the doctor or nurse-midwife and obtain an order for straight catheterization.

The presence of proteinuria may signal the onset of PIH, or it may indicate that the urine was contaminated with vaginal secretions, amniotic fluid, or perspiration. To aid diagnosis of PIH, check for other signs, such as elevated blood pressure, edema, and exaggerated deep tendon reflexes. If you detect these signs, notify the doctor or nurse-midwife.

Ketonuria may indicate dehydration or maternal exhaustion. If ketonuria is present, notify the doctor or nurse-midwife, and monitor the patient and fetus more closely. Be sure the patient has adequate fluid and nutrient intake. This requires extra effort when the patient does not have an I.V. infusion.

Provide comfort and support

During childbirth, the woman not only needs physical care but also a supportive human presence, pain relief, acceptance, information, and reassurance. By constantly providing for her physical comfort and emotional support, the nurse can meet most or all of these needs.

When caring for a woman in the first stage of labor, individualize her care by helping her select comfort and support measures that are most effective for her.

Tailor all comfort and support measures to the patient's condition and phase of labor. All of these measures help reduce her anxiety and prevent stress on the fetus.

As active labor begins, the patient becomes more serious and preoccupied with her contractions. She may become quiet and withdrawn or panicked and verbal; she may begin to doubt her ability to cope. Companionship and a relaxed, quiet atmosphere can aid her concentration and coping abilities and can promote rest between contractions. Breathing techniques may help her maintain self-control.

During transition, contractions grow more rapid and intense. The patient becomes self-absorbed, restless, irritable, and hypersensitive and may develop nausea, vomiting, hiccups, belching, or a natural amnesia. Increased perspiration with intermittent chills and hot flashes may sweep quickly over her. She may feel discouraged or panicky. During this phase, do not leave her alone. Provide constant reassurance, firm guidance in using modified breathing techniques, and steadfast physical and emotional support and comfort. Although transition is usually the most painful part of labor, it usually is very brief. At this time, analgesics are used with caution because if the medication is at the peak of action when the baby is born, the neonate could be depressed.

Create a supportive atmosphere. Be sensitive to the family's need to create a supportive environment. Intervene, as needed, to prevent a nursing diagnosis of *ineffective family coping: comprised related to patient's hospitalization, anxiety related to fear of childbirth,* or *anxiety related to the hospital environment.* Help the family personalize the environment to enhance the patient's comfort, security, and privacy and improve the labor progress by reducing anxiety and pain. (See *Involvement in labor,* pages 251 and 252.)

Promote good positioning and walking. During labor, a patient may be confined to bed because of concomitant procedures, such as labor induction, epidural anesthesia, or pain relief through analgesia or sedation; convenience in monitoring maternal and fetal well-being; or the policy of the health care facility. Such a patient may have a nursing diagnosis of *impaired physical mobility related to electronic fetal monitoring equipment.* For a patient who must remain in bed, help her maintain a lateral—rather than supine—position to enhance labor efficiency, comfort, and safety. The lateral position is commonly used to prevent maternal vessel compression and hypotension. This position promotes maternal and fetal circulation, enhances comfort, increases maternal relaxation, reduces muscle tension, and eliminates pressure points.

When allowed freedom of movement, most women will change positions many times to maximize comfort and enhance labor progress. If the patient is not confined to bed, help her find comfortable positions that allow adequate maternal and fetal surveillance. By using alternate positions, such as forward-leaning sitting, squatting, sitting, standing, or hands and knees, she can enhance her labor progress, comfort, and safety. These interventions will help a patient with a nursing diagnosis of *altered placental tissue perfusion related to maternal position.*

Also help the patient walk around, if possible. Although long walks may tire her, brief walks can decrease pain and improve comfort. They also can shorten labor by encouraging fetal descent using gravity.

Contraindications to walking include exhaustion, preterm labor, vaginal bleeding, medication administration, fetal distress, a presenting part poorly applied to the cervix, fetal malposition, and precipitous labor.

Maintain hygiene. During active labor, the patient perspires heavily and produces increased vaginal secretions with intact membranes or a constant flow of wet, sticky vaginal drainage with ruptured membranes. These activities can compromise her hygiene and add to her general discomfort.

Conserve energy and promote rest. Help the patient work with her body by using a conscious relaxation technique, especially if she has a nursing diagnosis of *knowledge deficit related to appropriate relaxation techniques.* This intervention not only will promote the pa-

FAMILY CARE

Involvement in labor

Traditionally, the focus of childbearing has been on the patient's role in pregnancy, labor, delivery, and parenting. Today, the patient may share the labor and birth with her partner or support person as well as other family members. The nurse can promote the effective involvement of these people using interventions tailored for them.

For the partner or support person

- Promote confidence in the ability to support the patient through this demanding period.
- Welcome the support person on admission, using the person's preferred name to encourage relaxation.
- Include the support person in the patient's history and physical assessment, if both desire this participation.
- Evaluate goals for the support person's involvement. Keep in mind that involvement may range from being present during the labor to active coaching throughout.
- Assess the support person's physical and emotional needs, and plan ways to address them during labor.
- Reduce anxiety and feelings of awkwardness by showing concern for the support person's interest and participation in childbirth.
- Make the support person feel important to the patient's comfort.
- Direct care and support measures if the person is hesitant and unprepared. Demonstrate or suggest the following comfort activities: hand holding, fanning, wiping the patient's face with a cool cloth, offering clear liquids or ice chips, providing a sacral counter-pressure massage, and helping her to walk or find a comfortable position.
- Reinforce the prepared support person's interaction and foster successful sharing. Encourage the support person's participation. Do not try to take over or intervene.
- Suggest appropriate times for the support person to take a break to eat, rest, or attend to personal hygiene. This prevents the person from feeling overwhelmed or trapped. Offer to stand in for the support person during breaks. Time these breaks to prevent disappointment and frustration if birth occurs while the support person is away.
- Help the support person listen to the fetal heart tones, whenever desired.
- Inform the support person of routine changes in the fetal heart rate patterns and their significance.
- Assure the support person that frequent monitoring does not indicate a problem.
- Keep the support person involved if a crises arises during labor. Help allay feelings of helplessness and fear by remaining calm and confident, sharing information, and providing reassurance that the health care team is doing everything possible.

FAMILY CARE

Involvement in labor (continued)

For the grandparents
• Be sensitive to the impact that unfamiliar and perhaps frightening modern birthing equipment and procedures may have on grandparents. Explain the equipment and procedures, as needed.
• Regularly inform family members outside the labor and delivery area of the patient's progress.
• Advise the family about necessary medical treatments or procedures. Reassure them that the health care team is doing everything possible to provide safe, high-quality care.

For the siblings
• Introduce yourself to the children and person who will be caring for them and answering their questions.
• Be aware that a child's response to childbirth depends on maturity and interest.
• Maintain a calm, matter-of-fact attitude to reassure the children that everything is proceeding normally. Most children will assimilate the information casually.

tient's self-esteem and sense of control, but also will conserve her energy and promote comfort. To promote rest between contractions, maintain a calm, quiet atmosphere and organize nursing tasks to minimize disturbances.

Based on the patient's preference, use gentle or therapeutic touch to promote relaxation. Some women find these techniques restful and reassuring and respond well even to simple hand-holding. Others find them offensive or intrusive, especially if they develop hyperesthesia.

Use massage to promote relaxation and help the patient remain in control. Teach the support person to perform a counterpressure massage on the lower back, sacrum, and buttocks to help ease labor discomfort. During transition, a back or foot massage can be especially effective. Show the patient how to use effleurage on her lower abdomen to decrease pain by providing distraction and increasing circulation. (See Chapter 5, The normal antepartal period.)

The use of visual imagery, quiet speech, eye contact, and appropriately timed analgesia also can promote rest and conserve energy. So may soft music and a cool breeze created by a hand-held fan, especially during transition.

Promote effective breathing. Effective breathing patterns help the patient work with her body efficiently and can break the anxiety-pain-hyperventilation cycle that may occur even in a prepared patient. They also can help prevent or correct a nursing diagnosis of *impaired gas exchange related to hyperventilation with increasing contractions.*

If the patient has learned certain breathing patterns in childbirth education class, reinforce her learning and support her efforts. If she has not attended classes, briefly teach her and her support person how to breathe effectively.

Relieve pain. Labor is physically demanding. Some women experience extreme pain and other intense physical sensations; others experience merely bothersome cramping. For a patient with a nursing diagnosis of *pain related to uterine contractions,* try different measures to relieve pain. Use progressive relaxation techniques, biofeedback, acupressure, or visual imagery, along with paced breathing, frequent repositioning, and the emotional and physical assistance of her support person. Or try alleviating her pain through analgesia and anesthesia, depending on safety considerations, labor progress, maternal and fetal well-being, and her preference and coping ability.

Care for the family
Throughout labor, provide care not only for the patient and fetus, but also for the family. Each family requires individualized interventions based on needs and childbirth goals. Keep in mind that some people choose not to participate in a family member's childbirth experience. The partner may prefer not to be involved; the patient may not want her partner to see her during labor. Respect each person's preferences and avoid imposing personal values.

Evaluation
To complete the nursing process, evaluate the effectiveness of nursing care by reviewing the goals attained and the family's involvement and satisfaction with the care. Remember that evaluation stimulates continued reassessment—and improvement—of the effectiveness of nursing care throughout the intrapartal period.

12 THE SECOND STAGE OF LABOR

The second stage of labor begins with complete cervical dilation and ends with delivery of the neonate. It requires exhaustive maternal efforts coupled with strong, effective uterine contractions. The patient will need substantial emotional support and encouragement. During this highly emotional and stressful period, the nurse must meet the needs of the patient, family, and fetus; monitor the progress of labor; prepare the environment and equipment needed for delivery; and evaluate the neonate's status after delivery.

CHARACTERISTICS OF THE SECOND STAGE OF LABOR

The transition from the first to the second stage of labor signals impending birth.

Onset

Several characteristics indicate this move from the first to the second stage of labor, including:
- an increasing urge to push, possibly accompanied by perineal bulging
- an increase in bloody show, caused by greater cervical dilation
- grunting
- gaping of the anus
- involuntary defecation
- bulging of the vaginal introitus
- spontaneous rupture of the membranes
- facial perspiration
- shaking of extremities
- abrupt onset of early fetal heart rate (FHR) decelerations, possibly caused by compression of the fetus's head during descent into the pelvic canal (report these FHR changes, although common, to the doctor or nurse-midwife).

Phases

Some authorities divide the second stage of labor into two distinct phases. The first phase lasts from complete dilation of the cervix until the presenting part reaches the pelvic floor. The second phase lasts from when the presenting part reaches the pelvic floor until birth.

During the first phase, the woman may not feel a strong urge to bear down. Typically, these urges are short and manageable and occur at the peak of each contraction. They may assist in the final retraction of the cervix before fetal descent. During the second phase, the woman typically feels an uncontrollable urge to push; during this phase, bearing-down efforts are most effective at expelling the fetus.

Duration

For primiparous patients, the second stage of labor averages 57 minutes, ranging from 48 to 174 minutes. For multiparous patients, the second stage averages 18 minutes, ranging from 6 to 66 minutes. The duration depends on the combined effects of fetal, maternal, psychological, and environmental factors. Add 1 hour to these times if regional anesthesia is used and will continue to be considered, within normal limits.

Fetal factors that may affect duration include physical condition, size, station, position, lie, presentation, molding, rotation, and rate of descent. Maternal factors include parity, labor position, fatigue level, age, degree of expulsive efforts, strength of uterine contractions, size and shape of the bony pelvis, resistance or relaxation of soft tissues, and such obstetric interventions as anesthesia and episiotomy.

Psychological factors that may affect duration include the patient's emotional readiness, degree of relaxation, and level of trust in her care providers. The patient's preparation for childbirth—from reading, childbirth education classes, information handed down from female relatives, and inner spiritual resources, for example—also affect her reaction to labor, which may influence its duration. Environmental factors, which include bright lights, noise, and hectic activity, may increase the patient's anxiety, lengthening labor. A quiet, relaxed environment can shorten labor.

This complex interplay of diverse factors may preclude an accurate prediction of how long the second stage of labor will last, even for a multiparous patient. Although we have little control over such physical factors as the size of the fetus or degree of pelvic resistance, we can influence other factors, such as the positions the patient assumes during labor.

While some authorities consider abnormal any second stage of labor that lasts longer than 2 hours, others have found no compelling reasons to intervene after 2 hours; in fact, one study showed that using forceps to decrease the length of the second stage led to more problems with the mother and neonate. Allowing the patient to progress at her own rate was found to be safe if all other factors were within safe parameters. Other studies show that although a prolonged second stage of labor (over 2.9 hours in a primiparous patient or 1.1 hours in a multiparous patient) may indicate a disorder and deserves careful monitoring, it does not necessarily give sufficient reason to terminate labor. If labor is progressing and the fetus displays no signs of distress, labor should continue until vaginal delivery occurs. The patient and fetus should undergo continual monitoring and documentation as labor progresses.

Assessment

During the second stage of labor, more frequent assessment focuses on the patient, fetus, and labor progress. As delivery nears, assessment becomes continuous, and the nurse will care for one patient exclusively. Beginning early in the second stage and continuing until delivery, the nurse assesses maternal vital signs, cervical dilation, contractions, bearing-down efforts, FHR, fetal descent, amniotic fluid, and the emotional response of the patient and support person.

Vital signs

Take vital signs at least every 15 minutes and more often if the patient has continuous epidural anesthesia, is hypertensive, or has other complicating conditions. Bearing-down efforts may increase the patient's blood pressure, pulse, and respirations. Take blood pressure as necessary between contractions, but use discretion if pressure has been stable and birth is imminent. A temperature rise of one degree may occur even in the absence of infection, but a temperature over 100° F (37.8° C) should be reported to the doctor or nurse-midwife. Dehydration or infection may play a role in temperature elevation.

Cervical dilation

When characteristics of the second stage appear, expect a vaginal examination to be performed to confirm dilation and assess the presenting part, fetal station, status of the fetal membranes, and color of the amniotic fluid.

Some women have a strong urge to bear down before the cervix dilates completely. This can cause cervical edema and tissue damage, and it may impede fetal descent. If examination reveals incomplete dilation and the woman has a strong urge, help the woman avoid bearing down. Help her onto her forearms and knees, a position that may decrease the urge to bear down by relieving pressure on the rectum. Instruct her to pant or blow through each contraction until examination reveals that the cervix has receded completely. To maintain her comfort as long as possible in this position, raise the head of the bed and place several pillows under her arms. Some facilities use a large bean bag to support women in this position.

In some women, incomplete dilation may be felt as an anterior "lip" on the cervix. This condition stems from uneven pressure of the presenting part on the cervix, such as when the fetus is occiput posterior; all of the cervix recedes except for a small anterior portion. The doctor or nurse-midwife may reduce an anterior lip of the cervix manually, using two fingers to ease the cervix over the fetus's head by pressing against it during a contraction. The woman can aid reduction by bearing down during the pressing. Keeping the fingers in place during the next contraction will help the doctor or nurse-midwife determine whether the lip has been effectively reduced.

Fetal bradycardia to 90 beats/minute may occur for 1 to 2 minutes after manual reduction of the lip. This may result from vagal stimulation and typically resolves on its own. If not, notify the doctor or nurse-midwife and initiate standard nursing care for fetal bradycardia.

Contractions

Assess the strength, frequency, and duration of uterine contractions every 15 minutes during the second stage. Contractions that have occurred every 2 or 3 minutes may extend to every 5 minutes during this stage, allowing the woman to rest between contractions. This may increase the length of the second stage. Some women have more frequent contractions and report unceasing pain. This pain may relate to increasing pressure from the presenting part and difficulty relaxing between contractions. If the woman has had epidural anesthesia, the support person or nurse may need to cue her when a contraction begins so that she can position herself to bear down. When the second stage lasts longer than 2 hours, uterine contractions may decrease in strength and frequency. The doctor or nurse-midwife should evaluate the need for oxytocin and assess for cephalopelvic disproportion or other abnormalities.

Bearing-down efforts

Assess the effectiveness of the woman's bearing-down efforts and her energy resources as the second stage progresses. Remind her to bear down at the peak of each contraction and to continue bearing down to the end of the contraction to facilitate fetal descent. After assessing the progress of the first few contractions in the second stage, notify the doctor or nurse-midwife of the woman's status. If descent is delayed, or if the woman complains of increased pain, fatigue, or frustration, the doctor or nurse-midwife should identify the problem and intervene appropriately.

Although epidural anesthesia can be useful in the first stage of labor, it may create problems for a patient in the second stage; the amount of sensory and motor block necessary to relieve pain may reduce, delay, or abolish bearing-down efforts. Moreover, epidural anesthesia may lengthen the second stage and increase the need for forceps or vacuum assistance. If the patient's bearing-down efforts produce little descent, even with direct coaching, then the anesthetic agent may have to wear off slightly or be administered in reduced amounts before she can bear down effectively. Reassure the patient that, although the pain will increase somewhat, her improved pushing efforts will help deliver the neonate more quickly.

Fetal heart rate

Assess the FHR more frequently during the second stage of labor than during the first, based on the patient's or fetus's risk status, underlying medical conditions, medications and anesthetic agent used, and any alterations in FHR patterns that arose during the first stage. For a low-risk patient, auscultate FHR every 5 minutes or use an electronic fetal monitor (EFM), depending on the patient's wishes, the doctor's or nurse-midwife's preference, and facility policy. Although a standard fetoscope may be used for manual auscultation of FHR, a Doppler ultrasound device typically is less obtrusive. If the woman finds repeated FHR auscultation disruptive, consider switching to EFM. A high-risk patient may require EFM, possibly with an internal scalp electrode to detect fetal distress or beat-to-beat variability.

Changes in the FHR become more difficult to interpret during the second stage because they occur more frequently and with more variation than during the first stage. In fact, 50% to 90% of healthy neonates display some abnormality in heart rate during the expulsive phase of labor. Variations in the FHR may result from umbilical cord compression, fetal descent, and maternal bearing-down efforts.

Although few studies focus on the outcomes of second stage FHR changes, one study found a correlation between a normal FHR pattern and a normal Apgar score.

Specific results of FHR alterations may not be obvious. Usually, accelerations pose little danger; decelerations and changes in variability should be monitored closely. (See *Assessing and managing fetal heart rate changes*.)

Descent

The fetus normally begins descent during active labor; if descent has not begun by 7 cm of cervical dilation, the nurse must suspect that an abnormality may exist. In one study, failure to descend occurred in approximately 4% of patients. Causes included:

FETAL STATUS

Assessing and managing fetal heart rate changes

Variability in the fetal heart rate (FHR) during labor is an indicator of fetal well-being. Yet variations can be difficult to interpret. Use the following basic guidelines to help interpret and manage FHR changes. Remember the definitions of fetal heart rate variations, as shown in *Variations of baseline fetal heart rate* on pages 201 and 202.

- Baseline FHR should remain within 20 beats/minute of the rate identified early in labor. A slight decline in this baseline is common, probably resulting from vagal stimulation from increased pressure on the fetus's head during descent into the pelvis.
- The FHR fluctuates more during the second stage of labor than during the first stage. Accelerations typically have no adverse effect on the neonate.
- Decreased FHR variability, especially if accompanied by bradycardia, decelerations, or lack of accelerations, may be cause for concern and further investigation. Decreased FHR variability has been associated with decreased umbilical cord blood pH, which reflects fetal distress.
- Second-stage FHR decelerations and bradycardia have been reported in 50% to 90% of all FHR tracings and usually produce no lasting adverse effects. Pronounced or prolonged decelerations require prompt delivery.
- Terminal bradycardia (FHR below baseline immediately before delivery) is common and probably stems from compression of the fetus's head, vagal stimulation, umbilical cord compression, and impaired uteroplacental perfusion. It typically lasts only a few minutes and produces no adverse effects.
- Scalp stimulation may help in evaluating fetal condition when bradycardia occurs. FHR acceleration in response to stimuli offers a reliable sign of fetal well-being. If the fetus develops bradycardia, the doctor or nurse-midwife may press the fetus's scalp with a finger while performing a vaginal examination. If the FHR rises, the fetus is not seriously acidotic. If delivery is not imminent, try raising the FHR by repositioning the patient, offering oxygen by mask, and encouraging her to breathe through contractions rather than push.

- large fetus (over 4,000 g)
- cephalopelvic disproportion
- fetal malposition, primarily persistent occiput transverse or occiput posterior positions
- short umbilical cord.

Begin assessing descent with each vaginal examination by measuring the relationship between the fetus's head and the patient's ischial spines. Suspect an abnormality if no descent occurs after a primiparous woman bears down for 1 hour or a multiparous woman bears down for one-half hour. Be careful to distinguish between actual descent and increased molding of the fetus's scalp, which may give the illusion of descent.

Amniotic fluid

Note any change in the color of the amniotic fluid during the second stage of labor because it may indicate fetal distress. When tainted with meconium, amniotic fluid becomes green and may range in consistency from thin (1+ or 2+) to thick (3+ or 4+). Thick amniotic fluid will contain particulate meconium. An increase in bloody show, which commonly occurs early in the second stage, may cause pink-tinged amniotic fluid. Port wine-colored fluid may indicate abruptio placentae. Notify the doctor or nurse-midwife of any of these changes.

Emotional responses

Assessment of the patient's emotional status and that of her support person becomes increasingly important as labor continues. Both may experience fatigue and frustration, especially early in the second stage. When told that she can push, the patient may feel relief and anticipation that labor will end soon. The support person and health care team may also feel a surge of renewed energy.

Patients respond in various ways to the sensation of bearing down. Some respond well because bearing down allows them to give in to the urge they feel and do something positive with the pain. Others respond poorly to bearing down, especially if the fetus is in a posterior position or if the patient fears spontaneous perineal lacerations.

Immediately after delivery, the patient may experience a range of emotions and reactions, including relief that the pain has diminished, a sense of achievement, exhaustion, and pleasure or disappointment in the appearance or sex of the neonate.

Nursing diagnosis

Based on continuous assessment and monitoring throughout the second stage of labor, the nurse formulates nursing diagnoses specific to the patient, fetus, support person, or other family members, as necessary. (See Appendix 1, NANDA taxonomy of nursing diagnoses.)

Planning and implementation

During the second stage of labor, the nurse must plan and act almost simultaneously. After detecting the onset of the second stage and assessing maternal and fetal well-being and labor progress, the nurse should notify the doctor or nurse-midwife of the patient's and fetus's status.

As the second stage progresses, the nurse should provide the patient with emotional support, coordinate her bearing-down efforts, assist with positioning, monitor hydration, facilitate delivery, and care for the neonate immediately after birth. Throughout this stage, the nurse should document any interventions used and note changes in the patient's condition. (See *Documentation checklist for the second stage of labor*.)

Provide emotional support
Especially for the primiparous patient, the second stage of labor may result in a nursing diagnosis of *anxiety related to duration of labor* or

---

Documentation checklist for the second stage of labor

Although documentation records vary among health care facilities, most require the nurse to document the following:

- vital signs
- vaginal examination findings (cervical dilation, station, position, crowning)
- uterine contractions (duration, frequency, intensity)
- bearing-down efforts
- amniotic fluid (color and amount)
- fluid intake and output
- emotional responses
- bloody show (amount and consistency)
- medication administered throughout labor and delivery
- fetal heart rate (variability, baseline, periodic changes, use of external or internal fetal monitor)
- presence of support person or others
- transfer to delivery room or birthing chair
- perineal preparation
- time of birth (full extraction of neonate)
- names of all people in the room at the time of birth
- episiotomy or lacerations and description of repairs
- positioning and behaviors
- Apgar scores
- resuscitation, if necessary
- passage of meconium or urine
- any neonatal abnormalities or umbilical cord variations
- initial parent-infant bonding.

ineffective individual coping related to exhaustion. Help resolve these problems by providing emotional support and reassurance. Provide general emotional support to the patient by assuring her if labor is progressing normally, that she will not be left alone, and that the doctor or nurse-midwife will be summoned. Depending on the support person's participation, the nurse's role can range from reassuring to active coaching during the second stage.

Reassure the patient that each expulsive effort helps to move her baby down and out. Suggest that she imagine herself opening and her baby moving down the birth canal and out.

Choose words carefully because patients in labor are highly vulnerable and sensitive to suggestions that they are not succeeding. Even mildly critical remarks intended to make the patient try harder may be hurtful.

The patient who becomes exhausted and discouraged during this stage of labor will want to know how much longer the effort must continue. Never try to estimate when birth will occur. Instead, suggest concentrating on and working with the contractions, perhaps by changing position or exhaling forcefully (blowing) instead of pushing through the next one. Encourage the patient to rest or doze between contractions. Affirm that labor is hard work that can seem to take forever, but that she is making progress and will get through it. Encourage her to draw energy from her supporters.

Especially during this stage, the patient's support person may need emotional support, a brief break, or gentle direction. If the patient's bearing down does not accomplish quick results, the supporter may need reassurance about these events. If necessary, suggest such concrete tasks as holding the patient's leg, supporting her body in selected positions, massaging her back, offering ice chips, or preparing a cool cloth for her forehead.

Coordinate bearing-down efforts

During painful periods, the patient may have a nursing diagnosis of *ineffective breathing pattern related to painful uterine contractions and bearing-down efforts.* Help resolve this problem by coordinating the patient's bearing-down efforts with active coaching as necessary.

As the second stage progresses, bearing-down urges become more intense and aid in expelling the neonate. Encourage the patient to bear down with each contraction as indicated. Encourage her to listen to you so that she can change her bearing down efforts to blowing out as needed. (See *Alternative ways of bearing down.*)

If bearing-down efforts produce inadequate results, give positive suggestions for change between contractions, help the patient into an alternative position, and encourage her to push through the pain rather

Alternative ways of bearing down

Traditionally, nurses have taught and reinforced the following method of bearing down: The patient takes a cleansing breath, exhales, bears down to a count of 10, inhales quickly three or four times between counts, and then takes a final cleansing breath. Typically, she assumes a C-shaped position curled around the fetus, holding her knees, with head bent to her chest.

Two alternative styles for bearing down include the open-glottis method and the urge-based method. In the former, the patient releases air through the glottis while bearing down. Theoretically, this reduces stress on the fetus. In the latter, the patient bears down as she feels the urge and in the manner that feels right to her.

Because childbirth educators teach all three bearing-down methods, the nurse should be familiar with each one and work to achieve the most comfortable and effective method for each patient. It may be necessary to alternate between methods throughout this stage of labor for increased comfort of the patient and to enhance the efficacy of each contraction.

than pull back from it. If she pulls back out of fear that she will hurt herself, try comfort measures and give continued encouragement and support. Remember that as the fetus descends and presses on the perineum, the patient will experience a strong burning sensation from the stretching of this tissue. Encourage her to push through the burning, which will eventually numb the area. Reassure her that this is the end of this stage of labor and her baby will soon be born. Also, applying warm washcloths to her perineum can decrease discomfort as well as increase the stretching capability of the perineal tissues.

Assist with positioning

Position changes may be especially helpful for a patient with a nursing diagnosis of *pain related to rapid delivery or fetal malposition*. Be sure to consider the advantages and disadvantages of a position before suggesting a change to the woman. The side-lying position helps slow a rapid delivery and may reduce perineal tension. The forearms-and-knees position can reduce back pain related to labor. When the fetus is in an occiput-posterior position or descends slowly, the patient may benefit from a squatting position. If she squats on the toilet, use a flashlight to maintain a steady view of the perineum.

If the patient assumes a lithotomy position for delivery, maximize her participation and bearing-down efforts by placing two pillows, a bean bag, or a backrest behind her shoulders or at the small of her back. Alternatively, she can lean against her support person to help maintain a more upright position.

For some patients, a birthing chair may help maximize comfort while meeting fetal needs and allowing the health care team to monitor maternal and fetal status. Used for bearing down and for delivery, the birthing chair is particularly suitable for primiparous patients because of the longer pushing phase. A tired patient who has tried several positions in bed may benefit from the birthing chair's hand grips and back support. The patient may assume a side-lying position in the birthing chair, as well as various degrees of upright and recumbent positions. Drawbacks to the birthing chair include a risk of increased blood loss and perineal edema; also, the forearms-and-knees and squatting positions are not feasible. The chair should not be used by a patient who has received an epidural block because she will lack the physical control needed to transfer to the chair.

Monitor hydration

A patient who shows decreased bearing-down efforts after a period of effective efforts may have a nursing diagnosis of *fluid volume deficit related to restricted fluid intake and fluid loss during labor efforts.* Continue to offer her juice, water, or tea. If bearing down lasts more than 2 hours, consider starting an I.V. line to deliver fluids, as prescribed.

Prepare for delivery

As delivery approaches, nursing responsibilities include making a judgment about when to summon the doctor or nurse-midwife, prepare the delivery area and the patient, and assist with delivery. Also, other personnel, such as the neonatologist or pediatrician, should be notified, especially if there is fetal distress or fetal anomalies detected prenatally, or if the patient has any medical complications necessitating further neonatal assessment. Making each of these decisions and determining when to summon the doctor or nurse-midwife are skills the nurse learns. Always consider the patient's labor history, current progress, and rate of descent when making your decision.

Many health care facilities feature combined labor and delivery rooms where the patient labors, delivers, and recovers in the same room with the same staff. This prevents having to move the patient when she is so uncomfortable and allows her to be taken care of by the same personnel throughout her labor and delivery.

Prepare the delivery area. Make all necessary physical preparations for the impending birth. This includes gathering and setting up needed equipment and reviewing the patient's and doctor's or nurse-midwife's wishes for the delivery.

If the patient plans to give birth in the labor bed, place extra pads under her buttocks to absorb the blood and amniotic fluid that emerge after delivery. If she will be transferred to a delivery room, ensure that the route contains no obstacles. Try to plan ahead for emergencies by checking needed supplies at the start of each day to ensure that all are present and within reach. Know how to operate the equipment. If delivery occurs en route, be sure the side rails of the bed are raised and that the patient remains draped.

Set up the instrument pack and delivery pack specified by the facility, gloves for the members of the health care team, and any special supplies or equipment requested by the doctor or nurse-midwife. Equipment should include the following: a sterile drape to go under the patient's buttocks, clamps and scissors for the umbilical cord, a bulb syringe, a dry sterile towel and warm blanket for the neonate, and a needle holder and syringes.

Additional supplies for the neonate may include a radiant heat unit, suctioning equipment with catheters (sizes 5, 8, and 10), oxygen bag and mask (sizes for premature and full-term neonates), laryngoscope with endotracheal tubes (sizes 2.5, 3.0, and 3.5), extra bulb syringes and neonatal suction (DeLee) catheters, feeding tubes, syringes and needles, and neonatal resuscitation drugs, such as naloxone hydrochloride (neonatal injection, 0.02 mg/ml), sodium bicarbonate, epinephrine, 50% dextrose in water, and glucose reagent strips.

Prepare the patient. Do not break the end of the delivery room bed (if this is to be done at all) until a nurse, doctor, or nurse-midwife is in position in case the fetus descends rapidly. Once the patient is positioned in the delivery room bed, prepare the perineum by swabbing with an antiseptic solution.

A patient in the lithotomy position may have to place her feet in the stirrups or leg holders. Align her knees at equal heights, and check that her legs are abducted at similar angles and that the stirrups are padded. All of this decreases the possibility of nerve compression in the legs. Open the drape pack for the doctor or nurse-midwife, and assist with draping, as needed. Follow universal blood and body fluid safety precautions throughout delivery.

Assist the preparation of the support person for delivery by giving instructions on hand-washing and assisting with gown or scrub suit, boots, cap, and mask, according to facility policy and Occupational Safety and Health Administration standards.

Assist with delivery. While the doctor or nurse-midwife scrubs and dons gown and gloves, adjust lighting as necessary to observe the perineum for the presenting part's imminent delivery. If the patient finds bright light distracting, dim the overhead lights but maintain perineal illumination.

As the fetus's head crosses the perineum, perineal tissue may lacerate spontaneously. According to one study, perineal damage extensive enough to require sutures occurs in two-thirds of primiparous patients.

To circumvent this potential problem, the doctor or nurse-midwife may perform an episiotomy, either midline or mediolaterally, or have the patient push down and blow out alternatively in order to slowly stretch the perineum. Possible benefits of episiotomy include:

- prevention of damage to the anal sphincter and rectal mucosa with third- and fourth-degree lacerations
- easier repair and better healing than a spontaneous laceration
- prevention of trauma to the fetus's head
- prevention of serious damage to pelvic floor muscles.

The nurse does not assist with the performance or the repair of an episiotomy but should communicate the patient's wishes to the doctor or nurse-midwife. However, the final decision is that of the health care provider based on the situation at the time. Further, the nurse should provide care and support during and after an episiotomy.

In theory, prenatal perineal massage by the partner may offer an alternative to episiotomy for reducing perineal damage. In addition, the nurse, doctor, or nurse-midwife can "iron out" the perineal tissue firmly with lubricated fingers as the fetus's head moves onto the perineum in conjunction with the patient pushing down and alternatively blowing out to increase slow perineal stretching. Some patients, however, may find touch disruptive, particularly because of edema and the increased vascularity of the perineal tissue.

Care for the neonate

Immediately after delivery, the doctor or nurse-midwife suctions the neonate and ensures an adequate airway and normal breathing. If the amniotic fluid contains meconium, the doctor or nurse-midwife suctions immediately after the head appears and before delivering the rest of the body, then assesses for aspiration of meconium. After delivery, nursing care shifts from just the patient to the patient and neonate. Complete the clamping of the umbilical cord, perform an initial assessment, dry and wrap the neonate continue to suction the upper airway as needed, and initiate bonding between the neonate and parents within the first few minutes after delivery.

Clamping the umbilical cord. The doctor or nurse-midwife holds the neonate at or below the level of the mother's uterus to facilitate transfer of blood until the umbilical cord is clamped. To cut the umbilical cord, the doctor or nurse-midwife may apply two Kelly clamps and cut between them. If the doctor or nurse-midwife and facility policy permit, ask the mother and support person if they would like to cut the cord. Assist with collection of cord blood using blood and secretion precautions as per the facility policy. Typically, the doctor or nurse-midwife draws blood from the umbilical vessels into a purple-top (heparinized) tube and stores it in the health care facility refrigerator in case further studies are needed. Blood type and a direct Coombs' test can be obtained from this sample if the mother is Rh negative.

Assessment. Note the time of birth and the condition of the neonate's airway, amount of mucus, and respiratory efforts. Mucus may be greater following fast descent or cesarean delivery because fetal thorax compression does not force fluid from the respiratory tract. Continue with assessment of the umbilical cord as well as heart rate, color, tone, and neonate's physical condition.

<u>Umbilical cord.</u> Inspect the umbilical cord for obvious abnormalities, and verify that it contains two arteries and one vein. The presence of only one artery and one vein has been associated with congenital kidney and cardiac problems. Note and document the total length of the cord. Notify the pediatric personnel of any abnormalities.

Physical examination. Assign an Apgar score at 1 minute and 5 minutes after delivery, preferably while the neonate lies on the mother's abdomen. (See *Assigning an Apgar score,* page 268.)

Explain the Apgar score's meaning to the mother and her partner. Just after the neonate's delivery, perform a quick physical examination to detect obvious congenital anomalies, birthmarks, or bruises associated with delivery. Make note if the neonate passes meconium or urine in the delivery room.

Initiate parent-infant bonding. As soon as the neonate's breathing has been established and the umbilical cord is clamped, lay the infant on the mother's abdomen and cover both with a warm blanket. Urge the mother and her partner to dry the neonate, if necessary, while maintaining skin-to-skin contact.

If the neonate's condition warrants placement in a radiant heat unit, position the unit and deliver care within the mother's view. Because radiant heat only warms outer surfaces and will not be effective if the neonate is wrapped in a blanket, place the dried neonate, unwrapped, on top of a dry blanket in the warmer. A modified Trendelenburg position will help drain mucus from the airways, if needed.

Assess the patient's and partner's response to the neonate. Many new parents feel insecure and will value the nurse's support and instruction. Assist parents if they ask how to hold their infant. Praise them for holding their neonate securely and for any other appropri-

Assigning an Apgar score

A method of indicating neonatal vigor, the Apgar score combines the results of five individual assessments: heart rate, respiration, muscle tone, reflex irritability, and color. The neonate is assessed by the nurse 1 minute and 5 minutes after delivery, and the scores assigned in each assessment category are added to arrive at the total Apgar score. The highest score possible is 10; the lowest is 0. The score may reveal the need for further intervention, confirm trauma during delivery, and indicate congenital anomaly, among other findings.

THE APGAR SCORING SYSTEM

Sign	Score		
	0	1	2
Heart rate	Absent	Slow—below 100 beats/minute	Above 100 beats/minute
Respiratory effort	Absent	Slow—irregular, labored, retracting, grunting, nasal flaring	Good crying
Muscle tone	Flaccid	Some flexion of extremities	Active motion
Reflex irritability	None	Grimace	Vigorous cry
Color	Pale blue	Body pink with acrocyanosis	Completely pink

ate behavior, such as talking to the infant or observing the infant's responses. Give feedback about the neonate's condition, such as, "The toes and hands are bluish right now but this is typical; they should change to pink within a few hours," or "It is normal for your infant's head to be molded after delivery. It will become more rounded over the next few days." With a Black neonate, reassure the parents that the infant's skin will darken to their approximate skin color within 3 to 7 days.

Evaluation

Examples of appropriate evaluation statements include:

- After adopting a forearms-and-knees position, the patient reported a decrease in the urge to push.
- The patient bore down productively during the final phase of the second stage of labor.
- The patient and her partner expressed appropriate bonding behavior with the neonate immediately after delivery.
- The patient and her partner each held the neonate properly shortly after delivery.

13

THE THIRD AND FOURTH STAGES OF LABOR

The third stage of labor begins with delivery of the neonate and ends with delivery of the placenta. It may last from a few minutes to 30 minutes. For most patients, this stage occurs without incident and produces a blood loss of less than 500 ml. However, postpartal hemorrhage may occur, signaling an obstetric emergency.

In this stage, the nurse assesses the mother for homeostasis, placental status and delivery, and perineal repair. The nurse also evaluates the neonate's adaptation to the extrauterine environment and assesses the family's response to the mother and neonate. The nurse must respond quickly to changing circumstances, resetting priorities.

The fourth stage of labor begins after delivery of the placenta and lasts about 1 hour. It marks the beginning of the "fourth trimester," during which the patient recovers from the stresses of labor and physiologically returns to a nonpregnant state. During this stage, the patient, her partner, and the neonate experience heightened awareness and sensitivity as they further their bonding.

During the third and fourth stages of labor, the patient's cultural beliefs can influence her self-care and health promotion measures, interactions with health care professionals, and care of and bonding with the neonate. To provide adequate care, the nurse should become acquainted with the patient's cultural beliefs and exercise care to avoid stereotyping her.

Nursing goals for the third and fourth stages of labor relate to the physiologic adaptation and changing needs of the patient and neonate. They typically include:

- documenting the patient's status and care as well as that of her neonate
- addressing the cultural needs of the patient and her family, and adapting nursing care to meet those needs.

NURSING CARE DURING THE THIRD STAGE

During this stage, the nurse may care for the mother and neonate simultaneously. To provide the best possible care, the nurse should apply the nursing process.

Assessment

Because the third stage of labor is brief, rapidly assess maternal vital signs and the status of the placenta, perineum, fundus, and neonate. Carefully document any drugs or fluids administered.

Maternal vital signs

During the third stage of labor the patient's vital signs typically return to prelabor levels: The blood pressure and pulse return to prelabor rates, the temperature is slightly increased, respirations are normal, gastrointestinal motility and absorption—if not impeded by drugs—return to normal. Assess vital signs frequently, reporting changes or abnormal findings to the doctor or nurse-midwife immediately. An increasing pulse rate followed by increased respirations and decreased blood pressure may be the first signs of postpartal hemorrhage and hypovolemic shock, which can occur rapidly. Frequently, the patient may state she feels "funny," light-headed, or in a dreamy state with a postpartal hemorrhage. These complications are relatively common and typically result from uterine atony and excessive blood loss during placental separation and delivery or from perineal lacerations.

Restlessness, tachypnea, and tachycardia may signal amniotic fluid embolism, another rare complication that may occur when amniotic fluid enters the maternal circulation during placental separation.

Placenta

After delivery of the neonate, watch for these normal signs of placental separation:

- a sudden gush or trickle of blood from the vagina
- increased umbilical cord length at the vaginal introitus
- change in the shape of the uterus from discoid to globular
- change in the position of the uterus to a location at or above the patient's umbilicus.

These signs indicate normal progress of the third stage of labor. They occur when the size of the uterine cavity decreases while the size of the inelastic placental tissue remains constant. As the placental tissue buckles and begins separating from the uterus, bleeding from open decidual arterioles forms a clot between the placental tissue and the uterine wall. This retroplacental clot further shears the placenta from the uterine wall and maintains hemostasis by controlling arteriolar blood flow.

When these signs occur, expect placental delivery shortly. After the placenta separates completely, it descends to the lower uterine segment. Myometrial contractions, which may have subsided temporarily, return at 4- to 5-minute intervals and propel the placenta into the vagina. At this point, the patient may push to help expel the placenta. The mechanism for pushing is similar to but less intense than that used during the second stage of labor.

Note the mechanism of placental expulsion. The Duncan mechanism occurs when the dark, rough, maternal side of the placenta appears first. The Schultze mechanism occurs when the glistening fetal side appears first. The mechanism of expulsion does not affect the patient's outcome.

Following expulsion, the placenta and cord are examined. Note the time, method, and completeness of the placenta's delivery. (See *Placental and umbilical cord variations*.)

Perineum

If the patient underwent an episiotomy or sustained lacerations, assist with surgical repair of the tissue by providing adequate light, suture material, a local anesthesia kit as needed, and patient support. The perineum is stitched in layers to maintain its structural integrity. After the repair, assess for an intact suture line, and note the degree of swelling, oozing, or discoloration caused by bruising or hematoma formation if present. Always document what is present immediately after the repair and any subsequent changes.

If the doctor or nurse-midwife did not perform an episiotomy, assist with inspection of the perineum for lacerations or edema. Also assist with inspection of the vagina and cervix for lacerations or retained placental fragments as needed. Generally, an ice pack is applied to the perineum for 2 to 3 hours to decrease edema and increase the patient's comfort by slightly numbing the area.

Fundus

Palpate the fundus to determine its location and consistency. After the placenta is delivered, the fundus normally is midline, 1 to 2 cm below the umbilicus, and firmly contracted. A soft, boggy, and poorly contracted fundus is a sign of uterine atony, a possible cause of postpartal hemorrhage.

The following factors commonly are associated with uterine atony and the potential for postpartal hemorrhage:

• history of postpartal hemorrhage with previous delivery
• delivery of a large-for-gestational-age neonate

Placental and umbilical cord variations

After delivery of the placenta, the nurse assesses it carefully, documenting any variations from the norm (such as a placenta that is not intact). The nurse also notes umbilical cord variations, such as unusual insertion into the placenta or an abnormal number of umbilical cord vessels. The illustrations below show some common variations and their significance.

Normal placenta

Normally, the placenta is delivered intact and no fragments remain in the uterus. It has many lobes with smooth, rounded edges and consistent color throughout, indicating adequate tissue perfusion. The placenta at term is flat, cakelike, round or oval, 6″ to 8″ (15 to 20 cm) in diameter, and ³/₄″ to 1¹/₄″ (2 to 3 cm) at its thickest parts. The maternal side is lobulated and the fetal side

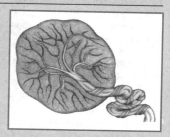

is shiny. It has no calcifications, discolorations, malformations, cysts, or other abnormalities. The umbilical cord inserts on the fetal side generally toward the middle of the placenta. The cord averages approximately 22″ (55 cm) in length. The amnion and chorion make up the fetal membranes that are attached to the fetal side of the placenta.

Placental variations

Battledore placenta
In this placental variation, the umbilical cord inserts in the margin of the placenta. This normal variation occurs in about 10% of gestations.

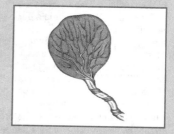

(continued)

Placental and umbilical cord variations
(continued)

Velamentous insertion

Occurring in about 1% of gestations, a velamentous insertion occurs when the cord vessels branch from the membranes to the placenta. A velamentous insertion poses a danger because if the membranes rupture, the cord vessels will rupture, leading to fetal hemorrhage. Blood vessels also may rupture, leading to hemorrhage between the amnion and chorion. Compression of the vessels during labor could explain fetal heart rate changes, indicating anoxia.

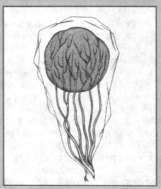

If velamentous insertion is detected when inspecting the delivered placenta, the danger to the fetus has passed.

Succenturiate lobe

A succenturiate lobe is an aberrant lobe or entire cotyledon that is separate from the placenta but connected to its main body by blood vessels. Occurring in less than 0.2% of gestations, a succenturiate lobe may tear away from the main portion of the placenta during separation and expulsion. If left in the uterus, a succenturiate lobe can cause postpartal hemorrhage or infection. It also may cause vasa previa (presentation of the cord's blood vessels in front of the fetus's head

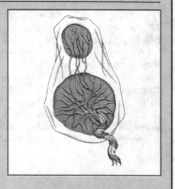

during labor and delivery). Vasa previa, which also may occur with velamentous insertion, endangers the fetus because the fetus's head can compress the unprotected vessels, reducing fetal oxygen supply. Also, the unprotected vessels may be ruptured easily, leading to life-threatening hemorrhage.

Placental and umbilical cord variations
(continued)

Umbilical vessels

Normal umbilical vessels
The normal umbilical cord contains three vessels: two arteries and one vein.

Abnormal number of vessels
Fewer than three umbilical vessels correlates with various congenital anomalies, such as cardiac and renal anomalies.

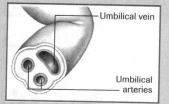

Umbilical vein

Umbilical arteries

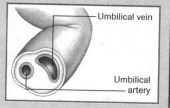

Umbilical vein

Umbilical artery

- polyhydramnios
- multiple gestation
- extended stimulation of labor with oxytocin
- bladder distention
- traumatic or difficult delivery
- grand multiparous patient
- anesthesia or excessive analgesia, history of prenatal anemia, prolonged labor, precipitous labor or delivery.

If uterine atony is not identified and corrected, postpartal hemorrhage can occur. (See *Uterine palpation and massage*, pages 276 and 277.)

Neonate

Depending on facility policy, the doctor, nurse-midwife, or nurse assesses the neonate immediately after delivery by assigning an Apgar score.

Continue to assess the neonate throughout the third stage of labor, focusing on evaluation of respiratory and cardiovascular status.

Nursing diagnosis

Based on assessment findings, formulate nursing diagnoses for the mother. (See Appendix 1, NANDA taxonomy of nursing diagnoses.) Then use the assessment findings and diagnoses to define care priorities during the postpartal period.

PSYCHOMOTOR SKILLS

Uterine palpation and massage

Through uterine palpation, the nurse can assess the location and firmness of the fundus. Uterine massage can help stimulate uterine contractions, which promote involution and prevent hemorrhage. Also, blood clots may be expelled during uterine massage. Before you begin, explain to the patient the procedure's steps and purpose; explain them again during the procedure.

To perform uterine palpation and massage, expose the lower abdomen and follow these steps.

1 Place one hand at the level of the symphysis pubis, cupping it against the abdomen to support the fundus and prevent downward displacement. Keep in mind that the elasticity of the ligaments supporting the uterus and the stretching experienced at term place the postpartal uterus at risk for inversion if it is not fixed in place during palpation and massage.

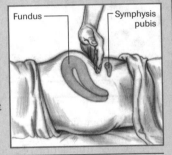

2 Place the other hand at the top of the fundus, cupping it against the abdomen.

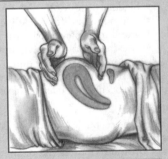

3 Gently compress the uterus between both hands. Note the level of the fundus above or below the umbilicus in fingerbreadths or centimeters. (One fingerbreadth equals about 1 cm). Also note the firmness of the fundus.

PSYCHOMOTOR SKILLS

Uterine palpation and massage *(continued)*

4 To massage the fundus, use the side of the hand above the fundus. Without digging into the abdomen, gently compress and release, always supporting the lower uterine segment with the other hand. Observe for lochia flow during massage.

5 Massage long enough to produce firmness. Because the fundus is tender, use only enough pressure to produce desired results without causing discomfort.

Planning and implementation

Routine care includes hygienic care, repositioning and transferring the mother to the recovery area (or assisting recovery in the labor-delivery-recovery area), providing neonatal care, and promoting bonding.

Provide hygienic care

At this stage, the mother may have a nursing diagnosis of *risk for infection related to perineal laceration* or *risk for infection related to episiotomy.* Immediately after the doctor or nurse-midwife has finished inspecting or repairing the perineum, help prevent infection by cleaning the patient's vulva with sterile water. Using a wet towel or gauze, wipe from the urethral area to the rectal area. Discard used gauze after each pass. Dislodge and remove dried blood or fecal material, leaving the perineal area free from bacterial contamination. Using a downward movement, apply a clean perineal pad.

Reposition and transfer the patient

To prevent hip joint dislocation if the patient's legs were in the stirrups and a nursing diagnosis of *risk for injury related to maternal positioning* or *altered tissue perfusion related to sudden change in pelvic or abdominal blood volume,* pay close attention to body dynamics and homeostasis when repositioning the patient. When helping her lower her legs from stirrups or from the flexed position, advise her to bring her legs together and lower them simultaneously.

If spinal or epidural anesthesia was used during delivery and the patient cannot control her legs, use a draw sheet or roller for the transfer and have other team members assist to ensure her safety.

After the patient has been repositioned, transfer her to the recovery area or allow her to remain in the labor and delivery area, depending on facility policy. Encourage her to move her legs around slowly and to rotate her feet at the ankles to increase circulation.

Care for the neonate

The nurse must also assess and provide care for the neonate during the third and fourth stages of labor. Assess the respiratory and cardiovascular status at 1 minute and 5 minutes of life, and then at 5-minute intervals unless the situation warrants closer, more frequent observation. Routinely evaluate the neonate every time the mother is assessed.

To assess the neonate's respiratory status, count respirations and note skin color. Respirations should range from 40 to 60 breaths/minute. Except for the hands and feet, which may have some acrocyanosis, the neonate's skin color should be similar to that of the parents.

To assess cardiovascular status, palpate the heart or auscultate it at the point of maximum impulse. The rate should range from 120 to 180 beats/minute. Palpate the femoral pulse for presence and quality. Lack of the femoral pulse may indicate aortic coarctation.

Nursing care. During this time, it is important to maintain the neonate's temperature, because neonates do not adequately control their body temperature until the second day of life. They can lose heat through four mechanisms: conduction, convection, evaporation, and radiation. (See *Preventing heat loss in the neonate*.)

Temperature regulation depends on metabolism of brown fat accumulated during the last 3 gestational months. The nurse must decrease all possible chances of cold stress by drying the neonate and keeping him warm.

Signs of cold stress include an accelerated respiratory rate, labored respirations, and an increased metabolic rate accompanied by greater use of glucose stores leading to hypoglycemia. If hypothermia does occur, the metabolic rate increases to produce heat; this can cause respiratory distress that can progress to metabolic acidosis, which requires quick, aggressive intervention.

In the neonate with a nursing diagnosis of **hypothermia related to cold stress,** check for signs of hypoglycemia, including tremors, seizures, irritability, lethargy (from breakdown of fats and proteins), and apnea or bradycardia (from changes in arterial oxygen saturation and a shift to anaerobic metabolism). A serum glucose level below 40 mg/dl before the first day or below 45 mg/dl on or after the third day indicates hypoglycemia. Neurologic immaturity may prevent homeostasis in the hypoglycemic neonate, leading to unstable vital signs.

If the neonate suffers cold stress, rewarm gradually to avoid hyperthermia and its complications; closely observe the neonate and check vital signs every 15 to 30 minutes. Hyperthermia may cause skin reddening, irritability, and an initial increase—then gradual drop—in the heart and respiratory rates, leading to apnea and bradycardia. To prevent complications, report any status changes immediately.

NEONATAL STATUS

Preventing heat loss in the neonate

Preventing heat loss is an important part of neonatal nursing care. Heat loss can occur through four mechanisms—conduction, convection, evaporation, and radiation. The nursing measures listed below help prevent heat loss by each mechanism.

Conductive heat loss
For loss of heat by skin directly touching a cooler object:
- Preheat the radiant warmer bed and linen.
- Warm the stethoscope before use.
- Wrap the neonate in a warm blanket or allow the mother to hold the neonate to provide the warming effect of skin contact.
- Pad the scale with paper or a preweighed, warmed sheet to weigh the neonate.
- Check the temperature of any surface before placing the neonate on it.

Convective heat loss
For loss of heat from the body surface to cooler surrounding air:
- Place the neonate's bed out of direct line with an open window, a fan, or an air-conditioning vent.
- Cover the neonate with a blanket when moving the neonate to another area.
- Raise the sides of the radiant warmer bed to prevent exposing the neonate to air currents.
- Avoid fans in the delivery room or nursery.

Evaporative heat loss
For loss of heat when fluids turn to vapor in dry air:
- Dry the neonate immediately after delivery.
- When the neonate is not in a warming bed, keep the neonate dry and swaddled in warmed blankets.
- Remove wet blankets.
- Delay the bath until the neonate's temperature is stable.
- When bathing the neonate, expose only one body part at a time; wash each part thoroughly and dry it immediately.
- When assessing the neonate, uncover only the specific area to be assessed.
- Place a cap on the neonate's head in the delivery room.

Radiant heat loss
For loss of heat due to the presence of a cooler solid surface near but not directly touching the neonate's body:
- Use a radiant heat warmer for initial post-delivery stabilization.
- Place the neonate in a double-walled incubator.
- Keep the neonate away from areas with cold surfaces (such as a cold formula bottle or a window in winter).

Other routine neonatal care. Routine neonatal care includes positive identification of the neonate by footprinting the baby and applying identification bracelets to the baby's ankle and wrist; a matching bracelet is placed on the mother's wrist. This is done as the facility policy dictates. Take two sets of footprints: one for the parents and one for the neonate's record.

In many facilities, the neonate is weighed and measured in the nursery and receives a vitamin K injection and ophthalmic prophylaxis. The nurse in the labor-delivery-recovery area may have to perform these tasks. Wherever these procedures are performed, encourage the support person to observe and bring back the news to the mother. Note the neonate's status during transfer to the recovery area or nursery.

Promote bonding

During the third stage of labor, the family may have a nursing diagnosis of *family coping: potential for growth related to neonate's birth.* For this reason, the neonate's introduction to the parents is paramount. Frequently, the doctor or nurse-midwife places the neonate in the mother's arms even before the cord has stopped pulsating or been cut. A neonate that must remain supine can lie on the mother's abdomen. Keep the mother and neonate together while assessments and procedures are performed.

Encourage both parents to touch and talk to the neonate immediately. If the parents are afraid to touch the neonate, reassure them. Upon hearing the parents' voices, the neonate should gaze in their direction and may open the eyes fully if they are shaded from the light.

Evaluation

Before the fourth stage of labor begins, evaluate nursing care provided during the third stage. In many facilities, the delivery nurse continues to care for the mother; in others, another nurse assumes care for the mother after transfer to the recovery area. In either case, note maternal status during transfer; evaluate maternal status by reviewing and comparing assessment data and considering the effectiveness of nursing interventions. The following examples illustrate appropriate evaluation statements:
- The patient's placenta was delivered intact.
- The patient's fundus was firm.
- The patient lost less than 500 ml of blood.
- The neonate adapted appropriately to the extrauterine environment, as shown by stable temperature, heart rate of 120 to 180 beats/minute, and respirations between 40 and 60 breaths/minute with no nasal flaring or grunting.
- The patient held and gazed at the neonate immediately after delivery.
- The father touched and talked to the neonate.

NURSING CARE DURING THE FOURTH STAGE

The nurse continues to use the nursing process to care for a patient during the fourth stage of labor. To interpret assessment data properly and make decisions about care, the nurse must understand the physiology of the recovery period, including shifts in internal pressures and changes in the cardiovascular, respiratory, urinary, reproductive, gastrointestinal, and musculoskeletal systems.

Assessment

Maternal status can change rapidly during the fourth stage of labor, and such life-threatening complications as postpartal hemorrhage can occur. Therefore, frequent assessments are necessary. Begin the assessment by reviewing subjective and objective data obtained during the previous stages of labor. A complete, concise verbal report from the previous nurse can assist the recovery nurse to understand the patient's labor and delivery course quickly and accurately. The recovery nurse must also review the patient's complete chart for all information pertinent to this labor course. Continue the assessment by collecting current data.

If the neonate stays with the mother during this period, continue to maintain the neonate's warmth and monitor cardiovascular and respiratory status.

Health history

First, review all data obtained on admission and throughout labor and delivery. The following elements of the patient's history help interpret fourth stage assessment findings.

Vital signs. Postpartal deviations from the patient's baseline can indicate hemorrhage, pregnancy-induced hypertension (PIH), dehydration, or infection.

Obstetric history. The patient's gravidity and parity help predict her uterine contractility and response to oxytocic medication. For example, a multiparous patient may have less muscle contractility because childbirth commonly causes a decrease in uterine muscle tone.

The patient's obstetric history can provide other clues about her probable postpartal recovery. For example, a woman who experienced postpartal hemorrhage after a previous childbirth has greater risk for hemorrhage after this one.

Labor duration and progress. Prolonged labor can lead to uterine atony, particularly if accompanied by many hours of oxytocic stimulation. It also may cause dehydration and exhaustion, which may result in circulatory and musculoskeletal problems. Precipitous labor and delivery can cause uterine atony, predispose the patient to hemorrhage, and produce lacerations or cervical tears that may increase blood loss. A full bladder can also lead to uterine atony and hemorrhage.

Physical assessment

Begin the maternal assessment after the neonate is stabilized and during or immediately after perineal repair. Assess the patient's vital signs and level of consciousness. After any perineal repair is completed and the patient has been helped into a more comfortable position, assess postpartal parameters and evaluate her discomfort, recovery from analgesia and anesthesia, and fatigue, hunger, and thirst. Also observe the family's response to the neonate's birth.

Postpartal parameters. During this assessment, evaluate vital signs, fundus, lochia (blood, tissue, and cells shed from the uterus immediately after delivery and continuing for several weeks), perineum, leg pain, and tremors. (See *Parameters of postpartal assessment*.)

Assess these parameters at least every 15 minutes during the fourth stage. In situations that deviate from the norm, such as a sudden drop in blood pressure or a large increase in bright red lochia, alert the doctor or nurse-midwife.

Discomfort. With each assessment during the fourth stage, determine the patient's discomfort. Determine the character, intensity, and source of discomfort, such as uterine contractions, laceration repair, or perineal hematoma.

Uterine contractions. Once the placenta has been delivered, the myometrial fibers contract to control blood flow from open vessels at the placental site. Sometimes called afterpains, each patient experiences these contractions differently. For example, the multiparous patient tends to need stronger and longer contractions to firm the uterus than the primiparous patient, and those stronger contractions produce more intense afterpains. Postpartal contraction pain also may intensify if oxytocic drugs have been administered to control uterine bleeding.

Episiotomy, laceration repair, or perineal hematoma. A patient who has undergone an episiotomy or laceration repair may experience a dull aching or burning sensation from edema and disruption of muscle and nerve tissue. Although some pain is inevitable, severe, throbbing, or increasing pain may signal a serious problem.

If the woman incurred minor sublabial tears that required no surgical repair, she may experience a burning sensation during voiding when acidic urine passes over open wounds. Fear of this burning may cause her to postpone voiding, leading to urine retention, bladder distention, and uterine displacement and atony. Have her rinse her perineum with warm water as she urinates. If the patient is having her

(*Text continues on page 288.*)

Parameters of postpartal assessment

For each postpartal assessment parameter, this chart describes assessment techniques, normal and abnormal findings, and related nursing interventions. During the fourth stage of labor, the nurse must assess these parameters at least every 15 minutes.

PARAMETER AND ASSESSMENT TECHNIQUE	FINDINGS	NURSING INTERVENTIONS
Vital signs Palpate the pulse for a full minute, observe respiratory rate and rhythm, and auscultate blood pressure; take temperature (usually 1 hour after birth)	*Normal findings* • Pulse within 4 to 17 beats/minute of predelivery rate • Respiratory rate within 2 to 4 breaths of predelivery rate • Systolic and diastolic blood pressure within 10 mm Hg of predelivery pressure • Temperature within 0.5 degrees of the normal 98.6° F (37° C)	*For a patient with normal findings* • Repeat assessments every 15 minutes until stable; then repeat according to facility policy or as prescribed. • Assess for orthostatic changes in blood pressure and increase in pulse if the woman reports light-headedness when rising or walking. Help the patient when getting up the first time by having her sit on the edge of the bed, waiting for 1 to 2 minutes, and then walking with her.
	Abnormal findings • Rapid pulse rate, characteristic of hemorrhage • Pulse rate more than 17 beats/minute slower than predelivery rate, which may indicate heart block or other postpartal cardiac anomaly	*For a patient with abnormal findings* • Notify the doctor or nurse-midwife. • Repeat vital sign assessments at least every 5 minutes along with other assessments. • Maintain fluid balance, as needed. • Be prepared to administer oxygen and medications as prescribed. *(continued)*

ASSESSMENT TIP

Parameters of postpartal assessment *(continued)*

PARAMETER AND ASSESSMENT TECHNIQUE	FINDINGS	NURSING INTERVENTIONS
Vital signs *(continued)*	• Depressed respiratory rate, which can result from medications or anesthesia • Tachypnea, which indicates oxygen need from hemorrhage or shock • Hypotension (less than 10 mm Hg between systolic and diastolic measurements), which may suggest extensive blood loss and impending shock • Hypertension (increase of 15 mm Hg in diastolic, 30 mm Hg in systolic), which may occur with pregnancy-induced hypertension (PIH) • Elevated temperature, which may be caused by dehydration, fatigue, or infection	• If hypertension is present, check the patient's reflexes. A patient with PIH who develops symptoms will show brisk reflexes with ankle clonus.
Fundus Palpate uterus to assess for size, consistency, and location of fundus.	*Normal findings* • Fundal height at the umbilicus or 1 to 2 cm below the umbilicus • Fundus midline, firm, and about the size of an average cantaloupe	*For a patient with normal findings* • Repeat fundal palpation every 15 minutes with other assessments. Measure position in fingerbreadths above or below the umbilicus. • Teach the patient the significance of a well-contracted uterus. Teach her to palpate her fundus and practice fundal massage.

Parameters of postpartal assessment (continued)

PARAMETER AND ASSESSMENT TECHNIQUE	FINDINGS	NURSING INTERVENTIONS
Fundus (continued)	*Abnormal findings* • Boggy, soft, poorly contracted uterus, deviated from midline and above the umbilicus, suggesting atony, clot retention, or a full bladder	*For a patient with abnormal findings* • Massage the fundus until it becomes firm and clots are expressed. • Reassess the fundus at least every 5 minutes. • Encourage the patient to void. • Encourage the patient who has chosen to breast-feed to begin because nipple stimulation causes release of oxytocin. • Administer oxytocic medications, if prescribed.
Lochia Inspect lochia flow and observe for clots at the perineum while assessing the fundus. Check to ensure that blood is not pooling under the patient.	*Normal findings* • Sanguinous fluid with no clots • Scant (1″ [2.5 cm] stain on perineal pad), light (1″ to 4″ [10 cm] stain), or moderate (4″ to 6″ [15 cm] stain) flow within 15 minutes	*For a patient with normal findings* • Repeat the assessment in 15 minutes. Remember to wear gloves and use good hand-washing technique.
	Abnormal findings • Heavy flow (saturation of one or more perineal pads) in 15 minutes or less, which indicates excessive bleeding and possible uterine atony	*For a patient with abnormal findings* • Evaluate for uterine atony. • Massage the fundus. • Notify the doctor or nurse-midwife, who may need to futher evaluate the patient's condition.

(continued)

Parameters of postpartal assessment (continued)

PARAMETER AND ASSESSMENT TECHNIQUE	FINDINGS	NURSING INTERVENTIONS
Lochia *(continued)*	• A steady trickle of bright red bleeding in a patient with a well-contracted uterus, which may indicate cervical, vaginal, or perineal laceration	
Perineum Inspect perineum. Remove the perineal pad, and use an adequate light source. Position the patient in the left or right lateral position with the upper leg flexed. Raise the upper buttock slightly to observe the perineum. Ask the patient to contract and relax the perineal muscles to assess muscle function. Place a clean pad on the perineum and help the patient into a comfortable position.	*Normal findings* • Intact perineum, possibly with slight edema, and painless contraction of perineal muscles • Incision with approximated edges, minimal swelling, no discoloration or bleeding from the incision, no discomfort on contraction of perineal muscles, and possible burning sensation in the incision area when voiding	*For a patient with normal findings* • Maintain cleanliness and comfort if the perineum is intact. • Assess the perineum every 15 minutes in a patient with an episiotomy. Place an ice pack on the perineum to increase comfort and decrease edema. Initiate perineal care after assessing the area. Begin sitz bath teaching as ordered. Teach and encourage Kegel exercises. Remember to wear gloves and use good hand-washing technique.
	Abnormal findings • Swelling and discoloration, which may indicate hematoma development • Bleeding, which may indicate unligated blood vessels • Dehiscence	*For a patient with abnormal findings* • Report edema, discoloration, or dehiscence immediately. • If signs of hematoma exist, monitor for signs of impending shock, such as restlessness

Parameters of postpartal assessment (continued)

PARAMETER AND ASSESSMENT TECHNIQUE	FINDINGS	NURSING INTERVENTIONS
Perineum (continued)	• Moderate to severe hemorrhoids	and changes in respirations, pulse, and blood pressure. For hemorrhoids, teach sitz baths, Kegel exercises, and hydrocortisone rectal suppository use as needed.
Leg pain and tremors Dorsiflex the foot. First, support the patient's thigh with one hand and her foot with the other. Then, bend her leg slightly at the knee, and firmly and abruptly dorsiflex the foot.	*Normal findings* • No discomfort in the calf or popliteal space • No ankle clonus	*For a patient with normal findings* • Encourage normal activity. • Repeat this assessment every 15 minutes.
	Abnormal findings • Pain in the calf or popliteal space, which may result from a thrombus • Ankle clonus, which may result from PIH	*For a patient with abnormal findings* • Report findings. • Obtain elastic stockings and advise the patient to wear them as prescribed. • Instruct the patient not to massage her legs. Encourage her to do ankle rotations and alternately extend and flex the feet to increase circulation and venous return. • Monitor for signs of embolism, such as shortness of breath, rapid drop in blood pressure, elevated heart rate, ashen coloring, and sweating. Teach patient to report any changes in her condition.

intake and output monitored, be sure to subtract the amount of water used at this time from the total volume of urine.

Dull aching or burning constitute normal episiotomy pain. Pain that throbs, increases, or does not respond to comfort measures may indicate an abnormality, such as perineal, vulvar, or vaginal hematoma.

A hematoma forms when blood seeps into the tissue because open blood vessels are not closed adequately during episiotomy repair. Characteristically, it swells gradually and reddens or becomes purple. Symptoms may include increasing and throbbing perineal pain, tachycardia, restlessness and, in severe cases, hypotension.

Cervical and vaginal hematomas pose potential problems during the fourth stage. They produce various discomforts, from a vague inability to achieve comfort to a throbbing sensation in the vagina that cannot be relieved by comfort measures. A hematoma may not be readily apparent on perineal inspection but does warrant further investigation by the doctor or nurse-midwife.

Other discomforts. During the fourth stage, the patient may experience other discomforts related to second-stage occurrences, such as the exertion and method of pushing, use of regional anesthesia, or positioning during delivery.

The patient may experience a dull ache in the sacral area caused by pressure from the fetus's head. If she pushed for an extended time, she may experience discomfort in her abdomen, arms, or upper shoulders and ribs. If she pushed from her upper chest while contracting her face and neck muscles, she may experience aching behind her eyes and a red or blotchy facial discoloration.

A woman who maintained an extended lithotomy position or braced herself with her legs may experience constant leg pain or aches. This pain must be differentiated from that caused by a thrombus or hypertension through assessment for Homans' sign, which is not found with muscular aches.

Recovery from anesthesia and analgesia. If the patient received an anesthetic or other medications during labor and delivery, evaluate her recovery with each assessment during the fourth stage. As the effects of the drugs begin to dissipate, evaluate the patient's condition and response to pain. As numbness from regional or local anesthesia diminishes, she may experience sudden and intense pain in the perineum and at the episiotomy site. Assess the character, intensity, and location of pain, and monitor response to measures such as repositioning and applying ice. These assessments will help distinguish between normal discomfort and pain that signals a problem.

If the patient had continuous regional anesthesia, assess the return of motor function to her legs. During each postpartal assessment, note the color and temperature of her legs and toes and her ability to move them.

When the doctor or nurse-midwife removes the epidural catheter after discontinuing regional anesthesia, observe and document catheter removal. If regional anesthesia was employed, observe the lumbar-area puncture site for drainage or bleeding.

If spinal anesthesia was administered, instruct the patient to remain supine until motor function returns. This reduces the risk of post-spinal headache.

Fatigue, hunger, and thirst. Depending on the duration of labor and the second stage, the patient may experience extreme fatigue or exhaustion immediately after delivery. Shaking or tremors may indicate muscle exhaustion, PIH, or infection. To differentiate normal postpartal tremors from those caused by PIH or infection, evaluate her blood pressure, temperature, and respirations; assess for ankle clonus; and assess deep tendon reflexes.

After the neonate is born, the patient may feel extremely hungry and thirsty, especially if she was restricted to ice chips or clear fluids during labor and if her labor was long. If the patient's labor was uncomplicated, honor her requests for food and fluids after delivery. Begin by administering sips of water or clear soda to assess for normal swallowing and for nausea.

Response to birth. Assess the parents' response to the neonate's birth at least once during the fourth stage of labor. Sensitive postpartal assessment of family interaction can provide valuable information that predicts future family interactions. The parents' first response to the neonate may be colored by their expectations for a perfect child, experience of pregnancy, culture, the consistency of the actual birth with expectations about it, and the child's normalcy.

Observe the new family as they experience one another. If they rely on another member, such as a grandmother or aunt, as the primary caregiver, include that member in the bonding experience.

Mother's response. One author describes the progress a mother makes in touching her child. She begins by touching the neonate with her fingertips and proceeds to use her entire hand. The en face position, in which the neonate's face turns toward the mother and they look directly at each other, indicates positive bonding. The mother may want to count the neonate's fingers and toes to assure herself of her child's normalcy. She may express concern about the neonate's color, breathing, crying, or lack of crying. These concerns reflect the mother's attempt to establish her child's reality and health.

Father's response. Researchers have described the relationship of a father's early contact with his child to his subsequent involvement with the child. The term "engrossment" defines positive bonding between father and child, characterized by tactile, visual, and verbal activities by the father that are directed to the neonate. Touching the neonate's skin, looking closely at the neonate, and expressing feelings of elation all indicate the father's engrossment.

Nursing diagnosis

Carefully review assessment findings and use them to develop appropriate nursing diagnoses. (See Appendix 1, NANDA taxonomy of nursing diagnoses.)

Planning and implementation

Although the fourth stage of labor is brief and focuses on assessment, planning is necessary and may occur during assessment. During this stage, interventions may include maintaining appropriate maternal positioning and activity, preventing hemorrhage, maintaining hygiene and comfort, maintaining fluid balance, meeting nutritional needs, and promoting bonding.

Maintain appropriate maternal positioning and activity

To prevent a nursing diagnosis of *pain related to maternal positioning,* position the patient for maximum comfort during her recovery. Adjust her position based on considerations such as the need to prevent postspinal anesthesia headache. Evaluate for presence or absence of ankle clonus or calf pain.

For fundal and perineal assessments, help the patient into the supine position. Between assessments, suggest that she assume a semi-Fowler's, high Fowler's, or lateral position, which may be more comfortable and give her a better position from which to view or breast-feed the neonate.

The events of labor and delivery determine the patient's activity during the fourth stage. If she experienced an uncomplicated labor and delivery, received little or no analgesia, delivered the neonate with her perineum intact, or delivered with a local anesthetic agent for an episiotomy, she may be able to walk and may appreciate this opportunity to move around under the nurse's observations. Even an uncomplicated delivery and labor warrant the ongoing evaluation by the nurse, according to facility protocol.

Before helping the patient out of bed for the first time, check her blood pressure. Some patients experience orthostatic hypotension after delivery and may require assistance. For this reason, help her rise slowly to prevent dizziness and weakness, and accompany her on her first walk to prevent a fall.

Expect a patient who experienced a long or difficult labor and delivery, received a regional anesthetic, or was heavily medicated during or after delivery to remain in bed and be less active.

Advise a patient who experienced postpartal hemorrhage to remain in bed until she stabilizes completely, which may take hours. Take special care to assist her when she first rises from bed.

Prevent hemorrhage

To help prevent a nursing diagnosis of **decreased cardiac output related to postpartal hemorrhage,** monitor the patient closely and take measures to prevent uterine atony and hemorrhage. Note the location and consistency of the uterus. Massage the patient's uterus gently during each assessment, and teach her to do so at regular intervals. If the fundus is boggy, continue massaging until it becomes firm and all clots are expressed.

To prevent uterine atony, administer oxytocin, as prescribed. (See *Drugs used in the fourth stage of labor,* pages 292 to 295.)

Encourage breast-feeding, which helps contract the uterus by stimulating the release of endogenous oxytocin. An ice pack on the abdomen, at the level of the fundus, has also been used to increase uterine contractility.

Encourage voiding to prevent bladder distention, which displaces the uterus and can cause atony. Note any changes in urinary status. Depending on the patient's condition, use the following interventions to prevent bladder distention—and postpartal hemorrhage:
- Provide a bedpan.
- Help the patient walk to a bathroom.
- Apply warm water over the perineum to encourage muscle relaxation.
- Use the sound of running water as a psychic stimulant.
- Catheterize the patient, if prescribed.
- Encourage fluid intake.

Maintain hygiene and comfort

The patient may have a nursing diagnosis of **pain related to severe uterine contractions, pain related to episiotomy, pain related to difficult labor and delivery,** or **risk for infection related to perineal trauma.** For such a patient, take measures that increase comfort, promote hygiene, and decrease chances of infection. Use the following general interventions to maintain maternal comfort and hygiene:
- Remove collected secretions, such as lochia and perspiration.
- Teach the patient self-care activities that ensure continued cleanliness.
- Provide clean, warm clothing and blankets.
- Change perineal pads and underpads after each assessment, or more frequently if appropriate.

(Text continues on page 295.)

292 THE THIRD AND FOURTH STAGES OF LABOR

SELECTED MAJOR DRUGS

Drugs used in the fourth stage of labor

Drugs commonly used during the fourth stage of labor include those listed here.

MAJOR INDICATIONS	USUAL ADULT DOSAGES	NURSING IMPLICATIONS
oxytocin (Pitocin)		
Ineffective uterine contractions after delivery of the placenta; heavy amount of lochia	10 to 40 units in 1,000 ml D_5W or normal saline solution I.V., infused at a rate to control bleeding, usually 20 to 40 milliunits/minute; many clinicians follow with ergonovine maleate or methylergonovine maleate I.M.	• Administer drug I.M. or by I.V. infusion, never by bolus injection. If possible, use an infusion pump or a drip regulator to ensure accurate delivery. • Monitor the patient's heart rate, central nervous system (CNS) status, blood pressure, uterine contractions, and blood loss every 15 minutes. • Watch for signs of hypersensitivity, such as blood pressure elevation. In a patient who had a long labor accompanied by infusion of oxytocin and large volumes of parenteral fluid, watch for signs of water intoxication, such as edema; oxytocin has an antidiuretic effect. • Use appropriate comfort measures to control pain caused by uterine contractions.
ergonovine maleate (Ergotrate) and methylergonovine maleate (Methergine)		
Prevent or control postpartal hemorrhage	For both drugs, 0.2 mg I.M. every 2 to 4 hours to a maximum of five doses	• Be aware that these drugs may be given if oxytocin does not control postpartal bleeding.

Drugs used in the fourth stage of labor *(continued)*

MAJOR INDICATIONS	USUAL ADULT DOSAGES	NURSING IMPLICATIONS

ergonovine maleate (Ergotrate) and methylergonovine maleate (Methergine) *(continued)*

| | | • Assess the patient's vital signs (especially blood pressure) before administration.
• Do not administer this drug if the patient is hypertensive.
• Do not administer this drug before delivery of the neonate because it can cause tetanic contractions.
• Watch for adverse reactions, which may include severe hypertension and signs of cerebral hemorrhage (such as loss of consciousness), myocardial infarction (such as chest pain), and retinal detachment (such as blurred vision).
• Monitor the patient's blood pressure, pulse rate, uterine contractions, and vaginal bleeding. Report sudden changes in vital signs, frequent periods of uterine relaxation, and any change in lochia character or amount.
• Use comfort measures to control pain caused by uterine contractions. |

acetaminophen (Tylenol)

| Relief of mild to moderate pain caused by episiotomy or uterine contractions | 325 to 650 mg P.O. every 4 to 6 hours as needed | • Assess the patient's need for analgesia. Her discomfort may increase with oxytocin administration and |

(continued)

Drugs used in the fourth stage of labor *(continued)*

MAJOR INDICATIONS	USUAL ADULT DOSAGES	NURSING IMPLICATIONS
acetaminophen (Tylenol) *(continued)*		
		• development of vaginal or perineal hematoma. • Monitor the patient's response to the drug; hypersensitivity may cause general malaise, rash, and sweating.
meperidine hydrochloride (Demerol)		
Relief of moderate to severe pain caused by uterine contractions	50 to 100 mg I.M., depending on the patient's weight and degree of pain	• Drug should be used only for short-term management of pain. • Assess the patient's need for analgesia. Evaluate the drug's appropriateness in relation to the patient's vital signs, history of drug sensitivity, and degree of discomfort. • Obtain the patient's baseline blood pressure and pulse and respiratory rates before administering this drug. Assess vital signs regularly to determine the patient's response to the drug. • Observe for adverse reactions, such as dry mouth, dizziness, and respiratory depression. • Keep naloxone hydrochloride (Narcan) readily available to reverse respiratory depression.

SELECTED MAJOR DRUGS

Drugs used in the fourth stage of labor (continued)

MAJOR INDICATIONS	USUAL ADULT DOSAGES	NURSING IMPLICATIONS
promethazine hydrochloride (Phenergan)		
Adjunct to narcotic administration to control nausea related to narcotic administration	12.5 to 25 mg P.O., I.M., or rectally every 4 to 6 hours	• Use with caution in a patient with hypersensitivity to this drug or with CNS depression. • Assess the patient's need for analgesia and nausea control. Evaluate the drug's appropriateness in relation to the patient's vital signs, history of drug sensitivity, and degree of discomfort. • Monitor the patient's vital signs and CNS status regularly. • Observe for adverse effects, such as transient hypotension, drowsiness, tinnitus, nervousness, hysteria, blurred vision, and seizures. • Advise the patient to rise slowly, and assist with ambulation.

- Clean the perineum at least once during the fourth stage with warm, clear water.
- Teach the patient perineal care techniques, including wiping from front to back after urinating or defecating and rinsing the perineal area regularly with warm, clear water.
- Offer a modified bed bath to remove perspiration and relax sore muscles.
- Offer a back and neck massage to relieve tension and stiffness caused by labor, pushing, or positioning.

Uterine contractions. To help relieve discomfort caused by uterine contractions, use the following interventions:
- Administer analgesic agents, as prescribed.
- Reduce the rate of continuous oxytocin infusion, as prescribed.
- Teach abdominal effleurage to ease the pain of contractions.

- Place a pillow over the patient's lower abdomen and help her assume a prone position, if her condition allows. The uterus should contract strongly several times and the pain should subside for a while. When the pain subsides, help her assume a comfortable position.

Episiotomy, laceration repair, hemorrhoids, or hematoma. Use the following interventions to help relieve perineal discomfort:
- Note the condition of the perineum.
- Apply an ice pack to the area.
- Apply witch hazel compresses to the area.
- Encourage the patient to contract and relax the perineal muscles (Kegel exercises).
- Administer analgesic agents, as prescribed.

Tremors. The following interventions may help relieve discomfort caused by tremors, such as those from chills (unrelated to PIH).
- Wrap warm blankets around the patient's feet or head.
- Provide warm oral fluids if the patient's condition warrants.
- Adjust the room temperature.

Maintain fluid balance and meet nutritional needs

During the fourth stage of labor, nursing diagnoses may include *fluid volume deficit related to fluid restriction during labor and delivery, fluid volume deficit related to fluid loss from perspiration during labor and delivery,* or *altered nutrition: less than body requirements related to food restriction and energy expenditure during labor and delivery.* If the patient has one of these nursing diagnoses, employ the following interventions:
- Monitor temperature, pulse rate, and blood pressure and compare them to baseline measurements to estimate the extent of the deficit.
- Provide oral fluids.
- Regulate I.V. fluids as directed by the doctor or nurse-midwife.
- Provide nourishment according to the patient's preference, if not contraindicated by complications. Assess the appropriateness of her food choices and recommend easily digestible alternatives, if necessary.

Promote bonding

The postpartal patient may experience at least 1 hour of heightened awareness and sensitivity to her surroundings, especially to the neonate, unless she received depressant medications. Bonding commonly begins at this time, unless the patient is distracted by pain or her environment. Typically, the neonate is quiet and alert during the first hour after delivery, and the mother experiences a surge of energy and heightened sensitivity at this time. Afterward, the neonate and mother may sleep or rest.

Once the neonate is stabilized, the patient may become increasingly concerned about herself. She may wonder why she still looks pregnant, why uterine contractions continue, and why she feels perineal discomfort. These personal concerns may delay bonding.

The first 1 or 2 days after childbirth have been described as a time of "taking in," when the mother exhibits dependent behavior and requires some "mothering" herself. Her needs relate to comfort, nutrition, and sleep, and she may focus on one or all of these during the first hour after delivery. Nursing interventions can help prevent a nursing diagnosis of *altered parenting related to unmet expectations about childbirth* or *altered parenting related to unmet expectations about the neonate's capabilities.*

The following methods have been suggested to promote family involvement and parent-infant bonding:

- Facilitate immediate, continuous mother-infant contact.
- Provide anticipatory guidance regarding the neonate's needs and abilities.
- Establish an emotionally warm and sensitive environment.

If the immediate postpartal situation does not permit extended contact, assist the family when bonding becomes practical. Note the parent's response to the neonate's birth and interaction with the baby.

Immediately after delivery, try promoting mother-infant bonding by encouraging the breast-feeding woman to hold the neonate to her breast. During breast-feeding, the mother and neonate face each other, have skin-to-skin contact, and interact as the mother responds to the feel, smell, and movement of her infant.

Help the woman breast-feed as long as the neonate desires because breast-feeding positively influences bonding, and unrestricted breast-feeding with correct latching on by the baby does not cause or increase nipple discomfort. Also, colostrum transmits immunoglobulins, fat-soluble vitamins, calories, and fluid to the neonate.

Evaluation

At the end of the fourth stage of labor, evaluate the effectiveness of nursing care while making a final assessment of the patient's stability. Appropriate evaluation statements include:

- The patient's fundus is firm and located 1 cm below the umbilicus.
- The patient's perineum is intact.
- The father and other family members held the neonate.
- The neonate opened both eyes fully and responded to the parents' voices.
- The patient used effleurage to reduce postpartal discomfort.
- The patient began breast-feeding her neonate.

After the fourth stage of labor, a facility with birth areas or units may transfer the patient from the birthing room to a room with an adjacent nursery where the neonate will be placed. A more traditional facility may transfer the neonate to a central nursery and move the patient to a postpartal room. Finally, if the family wishes to go home, the woman and neonate may be discharged a few hours after birth if they are both stable.

Before the transfer occurs, assess the woman's ability to leave the delivery area via stretcher or wheelchair and the neonate's stability for transfer in the mother's arms or by nursery personnel. Also check the mother's and neonate's name bracelets before they are moved. A patient who is drowsy from medication should not carry her neonate and may need to be transferred via stretcher with the side rails up.

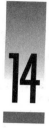

HIGH-RISK INTRAPARTAL PATIENTS

Over the past few decades, the definition of *high risk* in obstetrics has changed significantly to include old conditions with updated management perspectives and new conditions such as human immunodeficiency virus (HIV). Patients at high risk fall into two major groups: those with chronic disorders that predispose them to obstetric problems, such as cardiac disease, diabetes mellitus, and substance abuse; and those with pregnancy-related conditions that require special care, such as pregnancy-induced hypertension (PIH) and Rh isoimmunization. These patients are at high risk antepartally, which puts stressors on their bodies and the fetus' system. As the patient goes into labor, she and the fetus are continuously stressed; this stress can continue until delivery. (See *Intrapartal conditions and risks,* pages 301 to 304).

The high-risk intrapartal patient may not be well equipped to handle the emotional and physical demands of labor because of her struggle with the uncertainties of the pregnancy outcome. She probably was monitored closely during pregnancy and begins labor keenly aware of the risks for herself or her fetus. Indeed, she may be anxious or frightened about the effects of labor and delivery on her medical or obstetric condition. However, if the high-risk problem is diagnosed intrapartally, she may not have sufficient time, information, or energy to process and understand the severity of her condition.

Because high risk implies illness or disease, the patient may be unprepared for a positive childbirth experience, believing that cesarean delivery is inevitable. She may be concerned that she or her fetus may die during delivery.

Because the high-risk intrapartal patient may believe she is not healthy or normal, her anxieties about pain and the lack of control over labor and delivery may be exaggerated. This anxiety can compound her intrapartal problems because increased maternal anxiety is associated with labor dysfunction, delivery complications, fetal distress, and altered maternal-infant bonding.

In contrast to high-risk patients who invested extra time, expense, and care for a healthy pregnancy are those at high risk because of late—or no—prenatal care. Such patients and their neonates are at high risk due to socioeconomic status, poor health, or both. Lack of prenatal care increases the risk of perinatal morbidity and mortality.

A high-risk pregnancy has a much higher chance of perinatal complications. Many high-risk conditions create an unfavorable intrauterine environment that does not support normal fetal growth or oxygenation. The high-risk fetus is especially sensitive to hypoxia, stress, and trauma. Signs of fetal distress, such as fetal heart rate abnormalities and meconium-stained amniotic fluid, may develop more quickly during labor than during a low-risk labor and delivery.

For a high-risk neonate, perinatal concerns involve the significant increase in the morbidity and mortality associated with prematurity, postmaturity, or low birth weight. These conditions predispose the neonate to birth trauma, perinatal asphyxia, meconium aspiration, hypoglycemia, heat loss, polycythemia, and death.

Although the goal of care is a safe, satisfying delivery that produces a normal, healthy neonate, this goal may not be achieved. If a high-risk neonate is born seriously ill, disabled, or without hope for survival, the parents' worst fears are confirmed. If perinatal death or disability occurs, the family will need assistance with coping and grieving.

NURSING CARE

For the high-risk patient and her family, the nurse must provide basic intrapartal care. (See chapters 11, 12, and 13 for more information on the four stages of labor.) In addition, the experienced nurse must understand the complexities of high-risk labor and delivery and provide specialized care at a critical-care level of specialized practice.

To manage the nursing care of the high-risk intrapartal patient, the nurse must perform specialized maternal and fetal monitoring. This demands advanced knowledge and skills, a familiarity with the technology used to improve perinatal outcomes, and readiness to provide nursing care as an important part of a specialized perinatal team.

Every pregnant patient should be evaluated for medical and obstetric complications before the intrapartal period because early findings can assist health care professionals in correcting deficiencies and avoiding intrapartal complications. However, a high-risk patient may first be encountered during the intrapartal period, or a problem may develop late in the pregnancy that goes undetected until admission. In either situation, however, the nurse can use the nursing process to deliver high-quality care and reduce intrapartal complications.

(Text continues on page 305.)

Intrapartal conditions and risks

During the intrapartal period, the nurse should be alert to certain conditions that may pose risks for the patient and her fetus or neonate. These risks are described below.

CONDITION	MATERNAL RISKS	FETAL OR NEONATAL RISKS
Age (19 years old and younger)	• Psychosocial problems • Panic related to lack of control • Uterine dysfunction, which may cause prolonged labor or precipitous birth • Labor arrest • Abruptio placentae • Preterm labor • Increased incidence of maternal mortality from hypertension, ectopic pregnancy, and embolism	• Low birth weight (LBW) or intrauterine growth retardation (IUGR) • Prematurity • Fetal distress caused by reduced perfusion of the fetal-placental unit and insufficient oxygenation • Meconium aspiration • Perinatal asphyxia • Hypoglycemia • Neonatal respiratory or central nervous system (CNS) depression • Neonatal infection, especially with a sexually transmitted disease or prolonged rupture of membranes
Age (35 years old and older)	• Increased anxiety for neonate • Multiple gestation • Placenta previa • Preterm labor • Premature rupture of membranes (PROM) • Labor dysfunction and postpartal hemorrhage, especially in a woman with uterine leiomyoma • Prolonged or arrested labor, which can require oxytocin administration or cesarean delivery	• Chromosomal abnormalities, open neural tube defects, or cardiac defects • LBW or IUGR • Breech presentation • Small for gestational age (SGA) or large for gestational age (LGA) • Fetal distress • Meconium aspiration • Perinatal asphyxia • Neonatal respiratory or CNS depression • Stillbirth

(continued)

Intrapartal conditions and risks *(continued)*

CONDITION	MATERNAL RISKS	FETAL OR NEONATAL RISKS
Age (35 years old and older) *(continued)*	• Malpositioning • Cephalopelvic dispro-portion (CPD) • Placental abruption • Increased maternal mortality secondary to the increased incidence of medical conditions	• Shoulder dystocia sig-nificantly higher in this group
Cardiac disease	• Cardiac decompensa-tion • Heart failure • Pulmonary edema • Maternal death • Preterm labor, if cer-tain cardiac drugs were used • Decreased renal output	• Increased risk of con-genital heart defects • IUGR • Fetal hypoxia or as-phyxia • Premature birth
Diabetes	• Hyperglycemia • Diabetic ketoacidosis • Hypoglycemia • Hydramnios • Preterm labor • Excessive postpartal bleeding from uterine atony or birth trauma • Postpartal diabetes • Hypertension • Labor augmentation • CPD with subsequent cesarean section • Renal problems	• Congenital malforma-tions • Fetal distress • Fetal death, especially in a woman with dia-betic ketoacidosis • Macrosomia, shoulder dystocia • Neonatal hyperinsulin-ism leading to hypo-glycemia • Respiratory distress syndrome (RDS) • Polycythemia • Hyperbilirubinemia • Hypocalcemia • Cardiac hypertrophy
Infection	• PROM • Premature labor • Fever	• Premature neonate • Neonatal infection or sepsis • RDS • Fetal death

Intrapartal conditions and risks *(continued)*

CONDITION	MATERNAL RISKS	FETAL OR NEONATAL RISKS
Human immunodeficiency virus infection	• Increased maternal morbidity and mortality • Postpartal development of acquired immunodeficiency syndrome	• Perinatal transmission via transplacental route or at birth • Infection contracted through breastmilk • Fetal demise • Neonatal infection and death
Substance abuse	• Preterm labor • Precipitous birth • Abruptio placentae • Maternal infection • Psychosocial problems, such as isolation and anxiety • Poor pain tolerance • Interactions between abused substance and drugs administered during delivery	• IUGR causing LBW or SGA neonate • Neonatal infection • Congenital malformations • Neonatal withdrawal symptoms
Pregnancy-induced hypertension	• Insufficient perfusion of vital organs, including fetal-placental unit • Seizures, hypertonic uterine activity, and abruptio placentae, if the patient develops eclampsia • Hyperactive deep tendon reflexes • Disseminated intravascular coagulation (DIC) • HELLP syndrome • Maternal death • Preterm labor	• Premature neonate • Toxicity in neonate, if magnesium sulfate was administered to patient • IUGR causing SGA • Possible fetal demise
Rh isoimmunization	• Placental hypertrophy with uteroplacental insufficiency	• Fetal hypoxia and distress • Anemia *(continued)*

Intrapartal conditions and risks *(continued)*

CONDITION	MATERNAL RISKS	FETAL OR NEONATAL RISKS
Rh isoimmunization *(continued)*	• Chorioamnionitis • Abruptio placentae • Hydramnios, which may cause inefficient contractions • Preterm labor and delivery • Cord prolapse with ROM	• Jaundice • Liver, spleen, and heart enlargement • Anasarca • Myocardial failure
Multifetal pregnancy	• Preterm labor • Tocolysis • Increased risk of PROM • Increased risk of hypertension • Uterine overdistention with hydramnios • Ineffective labor secondary to overdistention of uterus • Uterine atony with increased risk of postpartal hemorrhage • Cesarean section • Increased risk of supine hypotension • Increased risk of cord prolapse with ROM	• Preterm labor or delivery • Difficult delivery of subsequent fetuses
Fetal demise	• Need for labor induction or augmentation • DIC • Postpartum grieving from unexpected loss with possible postpartum depression	• Fetal decomposition may complicate delivery

Assessment

As with any patient who seeks admission for labor and delivery, the nurse obtains the high-risk intrapartal patient's health history, conducts an abbreviated physical assessment, and assists in collecting specimens for appropriate laboratory tests. With a high-risk intrapartal patient, however, the nurse must make additional assessments and be prepared to notify the doctor of significant findings, as described below.

Health history

When taking a history, keep in mind that a patient may perceive a common, normal variation as a problem. Depending on the intrapartal patient's condition, adjust the approach to the health history, augmenting the basic interview with appropriate questions. These questions depend on the patient's age, disorder, and labor status, as well as the previous history taken.

Physical assessment

During the physical assessment, modify the standard examination to meet the high-risk intrapartal patient's needs, and note significant findings related to her high-risk condition.

Laboratory tests

Unless otherwise ordered, expect to collect all standard admission laboratory tests. Consider the patient's high-risk condition when reviewing the results.

Nursing diagnosis

The nurse reviews all health history, physical assessment, and laboratory test findings and then formulates nursing diagnoses appropriate for the high-risk intrapartal patient. (See Appendix 1, NANDA taxonomy of nursing diagnoses.)

Planning and implementation

Some nursing interventions for the high-risk intrapartal patient are the same as those for any other intrapartal patient. For example, the nurse must assess the patient and fetus, assist in labor management, promote comfort, assist with delivery, provide emotional support, promote bonding, teach the patient, and care for the patient's family. However, when caring for a high-risk patient, the nurse must be prepared to respond to intrapartal emergencies and may need to approach the usual labor and delivery tasks differently and modify normal intrapartal care.

Nursing care in high-risk obstetrics requires advanced nursing knowledge and skills. The nurse must be prepared to participate as an integral member of the perinatal team and work closely with the doctor to achieve optimal outcomes. For example, nursing care for the intrapartal patient with cardiac disease may require a one-to-one nurse-patient ratio. Care for the intrapartal diabetic patient focuses on maintenance of euglycemia (normal blood glucose levels) and prevention and identification of fetal distress. For an infected patient, intrapartal care calls for prompt, aggressive medical treatment of the infection and planning for immediate care of the neonate to help prevent illness. For a patient with PIH, care demands skills and expertise that seek to detect preeclampsia, prevent eclampsia, and deliver a healthy neonate.

The family of the high-risk intrapartal patient is likely to be very concerned about her and her fetus or neonate. The nurse must provide sensitive nursing care adapted to the family's needs. (See *High-risk intrapartal patients*.)

Evaluation

During the final step of the nursing process, the nurse evaluates the effectiveness of nursing care. The nurse should state all evaluations in terms of actions performed or outcomes achieved for each goal.

ADOLESCENT PATIENTS

The Centers for Disease Control and Prevention estimated in 1995 that 1 in 10 American girls ages 15 to 19 become pregnant and that 95% of those pregnancies were unintended. If an adolescent has a healthy pregnancy, is over age 15, is in good general health, and has had early and consistent prenatal care, adequate nutrition, and family support, she may progress through labor and delivery normally. Her risk for intrapartal problems may be no greater than that for the general population.

Even if she has maintained a healthy pregnancy, however, she is likely to be at risk for psychosocial problems during labor and delivery. These are especially common because of unfamiliar surroundings, a sense of isolation, heightened fears and fantasies about labor and delivery, and the forthcoming responsibilities of motherhood.

The adolescent patient may also be at risk for physical problems. A patient under age 15 or a multigravid adolescent patient over age 15 is at much higher risk for poor maternal, fetal, or neonatal outcomes related to birth. Compared to the general population, neonates born to adolescents under age 18 are twice as likely to weigh less than 1,500 g. Low birth weight (LBW) neonates have higher morbidity and mortality rates. Adolescents' generally smaller stature; lower preconception weight; tobacco, alcohol, and drug abuse; and insufficient antepartal weight gain from poor nutrition contribute to LBW neonates.

At one time, it was believed that adolescents had higher cesarean section rates than the general population. However, studies have shown no increased risk of prolonged labor or cesarean section in this group.

FAMILY CARE

High-risk intrapartal patients

The family of a high-risk intrapartal patient is likely to experience extreme anxiety for her and her fetus during the intrapartal period. Family members may feel left out, isolated from the patient, and intimidated by the setting, equipment, and staff. If they focus on the gravity of the patient's condition, they may lose sight of the impending celebration of birth.

To help reduce anxiety for the patient and her family, the nurse should be sensitive to their concerns and include a family member in her care if the patient chooses. When providing family-centered care, the nurse might use the following interventions:

- Encourage the family member to remain at the patient's bedside to provide reassurance.
- Encourage the family member to use touch or massage to reduce the patient's discomfort and anxiety.
- Teach the family member to help the patient with relaxation and breathing techniques.
- Instruct the family member to promote comfort by applying a cool cloth to the patient's brow or by providing mouth care.
- Allow the family member to fan the patient, as needed.
- Keep other family members informed of the patient's progress and provide reassurance to them.
- Explain unfamiliar equipment and procedures and the reasons for their use.
- Discuss choices about positioning, analgesia, and anesthesia with the patient and family member as appropriate.
- Clarify and interpret the prescribed treatment for the family, as needed.
- Discuss impending vaginal or cesarean delivery with the patient and family member.
- Encourage the family member to take frequent breaks to prevent fatigue and hunger.
- Incorporate the family's cultural preferences into the plan of care whenever possible.
- Attempt to establish realistic childbirth goals with the patient and her family. Support their decisions about care.
- Encourage open communication with active listening
- Encourage questions from the patient and her family and facilitate the discussions regarding her care.

Assessment

When caring for an adolescent intrapartal patient, the nurse obtains a health history, assists with a physical assessment, and collects laboratory test results as for any patient who seeks admission for labor and delivery. In addition, the nurse must make specific assessments and be prepared to notify the doctor or nurse-midwife of significant findings.

Health history

When assessing an adolescent patient, be aware that this may be her first experience in a health care facility. If she is in active labor, she may panic because she is unprepared and feels out of control. She may perceive history questions as unimportant and may be unwilling or unable to answer them because of fear or ignorance. To calm her and obtain the necessary information, include her support person in the interview and attempt to gain her trust and cooperation. If birth seems imminent, concentrate on the most important history questions and gather data quickly.

After determining her age, parity, and labor status, ask the patient about length of pregnancy, prenatal care received, and the presence of any complications. This information can direct the physical assessment. Be aware, however, that the adolescent may not know her last menstrual period (LMP), making gestational age assessment and subsequent prediction of intrauterine growth retardation (IUGR) or prematurity inaccurate.

When investigating her obstetric history, make particular note of complications that may recur, such as PIH, abruptio placentae, and postpartal hemorrhage. Typically, a young multiparous patient has closely spaced pregnancies, rapid labors, and small neonates, all of which predispose her to precipitous delivery.

Determine the patient's preconception weight and antepartal weight gain. Smaller maternal body size and poor gestational weight gain have been associated with LBW infants, who may not tolerate the stresses of labor well because of poor placental perfusion.

Discuss her use of tobacco, alcohol, or drugs—substances that are used by many adolescents. These substances can alter fetal and neonatal health.

When evaluating the adolescent patient's psychosocial status, be sure to assess her coping methods and support systems. Her ability to cope depends on her developmental stage, preparation for childbirth, family support, and flexibility of the health care team. She may need constant support during the intrapartal period. Determine whether or not the teen is giving the neonate up for adoption or has investigated other community support systems. Based on the adolescent's needs, determine whether any referrals are needed.

Physical assessment

An adolescent may feel embarrassed or shy about being examined by a "stranger." Her lack of control over her labor may make her feel vulnerable, restricted, and confused. To gain a sense of control over something, she may rebel against the physical assessment and other facility procedures. Provide reassurance, remain calm but firm, and explain each step of the assessment before performing it.

Measure the patient's vital signs as accurately as possible. Keep in mind that her anxiety may distort her initial vital signs. Nevertheless, her baseline blood pressure measurement will help detect PIH, and temperature and pulse rate will help detect infection or severe anemia.

Note fundal height, estimate fetal weight, and determine fetal presentation. These assessments can identify LBW, prematurity, malposition, and malpresentation. Alert the doctor or nurse-midwife to any suspicious findings for further evaluation.

Assist with a pelvic examination to determine labor progress, pelvic adequacy, the imminence of delivery, and the possibility of cephalopelvic disproportion (CPD). Gaining her trust is important for this examination. If the girl resists this evaluation, expect it to be delayed until she is more settled. Remember that she may perceive a forced pelvic examination as an assault and that she has the right to refuse any procedure.

Laboratory tests

During the pelvic examination, specimens to detect sexually transmitted diseases (STDs) and chorioamnionitis (which can cause neonatal complications) may be collected. Expect to obtain blood and urine specimens to test for anemia, STDs, hepatitis, rubella, Rh type and antibody screening, and urinary tract infections, especially if the patient has not received prenatal care. Because needles and blood can be frightening to an adolescent, provide reassurance and support when collecting specimens.

Nursing diagnosis

After evaluating the assessment findings the nurse formulates nursing diagnoses. (See Appendix 1, NANDA taxonomy of nursing diagnoses.)

Planning and implementation

Closely observe the adolescent patient for sudden onset of PIH. Pay careful attention to her blood pressure and other vital signs, urine protein levels, degree of edema, and deep tendon reflexes. (For more information, see "Pregnancy-induced hypertension" later in this section.)

If all parameters are normal, assess fetal status with intermittent external monitoring so the patient can get out of bed and be unrestricted. If she feels threatened by electronic fetal monitoring (EFM), explain that it helps determine her fetus's tolerance of labor. If the fetus shows signs of distress or IUGR, anticipate continuous EFM by internal fetal scalp electrode.

Labor management

During labor, an adolescent patient can become demanding if she fears abandonment and isolation. She may want and need constant support. She may bite, pinch, or cling to the nurse, especially during pelvic examinations. These actions are common in a teenager with a nursing diagnosis of *fear related to labor and delivery*.

To help the adolescent patient regain her composure, set limits and maintain a calm, confident approach. Also provide clear directions and descriptions. Teach her comfort and breathing techniques as you would any prenatal patient. Elicit the help of her partner or a family member to provide support. Keep in mind, however, that an adolescent may act out expected roles to gain her family's attention and become more hyperactive and helpless when they are present.

To enhance her coping ability, remain nonjudgmental and provide constant, positive encouragement about her progress and behavior. Direct her primary support person to provide comfort measures and labor coaching to help her through childbirth so that she may recall this event as an accomplishment.

For the adolescent, carefully assess labor progress and screen for such problems as uterine dysfunction or labor arrest. The adolescent's immature uterus may have an uncoordinated contraction pattern, and her labor may not progress without augmentation. Because her pelvis may not be fully developed, she may have a difficult labor with CPD.

Assist with delivery

To promote a positive childbirth experience for the adolescent girl, emphasize the normalcy of her experience and promote bonding, which ultimately may enhance the mother-infant relationship.

Throughout labor and delivery, provide supportive coaching and encouragement. Make every effort to decrease the trauma and enhance the intimacy and joy of the experience. A girl who fears trauma and mutilation from giving birth may have a nursing diagnosis of *knowledge deficit related to labor and delivery*. Such a patient may benefit from encouragement to "push the baby out so you can hold the baby in your arms." If she expresses concern that her body will never be the same and has a nursing diagnosis of *body image disturbance related to labor and delivery,* provide reassurance by explaining what she can expect as she goes through the postpartum period.

Promote bonding

The adolescent's experience of labor and delivery affects her bonding with her neonate. To promote bonding, express acceptance of, provide support to, and convey respect for the adolescent patient.

Adolescents seldom relinquish their neonates for adoption. However, if a patient chooses to do so, be sure to give her time with her neonate immediately after birth. This brief transition period helps the mother begin grieving and allows her to say goodbye to her neonate. It may help her resolve a nursing diagnosis of **decisional conflict related to offering the neonate for adoption.** It also may help her understand her accomplishment as a woman, her ability to manage labor, and her success. This fosters maternal bonding with the neonate and may affect her enjoyment of relationships with future children.

Evaluation

The nurse should state all evaluations in terms of actions performed or outcomes achieved for each goal. Examples of appropriate evaluation statements include:

- The adolescent had a labor and delivery free of complications.
- The adolescent expressed satisfaction with her decision to keep her neonate or to give up her neonate for adoption.
- The adolescent reported positive feelings and a sense of accomplishment related to her childbirth experience.

MATURE PATIENTS

Typically, mature primigravid women are in better health, better educated, better nourished, and have a higher standard of living than adolescent girls. Although they are at increased risk for some medical and obstetric complications, they typically proceed well through pregnancy and delivery.

Typically, the mature intrapartal patient has been screened prenatally for fetal chromosomal abnormalities, multiple gestation, gestational diabetes, PIH, appropriate fetal growth, placenta previa, and a tendency for premature labor. A healthy mature patient has similar intrapartal nursing needs to a younger patient.

For mature patients, aging or obesity are responsible for many intrapartal risks, including diabetes mellitus, gestational diabetes, PIH, chronic hypertension, thrombophlebitis, chronic renal disease, collagen disease, and uterine leiomyoma (benign neoplasm of the uterine smooth muscle), which can affect labor and delivery. Mature patients also are at higher risk for premature rupture of the membranes (PROM) and preterm labor and placental abruption.

The neonate of a mature patient is at increased risk for chromosomal abnormalities (including Down syndrome), open neural tube defects, and cardiac defects. This is especially significant to nursing care if the patient declined prenatal genetic screening or ultrasonography, because she may not be prepared for the birth of a neonate with a disorder.

If the mature patient has hypertension or PIH, her neonate is at risk for LBW or IUGR caused by uteroplacental insufficiency. Intrapartal risks for LBW include increased fetal distress, meconium aspiration, and neonatal depression. Hypertension also increases the risk of placental previa and abruption.

If the patient is obese or has gestational diabetes, her neonate may be born with macrosomia. Intrapartal concerns for a macrosomic fetus include stillbirth or birth trauma from shoulder dystocia.

One study of infant mortality and maternal age demonstrated that, compared to mothers ages 25 to 29, the risk of neonatal mortality was nearly equal in mothers ages 30 to 34; 18% higher in mothers ages 35 to 39; and 69% higher in mothers ages 40 to 49.

Assessment

When caring for a mature intrapartal patient, the nurse obtains a health history, assists with physical assessment, and collects laboratory tests as she would for any patient who seeks admission for labor and delivery. In addition, the nurse must make specific assessments and be prepared to notify the doctor or nurse-midwife of significant findings.

Health history

When taking a history, keep in mind that a patient may perceive a common, normal variation as a problem. Depending on the intrapartal patient's condition, adjust the approach to the health history, augmenting the basic interview with appropriate questions. These questions depend on the patient's age, disorder, educational level, and labor status.

Early in the interview, obtain the mature patient's LMP and estimated delivery date in order to screen for preterm labor, PROM and fetal distress (may have decreased fetal movements with fetal distress). As always, inquire about any medical or obstetric problems to help guide the plan of care.

Determine if the patient has a history of infertility. Infertility treatment with drugs that stimulate ovulation can predispose her to multiple gestation and accompanying risks, such as premature labor, malpresentation, and dystocia.

Also inquire if she has had any previous spontaneous abortions, has been trying to conceive for a long time, or conceived via artificial insemination. If so, she may be more anxious about this pregnancy outcome and may need close maternal and fetal monitoring during labor, if only to reassure her of normal progress.

Ask if she has had prenatal and genetic screening. For a patient who has not been screened, be prepared for the possibility of a neonate with serious chromosomal abnormalities, and plan to alert the neonatal team to the patient's history when delivery is imminent. Keep in mind, however, that genetic screening cannot detect all abnormalities; a patient who was screened may give birth to a neonate who needs intensive care.

Perform a psychosocial assessment to identify any needs that must be addressed in the plan of care. Determine if the patient is anxious about this birth or about other children at home. Find out if she has been managing a high-stress career. Anxiety and stress can affect fetal growth and can increase the risk of complications during labor and delivery. Also note the interactions between the patient and support person during labor.

Assess the patient's understanding of her condition and care. A mature primigravid patient is likely to have planned her pregnancy and may be knowledgeable about her prenatal health. Also evaluate the patient's coping skills. They may be well developed, and she may be better able to express her concerns or fears about labor and delivery than a younger patient. However, she may have a strong need to be in control. Such a patient may respond well to a nurse who encourages her participation in the plan of care, is sensitive to her needs for adaptation to labor, and supports her role transition.

Physical assessment
For a mature patient, establish baseline vital signs, fundal height and fetal position, deep tendon reflexes (DTRs), and fetal well-being and assess for hydramnios and vaginal bleeding. These can alert the nurse to potential problems that occur more frequently in mature women including PIH, small for gestational age (SGA), large for gestational age (LGA), hydramnios, multiple gestation, and malpresentation.

Laboratory tests
Unless otherwise noted, expect to collect all standard admission laboratory tests. Consider the patient's high-risk condition when reviewing the necessary test results.

Nursing diagnosis
After evaluating the assessment data the nurse formulates nursing diagnoses. (See Appendix 1, NANDA taxonomy of nursing diagnoses.)

Planning and implementation
Although every intrapartal patient and fetus should be assessed continuously, the high-risk intrapartal patient and fetus may require more frequent or additional types of surveillance, depending on the condition.

Assess vital signs and symptoms to detect impending problems. Identify evidence of fetal stress by initiating EFM and obtaining a baseline monitor strip. Early detection of fetal distress allows prompt intrapartal treatment.

Labor management

Labor dysfunctions are relatively common in mature patients. However, there has been a demonstrated relationship between advancing maternal age and increasing frequency of labor dysfunctions, labor protraction, and labor arrest. These dysfunctions may result from decreased efficiency of the aging myometrium or from increased incidence of CPD, uterine leiomyoma, and fetal malposition.

Because of the increased tendency of the mature woman to labor dysfunctions, carefully monitor the efficiency of contractions, which can affect her contraction pattern. Also assess fetal position, which can help determine the duration of labor.

If contractions cease and cervical dilation or fetal descent are arrested, anticipate assisting with I.V. fluids, oxytocin augmentation, and continuous EFM, unless signs of fetal distress or CPD exist.

Assist with delivery

For a healthy mature patient with no detectable intrapartal risks, expect a vaginal delivery. If labor dysfunction occurs or CPD is identified, prepare for a cesarean delivery, as prescribed.

An increased incidence of vacuum extractor and forceps deliveries has been documented among mature patients. This could result from decreased efficiency of the aging myometrium, decreased maternal stamina, and increased use of epidural anesthesia.

Maternal age is also a risk factor for cesarean section. Patients over 35 years of age are twice as likely to deliver by cesarean section than younger patients. Anticipate the complications that may arise in the labor and delivery area. If the patient has had oxytocin augmentation during a difficult labor, postpartal hemorrhage related to uterine atony may occur. Alert the neonatal team to attend an imminent delivery if assessments suggest neonatal abnormality.

Evaluation

Appropriate evaluation statements include:
- The patient had an uneventful labor and delivery without complications.
- The patient and her partner and family regularly received information about labor progress and fetal status.
- The patient began bonding with her neonate immediately after delivery.

CARDIAC DISEASE

Maternal cardiac disease has been noted to complicate nearly 1% of all pregnancies and is a major cause of maternal death in the United States. The intrapartal period poses the greatest risk for the patient with cardiac disease because the hemodynamic changes of pregnancy peak at this time.

Labor can produce sudden, profound changes in the cardiovascular system. During each contraction, pain and increased venous blood return from the uterus raise cardiac output 20%. Mean arterial pressure rises and is followed by a reflex bradycardia. Uterine contractions can compress the aorta and iliac arteries, forcing more blood to the upper torso and head.

Intrapartal management of the patient with a cardiac disease requires the expertise of an obstetrician, cardiologist, anesthesiologist, perinatologist, and obstetric nurse with critical care skills. The patient needs intensive obstetric and cardiac monitoring. Interventions are based on the patient's degree of cardiac decompensation. Even a patient with minimal activity limitation during pregnancy can experience sudden worsening of the disease during labor. The nurse should be familiar with the normal changes of pregnancy and with the maternal and fetal consequences of cardiac disease. (See Chapter 6, High-risk antepartal patients.)

Assessment

When caring for an intrapartal patient with cardiac disease, the nurse obtains a health history, assists with physical assessment, and collects laboratory tests as for any patient who seeks admission for labor and delivery. In addition, the nurse must make specific cardiac assessments and be prepared to notify the doctor of significant findings.

Health history

A patient with cardiac disease requires careful assessment of cardiovascular status. Inquire if she has recently had difficulty breathing, experienced chest pains or dizzy spells, or has felt increased fatigue. Severe dyspnea, chest pain on exertion, increasing fatigue, or syncope suggest significant cardiac disease or decompensation and should be reported promptly to the doctor.

Obtain a complete medication history. Any delay in medication administration during labor and delivery may affect the patient's cardiovascular status and general well-being.

Drugs used to treat cardiac disease potentially can harm the fetus and affect the perinatal outcome. Some cardiac medications may have teratogenic effects; others may precipitate preterm labor. Oral anticoagulants are potential teratogens when taken during the first trimester.

After the first trimester, they increase the risk of intrauterine bleeding. Subcutaneous heparin can be used in pregnancy.

Propranolol, a beta blocker used to treat hypertension and tachyarrhythmias, can cause a constantly high uterine tone and result in preterm labor. The drug may produce neonatal respiratory depression, sustained bradycardia, and hypoglycemia when taken late in pregnancy or immediately before delivery.

Thiazide diuretics can harm the fetus, especially when used in the third trimester or for extended periods. They may cause severe neonatal electrolyte imbalance, jaundice, thrombocytopenia, and liver damage. However, drugs such as quinidine and the digitalis glycosides are not known to have teratogenic effects or cause problems with use during the third trimester of pregnancy.

Physical assessment
When assessing the patient with cardiac disease, be especially alert for dependent edema, crackles in the lower lung fields, jugular vein distention, cyanosis, clubbing, diastolic murmurs, cardiac arrhythmias, and loud, hard systolic murmurs. Depending on their severity, these findings may indicate cardiac decompensation and must be reported immediately to the doctor.

Laboratory tests
Consider the patient's cardiac condition when collecting laboratory specimens and evaluating results. Frequently, such tests as cardiac enzymes and clotting studies are ordered depending on the patient's cardiac condition and its severity.

Nursing diagnosis
After evaluating the assessment data, the nurse formulates nursing diagnoses. (See Appendix 1, NANDA taxonomy of nursing diagnoses.)

Planning and implementation
Frequently check the maternal pulse, respirations, and blood pressure, and maintain strict fluid intake and output records, as prescribed. Expect continuous EFM as well as continuous maternal electrocardiogram monitoring; hemodynamic monitoring with an arterial line, central venous pressure, or indwelling pulmonary artery catheter may be ordered as well. Keep resuscitation equipment near the patient at all times.

Labor management
For the patient with cardiac disease, keep in mind that maternal position, contractions, and anesthesia can affect cardiovascular status during labor and delivery. Be sure to document any equipment or medications used.

Close observation is particularly important for a patient with cardiac disease with a nursing diagnosis of *altered renal tissue perfusion related to intrapartal blood loss.* Watch renal activity with intake and output and specific gravity checks every hour.

Keep close observation on and promote proper positioning for the patient with cardiac disease, especially if she has a nursing diagnosis of *altered cardiopulmonary tissue perfusion related to stress of labor on an abnormal heart.* She must avoid the supine position because it can decrease the heart rate and increase venous return, stroke volume, and cardiac output. During labor, encourage use of the lateral recumbent position, which improves cardiac emptying and promotes oxygenation. During delivery, do not elevate the patient's legs fully in the lithotomy position because this increases venous return and may overload the heart. The nurse must also watch for signs and symptoms of pulmonary edema in a patient with cardiac disease.

Promote comfort

For a patient with a nursing diagnosis of *pain related to labor and delivery,* keep in mind that labor pains can cause maternal tachycardia and elevate blood pressure, increasing the stress on the heart. Effective analgesia should minimize this effect.

Expect the patient to receive regional anesthesia such as epidural anesthesia to relieve pain during labor and delivery. Regional anesthesia is particularly useful in a patient with cardiac disease because it decreases cardiac output and heart rate and acts as a peripheral vasodilator that reduces venous return to the heart. However, it can cause hypotension, requiring close blood pressure monitoring.

Assist with delivery

During the second stage of labor, bearing down can reduce venous blood flow to the heart by increasing intrathoracic pressure. When the patient stops bearing down, cardiac output and blood pressure increase rapidly. Therefore, as indicated, instruct the patient to avoid bearing down in the second stage or expect the doctor to use epidural anesthesia, which eliminates the bearing down reflex. After the cervix is dilated fully, labor should progress naturally through the second stage. Uterine contractions usually produce fetal descent; the doctor allows it to proceed unless labor continuation would jeopardize the patient or her fetus. Keep in mind that some doctors prefer to shorten the second stage by using low forceps or vacuum extraction.

If the patient with cardiac disease delivers vaginally, expect her blood volume to be redirected to central circulation and cardiac output to increase dramatically. Monitor her closely and observe for abrupt changes in cardiac status.

For a patient who undergoes a planned cesarean delivery, expect a blood loss of about 1,000 ml, causing a temporary decrease in cardiac output and blood pressure. This patient has a nursing diagnosis of **decreased cardiac output related to intrapartal blood loss.** Be prepared to continue I.V. fluids and to increase as indicated.

Prepare for acute neonatal problems because the neonate of a patient with cardiac disease has an increased risk of morbidity and mortality. A patient with congenital heart disease has an increased risk of giving birth to a neonate with congenital heart disease. Antepartal maternal cyanosis is associated with preterm labor, resulting in LBW or a premature neonate. Maternal cyanosis and tachycardia also may cause hypoxia and fetal death. Keep the neonatal team advised and alert them when birth is imminent so that they can be present in the delivery room.

Plan to assess the patient continuously for at least 24 hours after delivery. Cardiac output increases immediately after delivery, when blood that had been diverted to the uterus reenters the central circulation. A patient with cardiac disease who cannot tolerate these postpartal changes may develop decompensation and heart failure. Prompt medical intervention may be required for such a patient. Therefore, the nurse must be able to recognize any change and report it immediately to the doctor.

Evaluation

Appropriate evaluation statements include:

- The patient assumed labor positions that supported cardiac function.
- The patient and her partner and family regularly received information about maternal and fetal status.
- The patient delivered successfully without further maternal or neonatal complications.

DIABETES MELLITUS

During pregnancy, a patient with diabetes mellitus requires close monitoring and management to prevent intrapartal problems. Prevention of hyperglycemia before conception and during pregnancy improves perinatal outcomes but does not remove all risks. Uncontrolled diabetes is associated with increased maternal, fetal, and neonatal morbidity and mortality. (See Chapter 6, High-risk antepartal patients.)

Uncontrolled diabetes can cause hydramnios. It also is associated with hypertensive disorders, such as chronic hypertension and PIH, which affect 15% to 30% of all pregnant patients with diabetes. Patients with diabetes also are at risk for preterm labor and, if associated with vascular changes, placental abnormalities.

Neonates of diabetic mothers whose diabetes has not been well controlled have a higher morbidity and mortality rate than those born to nondiabetic mothers. They also are at risk for neonatal hypoglycemia at birth and for macrosomia, which can lead to birth trauma. A neonate of a pregestational diabetic patient is at increased risk for congenital malformations, especially if the patient's glucose levels were uncontrolled during fetal organ development.

Assessment

When caring for a diabetic intrapartal patient, the nurse obtains a health history, assists with physical assessment, and collects laboratory tests as for any patient who seeks admission for labor and delivery. In addition, the nurse must make specific assessments regarding diabetes and be prepared to notify the doctor of significant findings.

Health history

When assessing a diabetic patient, determine when she last ate and took insulin. An omitted or reduced insulin dose can cause a surge in blood glucose levels. Insulin deficiency can lead to diabetic ketoacidosis (DKA), an acute complication of diabetes characterized by hyperglycemia, metabolic acidosis, electrolyte imbalance, coma, and possibly maternal and fetal death.

Physical assessment

When assessing the diabetic woman, be especially alert for signs of hyperglycemia, such as unusual thirst, increased urine output, fruity breath odor, and continuous, deep, rapid breathing. Also watch for signs of hypoglycemia, such as faintness, trembling, impaired vision, and changes in level of consciousness, vital signs, and urinary output.

Laboratory tests

For a diabetic patient, carefully check blood glucose levels, as prescribed. (See chapter 6 for more information on levels indicating gestational diabetes.) The insulin-dependent diabetic patient is at risk for DKA when blood glucose levels approach 300 mg/dl.

If an elective induction or repeat cesarean delivery is planned, the doctor may perform an amniocentesis to determine the lecithin/sphingomyelin (L/S) ratio and phosphatidylglycerol (PG) level. These test results provide information about fetal lung maturity, which helps determine whether a vaginal delivery is possible or cesarean delivery is necessary as well as the timing of delivery.

Nursing diagnosis

After evaluating the assessment data, the nurse formulates nursing diagnoses. (See Appendix 1, NANDA taxonomy of nursing diagnoses.)

Planning and implementation

For an intrapartal patient with diabetes, expect to observe and report on her fetus, renal and cardiovascular functions, vital signs, glucose levels, and insulin and glucose infusions. Include any signs and symptoms of complications in your documentation.

Assess the fetus

To detect fetal distress, assess the fetus continuously through EFM and evaluate maternal blood glucose levels hourly. Glucose levels should range from 60 to 100 mg/dl. Even short periods of maternal hyperglycemia during labor can lead to neonatal hypoglycemia.

Assess renal and cardiovascular functions

Keep in mind that chronic hypertension and PIH are common among diabetics. If the patient has diabetes-related renal disease, anticipate strict recording of her fluid intake and output during labor and delivery. When administering I.V. fluids, expect to use an infusion pump to regulate the exact dosage. Because chronic hypertension usually accompanies renal disease, closely monitor her blood pressure. Frequently assess for edema, proteinuria, pulmonary edema, and hyperactive DTRs. Carefully evaluate and document these findings and report abnormal findings promptly to the doctor.

A patient with a history of cardiovascular complications caused by diabetes requires close cardiac monitoring. Such a patient is at high risk for complications and may need follow-up by the critical care team.

Assess glucose levels and infusions

Expect to check the diabetic patient's blood glucose levels carefully during and immediately after the intrapartal period. The doctor will attempt to maintain her glucose levels within the target range using a continuous I.V. insulin and glucose regimen. This range is determined by her prenatal and labor needs and is decided upon by her doctor. Regimens vary from minimal glucose and no insulin to 5 g of glucose/hour and 1 to 2 units of insulin/hour, adjusted according to glucose levels that can be checked by hourly fingersticks. Regardless of the insulin regimen used, glucose is necessary to compensate for the energy expenditure of labor. (See *Administering insulin to high-risk intrapartal patients.*)

Insulin infusion may be needed until delivery of the placenta; glucose infusion, until the patient consumes food.

Administering insulin to high-risk intrapartal patients

During the intrapartal period, monitor the patient's blood glucose levels closely. Administer insulin and glucose via I.V. fluids, according to the patient's needs. Every 1 to 2 hours, perform a fingerstick glucose test and adjust the insulin pump and I.V. solution accordingly. Administer insulin and glucose as ordered, based on the guidelines below.

BLOOD GLUCOSE LEVEL (MG/DL)	INSULIN DOSAGE (UNIT/HOUR)	FLUIDS (125 ML/HOUR)
Less than 100	0	Dextrose 5% (D_5) in lactated Ringer's solution
100 to 140	1	D_5 lactated Ringer's solution
141 to 180	1.5	Normal saline solution
181 to 220	2	Normal saline solution
More than 220	2.5	Normal saline solution

The patient who is to have a planned cesarean delivery or induced labor the following morning should be instructed to take nothing by mouth after midnight and to skip her morning dose of insulin.

Check the patient's blood glucose levels immediately after delivery and at least every 4 hours thereafter. After the patient begins eating, the doctor may reinstitute insulin administration when hyperglycemia recurs. The patient's antepartal insulin dose serves as a guide to her postpartal dose. Be aware, however, that a lower dose may be prescribed after delivery because of the rapid declines in placental hormones and cortisol, which reduce opposition to insulin.

Labor management

In a patient with hydramnios, anticipate a large gush of fluid when her membranes rupture. This can precipitate umbilical cord prolapse. Be prepared to intervene appropriately. (See Chapter 15, Intrapartal complications and procedures.)

Assist with emergencies. In a patient with insulin-dependent diabetes mellitus, poorly controlled blood glucose levels and insulin deficiency can lead to DKA, which can cause intrauterine fetal death.

DKA produces maternal acidosis, which causes fetal acidosis and fetal distress. Until prompt treatment restores maternal homeostasis, the patient and her fetus will remain in jeopardy. (See *Diabetic ketoacidosis.*)

The diabetic patient with preterm labor should not be given tocolytics unless the benefits outweigh the risks. The risks include decreased glucose control leading to ketoacidosis.

Assist with delivery

If the diabetic patient has controlled blood glucose levels during pregnancy and shows no signs of placental insufficiency, anticipate a vaginal delivery after the onset of spontaneous labor. Vaginal delivery at term is preferred with a normal L/S ratio and PG level, indicating fetal lung maturity, and if the fetus shows no evidence of macrosomia or compromise.

Anticipate a difficult delivery if the fetus has macrosomia because it can be a cause of shoulder dystocia and lead to maternal and neonatal birth trauma. If the patient experiences a difficult delivery, she may have vaginal and perineal lacerations and excessive postpartal bleeding.

If fetal distress or maternal problems occur, assist with a cesarean delivery if needed. The delivery should be planned carefully to minimize maternal and neonatal morbidity and mortality. The neonatal team should be present at the delivery. (See *Indications for planned delivery for the diabetic patient,* page 324.)

A heel stick of the neonate to obtain a blood sample for glucose testing may be performed in the delivery area. During the intrapartal period, maternal hyperglycemia may lead to neonatal hyperinsulinism and hypoglycemia, causing a rapid drop in the blood glucose level in the first 30 to 60 minutes after birth. Neonatal hypoglycemia may be asymptomatic or produce such signs as twitching, jitteriness, hypotonia, apnea, and seizures. If hypoglycemia is detected, keep the neonate warm until treatment can begin, probably in the neonatal intensive care unit.

Evaluation

Appropriate evaluation statements include:
- The patient's blood glucose levels remained within acceptable limits.
- The patient displayed no signs of hypoglycemia or hyperglycemia.
- The patient delivered a stable neonate.
- The patient experienced spontaneous labor at term.
- The patient and her family regularly received information about maternal, fetal, and neonatal status.

EMERGENCY ALERT

Diabetic ketoacidosis

For a patient with diabetes, the stress of labor can trigger ketoacidosis. This form of acidosis is accompanied by ketone accumulation in the blood and can lead to coma and death if not treated promptly. It also can compromise the fetus. The following chart will help the nurse identify the signs and symptoms of diabetic ketoacidosis (DKA) and prepare to intervene or assist. Correction of maternal DKA should reverse fetal compromise.

Signs and symptoms
- Hyperglycemia and ketonuria
- Signs of dehydration, such as poor skin turgor, flushed dry skin, oliguria, and confusion
- Hypotension
- Deep, rapid respirations
- Decreased level of consciousness, possibly leading to coma
- Fruity or acetone-like breath odor
- Nausea and vomiting

Nursing considerations
- Confirm DKA by obtaining arterial blood gas levels, as prescribed; using a reagent strip to evaluate the patient's urine for ketones; using a reflectometer to monitor blood for a glucose test; and sending for baseline laboratory studies, such as electrolyte and serum blood glucose levels.
- Summon health care team members, including the obstetrician, endocrinologist, and internist.
- Record hourly fluid intake and output on a flowsheet.
- Document all laboratory test results, maternal vital signs, and fetal heart rate (FHR).
- Start an I.V. line with an isotonic solution, such as normal saline solution, as prescribed.
- Monitor the patient's cardiac status with a bedside electrocardiogram (ECG) monitor, if possible. On an ECG strip, hyperkalemia may produce small P waves, a prolonged PR interval, widened QRS complex, and tall, peaked T waves. It can precipitate cardiac arrhythmias and typically occurs in DKA when potassium is pulled from cells into the blood. Attempt to maintain serum potassium in the 4 to 5 mEq/L range. Expect to draw blood to check serum potassium levels every hour.
- Administer short-acting, regular insulin, as prescribed. Before administering insulin, however, ensure that fluid replacement has been initiated.
- Monitor blood glucose levels every hour.
- Administer I.V. glucose only after the patient's blood glucose level is at 150 to 200 mg.
- Assess the FHR and variability continuously with electronic fetal monitoring.

Indications for planned delivery for the diabetic patient

For a diabetic patient, the following assessment findings may indicate the need for a planned delivery. Depending on the severity of these findings and the patient's condition, planned delivery may include an induced vaginal delivery or a cesarean delivery.

- Fetal distress as identified on electronic fetal monitoring or by patient report of markedly decreased fetal movements (less than 10 per day)
- Signs of intrauterine growth retardation, including inadequate fundal height and abnormal findings on ultrasonography
- Estimated gestation duration greater than 42 weeks confirmed using serial ultrasonography, last menstrual period, and regular prenatal assessments
- Pregnancy-induced hypertension
- Signs of markedly failing renal function, such as decreasing urine output
- Macrosomia with a fetus greater than 4,000 g shown by fundal heights greater than gestational age, ultrasonography, and hands-on fetal weight estimate

INFECTION

Infections are a major cause of maternal, fetal, and neonatal death. During the intrapartal period, they are more common in patients with premature labor, PROM, fever, or fetal death.

The primary perinatal infections are bacterial or viral and are caused by such organisms as group B beta-hemolytic streptococcus, herpes simplex virus (HSV), hepatitis B virus, chlamydia, or other STDs. They may be transmitted to the fetus through an infected uterus or birth canal and can lead to morbidity or mortality because the fetus's immature immune system cannot fight off these life-threatening organisms. Fungal (candidiasis) or protozoal (trichomoniasis) infections are not potentially fatal.

Many factors can predispose a patient to intrapartal infection, including obesity, severe anemia, poor hygiene, uncontrolled diabetes, chronic renal or respiratory disease, and a depressed immune response. Women at increased risk for STDs, which are the most common intrapartal infections, constitute a large and varied population, including:

- unmarried women
- women under age 24
- women with multiple sex partners, especially with a history of treatment for STDs
- women treated for recurrent vaginitis or a previous STD.

During labor, predisposing factors to infection may include preterm labor, prolonged labor, prolonged rupture of membranes (rupture that occurs more than 24 hours before labor onset), use of such invasive equipment as internal fetal scalp electrodes or intrauterine pressure catheters, and multiple vaginal examinations.

Assessment

When caring for an intrapartal patient with infection, the nurse obtains a health history, assists with physical assessment, and collects laboratory tests as for any patient who seeks admission for labor and delivery. In addition, the nurse must make specific assessments and be prepared to notify the doctor of significant findings.

Health history

Because any patient may contract an infectious disease and because it may have grave consequences, assess all intrapartal patients for infection, noting symptoms of and risk factors for infection. Early recognition of intrapartal infection allows prompt treatment and helps prevent its spread.

During the admission interview, review the patient's history of antepartal illness, possible exposure to STDs, and any treatments received. This information may point to a serious infection that may be asymptomatic when the disease is most virulent.

Ask the patient about recent exposure to colds or viruses or whether she has a persistent cough or fever. Inquire about past or current urinary tract infections, which typically recur during pregnancy. These questions also may uncover evidence of infection.

Also inquire about general signs and symptoms of infection, such as fever, chills, fatigue, and anorexia as well as specific signs and symptoms of upper respiratory, genitourinary, and other infections.

When taking the patient's obstetric history, rule out prolonged PROM, which can lead to chorioamnionitis. Note the onset of labor to be able to determine prolonged labor, which can predispose the patient to infection.

Physical assessment

When assisting with the physical assessment, be alert for signs of dehydration, maternal or fetal tachycardia, fever, chest congestion, uterine or other abdominal tenderness, costovertebral angle tenderness, perineal lesions, and purulent, malodorous vaginal secretions. These signs suggest infection.

Even if the patient displays no obvious signs of infection, be vigilant about following infection control guidelines. Assume that any woman may be infected with the HIV or hepatitis B virus, and observe standard precautions with every patient. A careful, gentle vaginal exam should be done on admission of a patient with a recent history of HSV.

Laboratory tests

Anticipate the laboratory tests ordered for the patient with an infection, which may include a complete blood count with differential; erythrocyte sedimentation rate; HIV, with proper consent obtained, and venereal disease research laboratory as indicated; blood culture; urinalysis; urine culture and sensitivity test; cervical, vaginal, and lesion cultures; chest X-rays; and culture and microscopic evaluation of amniotic fluid. These tests help pinpoint the type and degree of infection.

Nursing diagnosis

After evaluating the assessment data, the nurse formulates nursing diagnoses. (See Appendix 1, NANDA taxonomy of nursing diagnoses.)

Planning and implementation

Expect to administer I.V. fluids immediately to improve hydration, reduce fever, and prevent maternal exhaustion. Use external EFM to avoid further contamination of the fetus. Assess and document maternal vital signs, including temperature changes. After collecting blood or vaginal cultures to identify the infecting organism, administer broad spectrum I.V. antibiotics, as prescribed. Carefully assess maternal and fetal responses to infection treatments during the intrapartal period.

Assist with delivery

Once an intrapartal bacterial infection is identified, labor induction or augmentation with oxytocin may be prescribed to shorten the diagnosis-to-delivery time to less than 12 hours. The number of vaginal examinations should be limited and amniotomy should be avoided. Provide meticulous perineal care. Document the character of vaginal secretions, especially color and odor. Anticipate spontaneous vaginal delivery, depending on the severity of the infection and the maternal and fetal tolerance to labor.

Expect to avoid cesarean delivery in the infected patient because it significantly increases the risk of maternal morbidity and postpartal endometritis. However, if the patient has active lesions from HSV infection or in some settings has had an HSV genital infection up to 2 weeks before delivery, anticipate a cesarean delivery. If rupture of membranes occurs 4 to 6 hours or less before the patient is admitted, anticipate a cesarean delivery to prevent the fetus from coming into contact with lesions in an infected birth canal. It has been a practice to avoid cesarean section for women who had evidence of recent infection and rupture of membranes for more than 4 hours prior to delivery, based on the belief that the infection would have ascended to the fetus during that time. However, in the absence of digital examination or instrumentation there is no evidence that ascending infection occurs. The American College of Obstetricians and Gynecologists has adopted the position of: 'No lesions, no cesarean section.' This basically supports vaginal deliveries as long as no lesions are visible.

When anticipating delivery for an infected patient, summon the neonatal team so that they are ready for the potentially ill neonate. The neonate may be premature and at increased risk for sepsis as well as for lung immaturity, with such problems as respiratory distress syndrome. If the patient received adequate antibiotics for sepsis during labor, the neonate is less likely to have respiratory depression at birth; if not, the neonate may require resuscitation.

Coordinate family care and communicate all pertinent information to the nursery and postpartal teams. After delivery, collect specimens for culture from the mother, neonate, and possibly the placenta, and send them to the laboratory, as prescribed. These cultures may reveal previously undetected infection in the mother and infection transmission to the neonate.

Provide emotional support

An intrapartal patient with an infection will need emotional support because of anxiety for herself and her neonate. She may have a nursing diagnosis of **anxiety related to unexpected fetal outcome** or **social isolation related to isolation precautions.** For such a patient, provide emotional support and reassurance.

If she has an active HSV infection, she and her partner may be concerned about cesarean delivery and the chance of having a neonate with a potentially fatal infection. While preparing the patient for cesarean delivery, provide reassurance and teach her and her partner about the virus and the rationale for surgery.

Also be aware that the patient and her partner may harbor guilt, resentment, or embarrassment because of the stigma of this STD. Reassure the patient that only the staff responsible for her care will be aware of her diagnosis. Such a patient may have a nursing diagnosis of **denial related to socially unacceptable infection.** If so, maintain her confidentiality and respect her preferences.

For any patient with an infection, explain the disorder and its ramifications, which may include separating her from her neonate at birth. If so, encourage her to express her frustration and sadness at this prospect.

Evaluation

Appropriate evaluation statements include:

- The patient verbalized an understanding of the need for infection control techniques.
- The patient's family expressed support and concern for her.
- The patient safely delivered a stable neonate.

SUBSTANCE ABUSE

During pregnancy, substance abuse can lead to serious perinatal risks. Substance abusers tend to have unplanned pregnancies or may be uncertain when the pregnancy began. They may have inadequate nutrition, smoke heavily, abuse multiple drugs, and seek prenatal care late, if at all.

These actions put the substance abuser and her fetus at risk during the intrapartal period. For example, cocaine use during pregnancy causes maternal and fetal vasoconstriction, tachycardia, and elevated blood pressure. These effects reduce blood flow to the fetus and can induce uterine contractions. Cocaine use also increases the risk of preterm labor, abruptio placentae, and delivery of an LBW or SGA neonate.

Substance abuse also can cause problems that may affect the antepartal period and lead to intrapartal problems. For example, severe nutritional deficiencies, STDs, and social isolation can decrease the patient's ability to cope with labor. Use of nonsterile needles can cause maternal infection or embolization. All of these can affect maternal and fetal health.

Some states have strict laws regarding substance abuse and child protection. For example, if the patient used or tested positive for drugs during the antepartal or intrapartal periods, some states have laws that mandate home environment evaluation and referral of the patient for drug treatment before the neonate can be discharged. Keep in mind that laws like this may prevent patients from being totally candid with health care providers.

Assessment

When caring for a substance-abusing intrapartal patient, the nurse obtains a health history, assists with physical assessment, and collects laboratory tests as for any patient who seeks admission for labor and delivery. In addition, the nurse must make specific assessments regarding substance use and abuse and be prepared to notify the doctor of significant findings. The nurse should also assess the need for any referrals.

Health history

The admission interview is the ideal time to assess the patient for substance use, abuse, or withdrawal. With careful questioning, probe sufficiently to discover if substance abuse is a problem and, if it is, determine the patient's current status. This is especially important because the substance abuser may enter the health care facility without revealing her problem.

Explore past and present substance use in a nonjudgmental manner. Remember that the substance abuser is likely to be anxious or depressed and to display abrupt behavior changes. When you begin to ask questions, reassure the patient that the reason you need to know this information is to ensure that you can give her and her baby the best and safest care possible.

Begin the history by determining the patient's first use of tobacco, alcohol, and drugs, and then lead to a current substance abuse history. To evoke honest responses, ask nonthreatening questions, such as, "Do you currently drink alcohol or use drugs?"

Review the patient's medical history for clues to prior substance abuse, such as serum hepatitis, venous thrombosis, thrombophlebitis, cellulitis, abscess, hypertension, STDs, and HIV infection. Such complications are associated with substance abuse and use of drug equipment.

The patient who abuses substances may experience menstrual irregularities or amenorrhea. As a result, she may be unaware of her pregnancy until she begins to look pregnant or feel fetal movement. Because of this, determination of gestational age may be difficult, especially if she has not had prenatal care. Maternal nutritional deficiencies and drug exposure in utero can cause IUGR, further complicating gestational age determination.

Pay close attention to the patient's complete obstetric history. Substance abuse may have complicated previous pregnancies and may cause problems in this one. Illicit drug use during pregnancy can affect the patient and her fetus or neonate.

During the history, evaluate the patient's feelings about her pregnancy. The substance abuser may have ambivalent feelings about pregnancy. Carefully document her responses and bonding behaviors, such as talking about the fetus and touching her abdomen. This information can help health care professionals make decisions about the neonate's safety.

Physical assessment

Observe the patient's physical appearance for signs of substance abuse. Note drowsiness, lethargy, or a malnourished, gaunt, or untidy appearance. Also note extremely dilated or constricted pupils; track marks, abscesses, or edema in the arms or legs; and inflamed or indurated nasal mucosa or nasal septum abnormalities.

Laboratory tests. Because of the patient's lifestyle, she may have multiple infections and diseases. Expect to perform all routine intrapartal tests as well as tests for hepatitis, tuberculosis, STDs, and HIV infection, as prescribed. If the patient admits to substance abuse or shows its clinical indications, expect a urine toxicology screen to be performed for confirmation, as prescribed. If you suspect substance abuse but the patient denies it, suggest to the doctor that he obtain a urine toxicology screen. Inform the patient about the screen and its purpose. Be sure to document the results of the screen.

Nursing diagnosis
After evaluating assessment findings, the nurse formulates nursing diagnoses. (See Appendix 1, NANDA taxonomy of nursing diagnoses.)

Planning and implementation
For a substance abuser, closely assess vital signs for maternal or fetal tachycardia, depressed maternal respirations, and elevated blood pressure.

Labor management
After labor begins, the substance abuser may delay coming to the facility because of fear or may use drugs to ease her labor pains and not realize that delivery is imminent. For these reasons, she is at risk for giving birth outside the facility or en route. When she does arrive, carefully monitor the patient's labor progress. Because the substance abuser is at increased risk for precipitous birth, evaluate her labor progress quickly and be prepared for a rapid delivery. Frequently assess maternal vital signs and contractions.

Keep in mind that labor management for a substance abuser is the same as for any other patient. Medical management may include early artificial rupture of the membranes. Illicit drug use shortly before delivery increases the risk of fetal distress. Therefore, the nurse must evaluate the amniotic fluid for color (such as meconium staining or blood) and quantity. Anticipate continuous EFM to assess fetal well-being.

Promote comfort
Analgesia for the substance abuser's labor pain will not contribute to her drug problem. Document her response to analgesia and observe her for interactions between analgesics and illicit drugs. Because the substance abuser commonly is not accompanied by friends or family, provide nonpharmacologic comfort measures and coach her through labor to reduce her feelings of isolation.

Assist with delivery

Work closely with the neonatal team to ensure continuity of care. The neonate of a substance abuser is at increased risk for congenital malformations, prematurity, and IUGR. About two-thirds of neonates born to heroin or methadone users are born with withdrawal symptoms; cocaine-dependent neonates commonly experience painful withdrawal symptoms that may last up to 3 weeks. Anticipate the need for a neonatologist or pediatrician at delivery because the neonate may require resuscitation and intubation.

Provide emotional support

The substance abuser who is aware of child protection laws may fear prosecution or worry that her neonate will be taken from her. She may have a nursing diagnosis of *ineffective individual coping related to prospect of prosecution* or *fear related to removal and loss of neonate by statute.* If so, try to understand her fears and the difficulty of her decision to seek intrapartal care at the health care facility. Express acceptance of and patience with the patient.

The substance abuser who gives birth without the support of her family or friends may have a nursing diagnosis of *social isolation related to substance abuse* or *ineffective individual coping related to lack of family support.* If so, stay with her as much as possible, coach her through labor, and provide reassurance and support.

Promote bonding

State laws and social service representatives may determine if the substance abuser can take her neonate home. While her home environment is evaluated, promote bonding and offer information about the neonate's needs. To help foster early bonding, follow these guidelines:

- Accept the patient's condition in a nonjudgmental manner. Prepare the mother for potential signs of withdrawal in the neonate, especially those that might be frightening or require special handling or referrals.
- Offer information about the neonate's condition.
- Explain facility policies briefly and directly.
- Encourage contact such as holding the neonate after birth and planning for nursery visits.

Evaluation

Appropriate evaluation statements include:

- The patient received analgesia to relieve labor pain.
- The patient expressed an understanding of her labor progress.
- The patient demonstrated signs of bonding with her neonate by holding him and gazing at him after birth.

PREGNANCY-INDUCED HYPERTENSION

A hypertensive syndrome that occurs during pregnancy, PIH has two forms: preeclampsia (characterized by hypertension, proteinuria, edema, rapid weight gain, headache, blurred vision, and increased DTRs) and eclampsia (characterized by all of the signs above plus seizures). Affecting about 5 to 10% of all pregnancies, preeclampsia may progress to eclampsia suddenly or gradually. Therefore early detection and treatment are imperative. Major predisposing factors are nulliparity, family history of preeclampsia or eclampsia, multiple fetuses, diabetes, chronic vascular disease, renal disease, hydatidiform mole, fetal hydrops. The patient with PIH may be very ill. Failure to recognize and appropriately manage PIH accounts for about 18% of maternal deaths in the United States.

PIH is characterized by insufficient perfusion of many vital organs, including the fetal-placental unit. It is completely reversible with pregnancy termination, but symptoms and the dangers involved with eclampsia may remain for 24 to 48 hours after delivery. The patient may report warning signs of impending preeclampsia including sudden weight gain, varying degrees of edema, numbness in her hands or feet, headache, or vision problems.

The major goal of preeclampsia management is prevention of eclamptic seizures. To achieve this goal, the nurse must understand the pathophysiology, progression, and prognosis of the disorder, and must recognize and immediately report to the doctor the classic signs of preeclampsia. (See Chapter 6, High-risk antepartal patients.)

Assessment

When caring for an intrapartal patient with PIH, the nurse obtains a health history, assists with physical assessment, and collects laboratory tests as for any patient who seeks admission for labor and delivery. In addition, the nurse must make specific assessments for PIH and be prepared to notify the doctor of significant findings.

Health history

Assess the patient for signs and symptoms of PIH especially those of increasing severity. Expect her to complain of symptoms in various body systems because PIH reduces perfusion to nearly all tissues.

Inquire about the patient's pattern of weight gain during pregnancy. A sudden gain of 2 pounds in one week or 6 pounds in one month is a warning sign of preeclampsia. Ask about edema of the hands, feet, or face, as edema is a common, early sign of preeclampsia. If edema is severe, the patient will require further evaluation for other signs of preeclampsia.

Ask about other signs and symptoms that may suggest PIH. A patient's complaints of tightness from edema or intermittent numbness in her hands may indicate ulnar nerve compression from edema. Complaints of epigastric pain or stomach upset may signal hepatic distention, a warning sign of impending eclampsia. Headache and mental confusion indicate poor cerebral perfusion and may precede seizures. Visual disturbances such as scotomata indicate retinal arterial spasm and edema. The nurse should thoroughly review the chart to ascertain the patient's prenatal course, and to determine if the patient has had slight increases in blood pressure, edema, and proteinuria that have been addressed or that have gone unnoticed.

Physical assessment

The patient's prenatal blood pressure should be compared to her current readings. In preeclampsia, blood pressure increases by at least 30 mm Hg systolic and 15 mm Hg diastolic were the parameters for many years. However, a blood pressure of 140/90 mm Hg after 20 weeks' gestation has been noted to suggest PIH. This would warrant closer observation and inquiry. Severe preeclampsia exists when blood pressure is 160 mm Hg or more systolic or 110 mm Hg or more diastolic and significant edema and proteinuria are present. However, eclampsia can occur with much lower blood pressure.

Laboratory tests

For all intrapartal patients, test a random urine specimen with a protein-sensitive reagent strip to screen for proteinuria. Be aware that urine contamination with blood or amniotic fluid will cause a false-positive result because these fluids contain protein. Also, a urinary tract infection can cause proteinuria.

If results indicate proteinuria, expect to collect a 24-hour urine specimen for quantitative analysis, as prescribed. Severe preeclampsia exists when urine protein measures 3+ or 4+ on a reagent strip or 5 g or more (or 300 mg/L) on a quantitative analysis. Urine specific gravity may decrease due to renal insufficiency with PIH also. Frequent blood work will be conducted to evaluate coagulation, liver functions, hemoconcentration, and renal functions. The nurse must promptly document and report these results to the doctor.

Nursing diagnosis

After evaluating assessment findings, the nurse formulates nursing diagnoses. (See Appendix 1, NANDA taxonomy of nursing diagnoses.)

Planning and implementation

Before delivery, the patient must be stabilized and the fetal-placental unit closely monitored. All facilities have a PIH protocol to follow. The obstetric team will determine what to use for each individual. Vital signs must be monitored frequently. Cardiovascular monitoring with an indwelling pulmonary artery or central venous pressure catheter for the patient with severe PIH may be prescribed, especially if she is oliguric. This allows closer monitoring of blood pressure and intravascular volume, which is particularly important with a nursing diagnosis of *altered renal tissue perfusion related to elevated blood pressure*. Furthermore, an indwelling urinary catheter will be inserted to monitor kidney output.

Determine the patient's level of consciousness. As a result of drugs used to treat PIH, she may show depressed blood pressure and respirations and may sleep between contractions. As long as her respiratory rate is normal, do not be alarmed but continue to monitor her closely.

The woman will require continuous EFM to detect signs of placental insufficiency and evaluate fetal well-being. Keep in mind that the seizures of eclampsia cause maternal hypoxia and can produce fetal bradycardia. After seizures stop, fetal heart rate should return to baseline.

Labor management

A woman with preeclampsia may be put on magnesium sulfate ($MgSO_4$) or antihypertensives to reduce the chance of eclampsia. These medications can decrease uterine tone and slow labor; oxytocin augmentation may be necessary. DTRs should be less hypertonic as well. $MgSO_4$ can be toxic and blood levels must be checked regularly. Toxic levels can also be suggested by the absence of active DTRs. Because a patient with eclampsia is likely to be lethargic or semicomatose, she may have a reduced response to uterine contractions. Therefore, expect to monitor her uterine contractions closely, palpating the abdomen frequently.

The patient may display hypertonic uterine activity and develop vasospasm, which increases the risk of abruptio placentae. A sustained rigid abdomen with severe pain indicates possible abruptio placentae and must be reported to the doctor immediately. As in most labor situations, the patient should be on her left side to increase venous return and placental perfusion.

Assist with emergencies

A patient with PIH is always at risk for eclampsia; prepare to carry out the doctor's orders for management. About 5% of patients with preeclampsia develop eclampsia. Most seizures occur during the intrapartal period but can occur 24 to 48 hours postpartum; in some cases seizures have occurred up to 10 days postpartum. The number of seizures a patient experiences can vary from 1 to 20.

Patients most at risk for seizures are those who have not received adequate prenatal care and those with unrecognized PIH of increasing severity. However, no specific signs and symptoms can be used to predict the development of seizures. Therefore, treatment of all patients with preeclampsia is based on concerns for the few who may develop eclampsia.

For any patient with PIH, nursing care includes taking seizure precautions, assisting with prevention or treatment of seizures, assessing maternal and fetal response to treatment and related disorders.

Taking seizures precautions. To avoid general injury to the patient, pad the side rails of her bed. This precaution is particularly important for a patient with a nursing diagnosis of **risk for injury related to seizures.** Never use a padded tongue depressor to keep the patient from biting her tongue during a seizure—it is ineffective and may cause further injuries. It is important however, to have an airway at the patient's bedside.

If necessary, establish an airway and administer oxygen. To prevent aspiration of secretions, position the patient on her side. If she is oliguric, position her on her left side to increase urine excretion and uterine perfusion.

To reduce the nervous system irritability that usually precipitates seizures, dim the lights and reduce unnecessary noise. Organize care to avoid frequent disturbances. Keep the number of people at the patient's bedside to a minimum, but allow a family member to remain with her. This may help reduce her anxiety and help keep the family informed and involved in her care.

Assist with prevention or treatment of seizures. $MgSO_4$ is the treatment of choice for seizures because it is effective and relatively safe, although it can be toxic for the patient and fetus. It depresses neuromuscular transmission, which diminishes hyperactive reflexes and prevents seizures. It also reduces cerebral edema and intracranial pressure, which cause mild vasodilation.

Expect to administer $MgSO_4$ I.V. or I.M. For I.V. use, initially give 4 g in a 20% solution slowly over 20 minutes. (To treat seizures, expect to administer 4 g of $MgSO_4$ I.V. over 20 minutes.) Follow this I.V. bolus infusion with continuous I.V. infusion of 1 to 2 g/hour, as prescribed.

Assess maternal and fetal response to treatment. The therapeutic blood level of $MgSO_4$ is 2.5 to 7.5 mEq/L; signs of toxicity may appear when the level exceeds 7 mEq/L. Monitor the patient closely to detect signs of $MgSO_4$ toxicity, such as hypotension, respiratory paralysis, and reduced reflexes. Monitor and document DTRs every hour for the patient receiving $MgSO_4$. Assess the patellar reflex (which is at best a gross measure of plasma concentration) or, if the patient has received epidural anesthesia, the biceps reflex. Alert the doctor if the reflex is absent, which may indicate that $MgSO_4$ is approaching toxic levels. However, $MgSO_4$ therapy is not based solely on this observation because these reflexes may be absent with concentrations lower than the therapeutic level.

Monitor and document the patient's respiratory rate every 15 minutes, and inform the doctor if the respiratory rate is depressed. $MgSO_4$ is excreted by the kidneys, and any renal impairment may lead to magnesium retention and toxicity. Expect to insert an indwelling urinary catheter for accurate monitoring. Monitor the patient's fluid intake and output every hour. Carefully measure and document urine output each hour and before administering a dose of $MgSO_4$. Note a urine output of less than 25 ml/hour.

Because $MgSO_4$ is not an antihypertensive drug, expect to continue to monitor the patient's blood pressure closely, and record these measurements every 15 minutes. If the blood pressure remains significantly elevated, expect to give a drug such as hydralazine (Apresoline) to control hypertension.

Several drugs may be used in combination to lower blood pressure, induce or augment uterine contractions, and relieve pain. Monitor the patient's response to this multiple drug therapy to assess its effectiveness and detect any adverse reactions.

Keep calcium gluconate at the patient's bedside in case of $MgSO_4$ overdose. As prescribed, administer 1 g of calcium gluconate in 10 ml of a 10% solution I.V. over 3 minutes.

Expect to continue administering $MgSO_4$ throughout labor and delivery and for at least 24 hours afterward. Document the infusion dosage so that the recovery nurse can continue therapy properly.

Fetal levels of $MgSO_4$ correlate with maternal blood levels. Anticipate continuous fetal monitoring during the intrapartal period. Be aware that $MgSO_4$ therapy may cause a transient loss in beat-to-beat variability with internal fetal monitoring.

Assess for related complications. A small percentage of patients with eclampsia develop pulmonary edema with a nursing diagnosis of **altered cardiopulmonary tissue perfusion related to elevated blood pressure.** To detect this complication, auscultate the patient's lungs at least every half hour for crackles or other abnormal sounds and monitor her fluid intake and output at least every hour.

About 20% of women with PIH are at increased risk for disseminated intravascular coagulation (DIC). Therefore, expect to obtain specimens for clotting studies, and carefully observe all orifices and puncture sites for increased serosanguineous drainage. Report and document any abnormal findings immediately. If the patient shows signs of DIC and spontaneous hemorrhage, prepare for expeditious vaginal or cesarean delivery.

The HELLP syndrome is a very serious complication of PIH and indicates liver involvement. It stands for: Hemolysis, Elevated Liver enzymes and Low Platelets. A potentially life-threatening situation, it must be watched for constantly in PIH.

Assist with delivery

Although PIH resolves shortly after delivery, delivery usually is not desirable until the fetus reaches sufficient maturity. However, delivery will be mandatory in a patient whose blood pressure cannot be controlled, whose weight gain from edema continues despite bed rest, and whose proteinuria increases. In such a patient, delivery is justified even when the estimated gestational age falls below 30 weeks.

In an unstable patient, cesarean delivery is undesirable because it could contribute to maternal stress and complications. Ideally, the fetal-placental unit is monitored closely, the patient is stabilized and monitored closely, and she delivers vaginally.

After the patient is stabilized, prepare for vaginal or cesarean delivery, depending on her condition and doctor management. Ideally, she would deliver vaginally to avoid the complications of surgery. If the cervix is likely to respond to oxytocin—that is, if it is soft, open, and not posterior in position—and the patient and fetus are stable, induced vaginal delivery is preferred. If assessments reveal fetal distress or an estimated fetal weight of less than 1,500 g, cesarean delivery is preferred.

As a result of the stress of PIH, the patient may have a shorter labor and a precipitous delivery. Prepare to intervene quickly in this situation.

Alert the neonatal team to be present for delivery, especially if the neonate is premature, which is common in patients with severe preeclampsia. Work with the neonatal team and prepare for care of the neonate.

If the patient received $MgSO_4$ during labor, prepare for potential neonatal effects. $MgSO_4$ toxicity may occur in the neonate, producing respiratory depression, hypotonia, and hypotension.

Evaluation

Appropriate evaluation statements include:

- The patient's blood pressure was stabilized.
- The patient's fluid intake and output were balanced.
- The patient delivered a stable neonate.
- The patient did not develop seizures.
- The patient and her neonate remained free of further complications.
- The patient and family have been given information regarding what is occurring.

RH ISOIMMUNIZATION

Rh isoimmunization refers to sensitization and immune response of maternal blood antibodies to fetal blood antigens, which can create a serious blood incompatibility between the mother and fetus during pregnancy. This can lead to erythroblastosis fetalis (hydrops fetalis or hemolytic disease of the newborn).

Erythroblastosis fetalis or hemolytic disease of the newborn is a serious hemolytic disease of the fetus and neonate that may lead to myocardial failure. It produces anemia, jaundice, anasarca, and liver, spleen, and heart enlargement. Marked edema of the placenta has been noted to be characteristic of hydrops, the most severe manifestation of erythroblastosis. Hydrops is thought to result from profound anemia leading to circulation failure, hypoproteinemia and changes in the vascular and extravascular fluid compartments.

Rh isoimmunization results when a patient has Rh-negative blood and her fetus has Rh-positive blood. However, this is becoming more rare because most Rh-negative women now receive $Rh_o(D)$ immune globulin (RhoGAM) during antepartal and postpartal care, which provides passive immunization against the Rh antigen. Now, it is generally seen in patients who had an abortion or a birth without receiving RhoGAM.

Today, hemolytic disease of the newborn occurs more commonly when the patient develops a sensitivity to other foreign blood antigens. This sensitization is known as nonimmune hydrops fetalis. Maternal factors that contribute to development of nonimmune hydrops include multiple gestation, previous transfusion of blood that contained foreign antigens, diabetes mellitus, thalassemia, PIH, or perinatal infections, especially syphilis or cytomegalovirus infection. (See Chapter 7, Antepartal complications.)

Unlike other high-risk intrapartal patients, the patient with Rh isoimmunization does not feel ill. However, if she knows the consequences of isoimmunization, she may experience extreme guilt and anxiety because of her body's actions against her fetus. She may have endured frequent invasive tests and close fetal monitoring to prevent fetal death. She may view the intrapartal period as the culmination of a trying time.

Assessment

When caring for a patient with Rh isoimmunization, the nurse obtains a health history, assists with physical assessment, and collects laboratory tests as for any patient who seeks admission for labor and delivery. In addition, the nurse must make specific assessments for Rh isoimmunization and be prepared to notify the doctor of significant findings.

Health history

When collecting history data from an isoimmunized patients ask about the antepartal progression of the disorder. The patient may be extremely knowledgeable or may require teaching about the frequent surveillance of her fetus. She may have had a prenatal intrauterine blood transfusion.

Inquire about her obstetric history, which may provide information about Rh problems. For example, her fetus may be at increased risk for developing erythroblastosis fetalis if she did not receive $Rh_o(D)$ immune globulin during her previous pregnancy. Also, determine the patient's expectations for and concerns about her pregnancy. This information may help guide the nursing plan of care.

Physical assessment

An isoimmunized patient may develop chorioamnionitis if her amniotic fluid becomes contaminated during intrauterine blood transfusions or amniocentesis, which commonly is performed in pregnant patients with Rh problems. During the physical assessment, observe for signs of chorioamnionitis, such as maternal or fetal tachycardia, fever, uterine or other abdominal tenderness, and purulent vaginal secretions with rupture of the membranes.

Other obstetric conditions associated with isoimmunization include signs of abruptio placentae, such as a painful, taut abdomen, or signs of hydramnios, such as excessive abdominal distention and dyspnea.

Laboratory tests

Lung maturity studies, such as L/S ratio and PG level, may guide plans for an isoimmunized patient to have a premature delivery.

Nursing diagnosis

After evaluating assessment data, the nurse formulates nursing diagnoses. (See Appendix 1, NANDA taxonomy of nursing diagnoses.)

Planning and implementation

Because abruptio placentae is more common in isoimmunized patients, observe carefully for signs of vaginal bleeding or uterine tetany. Monitor maternal vital signs especially temperature measurements.

Depending on gestational age and delivery options during labor, use continuous internal EFM with a fetal scalp electrode to monitor fetal heart rate (FHR) and EFM with an intrauterine pressure catheter to monitor uterine contractions if the membranes are ruptured and the presenting part is engaged. Closely observe the FHR for signs of fetal distress or hypoxia. Fetal distress in Rh isoimmunized premature fetuses, especially in the absence of labor, indicates the need for cesarean delivery. Severe fetal hemolysis may lead to heart failure in the fetus. If an abnormal FHR emerges, expect to assist the doctor with fetal scalp sampling to estimate fetal tolerance of labor and to determine if cesarean delivery is required.

Labor management

If the patient has hydramnios, her uterine contractions may be inefficient, producing uncoordinated labor patterns with coupling or hypotonic contractions. For such a patient, the doctor may rupture the membranes by needling them slowly and carefully. This helps prevent a sudden gush of amniotic fluid, which can cause cord prolapse or vertex malpositioning of the fetus on descent. Continue to monitor the patient's labor pattern.

Promote comfort

Know that analgesia and anesthesia may be restricted during labor because of fetal immaturity and instability. Be prepared to use nonpharmacologic pain relief measures and to offer labor coaching to the patient.

Evaluation

Appropriate evaluation statements include:

- The patient expressed an accurate understanding of her condition and that of her fetus.
- The patient delivered a stable neonate. The patient remained nonsensitized following the pregnancy through the use of RhoGAM.

MULTIFETAL PREGNANCY

Multifetal pregnancy is the presence of more than one fetus in the uterus simultaneously. Generally, this refers to a twin pregnancy and less commonly, a triplet, quadruplet, or quintuplet pregnancy. Since the introduction in the 1960s of fertility drugs that induce ovulation, the incidence of multiple births has had a marked increase.

Multifetal pregnancies result from either the division of one fertilized ovum into multiple fetuses or the simultaneous fertilization of more than one ovum. For example: twins can develop from one ovum dividing in half, producing identical twins who share the same placenta and amniotic sac. Other variations in the development of identical twins have been described based on when the fertilized ovum divides in the fetal developmental stages. The other possibility is the simultaneous fertilization of two ovum producing fraternal twins who have separate placentas and amniotic sacs.

The major goal of a multifetal pregnancy is to prevent preterm labor and delivery. The nurse must be alert to the dangers and risks of this condition and evaluate and act accordingly. (See *Intrapartal conditions and risks*, pages 301 to 304.).

Assessment

When caring for a patient with multiple fetuses, the nurse obtains a health history, assists with the physical assessment, and collects laboratory tests as for any patient seeking admission for labor and delivery. In addition, the nurse must make specific assessments for multifetal pregnancies and be prepared to notify the doctor of significant findings.

Health history

When collecting historical data from the patient, assess for signs and symptoms of preterm labor, problems with hydramnios and uterine overdistention. Make notes regarding previous laboratory test results, including ultrasound findings. Evaluate all prenatal findings and occurrences that may affect the nursing plan of care.

Physical assessment

During the physical assessment, evaluate for signs of uterine overdistention including dyspnea and orthostatic hypotension.

Encourage the patient to sit up or remain in a semi-Fowler's position with a wedge behind her right hip to prevent these problems. Check for signs of premature labor by palpating for contractions and applying an EFM for each fetus.

Laboratory tests

Ultrasound may be done upon admission to confirm fetal number, sizes, presentations, and amniotic fluid quantity. Lung maturity studies may be done as well.

Nursing diagnosis

After evaluating assessment findings, the nurse formulates nursing diagnoses. (See Appendix 1, NANDA taxonomy of nursing diagnoses.)

Planning and implementation

Because preterm labor and delivery are major complications of multifetal pregnancies, they should be managed with a team approach including nurses, perinatologist, neonatologist, and obstetrician. Document the notification and arrival of the neonatal team. (See Chapter 6, High-risk antepartal patients.) The major concerns in labor include prevention of cord prolapse and fetal compromise.

Frequently monitor maternal and fetal vital signs and overall status. Be prepared for a vaginal delivery or possible cesarean delivery. The chance does exist that after one fetus delivers vaginally that the other fetus or fetuses may become malpresented and necessitate a cesarean section. Be sure to document all labor and delivery occurrences and outcomes.

Evaluation

Appropriate evaluation statements include:
- The patient delivered stable neonates.
- The patient was comfortable in the semi-Fowler's position.
- The patient stated that she understood the occurrences of the delivery.
- The patient remained stable, even with the risk of hemorrhage, during the intrapartum.

15

INTRAPARTAL COMPLICATIONS AND PROCEDURES

Many intrapartal complications are caused by reproductive system disorders that can arise from uterine, pelvic, placental, membrane and amniotic fluid, or umbilical cord factors. To assist the doctor, the nurse must understand both the physiologic changes associated with these disorders and the medical treatment required. Intrapartal complications may also arise from fetal factors such as malpresentation or malposition.

UTERINE FACTORS

Many uterine factors can affect the progress of labor. Uterine contractions play a critical role in determining whether labor is normal or dysfunctional. (See *Dysfunctional labor,* pages 344 and 345.) Other intrapartal complications related to the uterus include postterm labor, precipitate labor, uterine rupture, uterine inversion, and congenital or structural uterine anomalies.

Uterine dysfunction may be classified as hypotonic or hypertonic. In hypotonic dysfunction, the more common of the two, contractions are weak and have a normal gradient (greatest in the fundus and weakest in the lower uterine segment and cervix). These contractions do not generate enough pressure to dilate the cervix. Hypotonic dysfunction typically occurs during the active phase of labor and can be precipitated by maternal dehydration, exhaustion, and fear or stress.

Hypertonic dysfunction, which typically occurs during the latent phase of labor, is characterized by intense, painful contractions unaccompanied by normal cervical dilation. This is due either to an elevated intrauterine resting tone or an abnormal contraction gradient (uterus may contract most strongly in its midsegment). This can lead to maternal exhaustion and fetal distress.

When pregnancy lasts 42 completed weeks or longer, labor is considered postterm and may cause difficulty if the fetus is large for gestational age—a condition that could result in cephalopelvic disproportion (CPD).

Dysfunctional labor

When a fetus fails to move out of the uterus and through the birth canal, or when this progression takes an abnormally long time, the patient is in dysfunctional labor. Other terms used to describe dysfunctional labor include dystocia, prolonged labor, and failure to progress. Dysfunctional labor is estimated to occur in 1% to 7% of all patients. Depending on the circumstances involved, it may threaten the health or life of the patient and fetus.

Dysfunctional labor has several causes. Altered uterine muscle contractility can prevent cervical dilation and effacement, blocking fetal descent. Altered muscle contractility may result from abnormalities of the uterus or bony pelvis or fetal position and presentation. Other causes include administration of narcotic or anesthetic agents, primiparity, and maternal exhaustion. In many cases, the cause cannot be identified with certainty. The latent phase can be considered prolonged if it exceeds 14 hours for a multiparous patient or 20 hours for a nulliparous patient.

The most important factors in assessing labor progress are cervical dilation and fetal descent. Without cervical dilation, descent cannot occur. Most nulliparous patients show cervical dilation of at least 1.2 cm per hour during active labor; most multiparous patients dilate by at least 1.5 cm per hour during active labor. Dilation of less than these rates constitutes a prolonged active phase. The active phase is divided into three phases. The acceleration phase occurs when the rate of cervical dilation begins to increase; the phase of maximum slope, when cervical dilation is almost complete; and the deceleration phase, when the rate of cervical dilation slows.

Progression of labor can be depicted by plotting cervical dilation in centimeters against elapsed time. In normal labor, the resulting graph will form an S-shaped curve, as shown. In dysfunctional labor, the dilation curve will become flattened or elongated. The accompanying graph compares normal labor with one type of dysfunctional labor—prolonged latent

Characterized by rapid progression, precipitate labor typically lasts less than 3 hours. It may result from decreased resistance of soft tissue in the birth canal or by abnormally strong uterine contractions. Although recent studies suggest that precipitate labor poses no greater risk to the patient and fetus than normal labor does, many experts believe that precipitate labor increases the risk of maternal lacerations and fetal intracranial hemorrhage and asphyxia. Additional risks include unattended delivery, fetal hypoxia from intense uterine contractions, and decreased uterine tone after delivery leading to postpartal hemorrhage.

Rupture of the uterus is a serious medical emergency that may occur before or during labor. A complete rupture tears all layers of the uterus, establishing direct communication between the uterine and

Dysfunctional labor (continued)

phase. Effects of prolonged labor on the patient include exhaustion, dehydration, increased risk for postpartal hemorrhage, increased risk for assisted or cesarean birth, and feelings of inability to deliver in a timely fashion. Effects of prolonged labor on the fetus may include hypoxia, asphyxia, and physical injuries sustained during descent. In many cases, dysfunctional labor is an indication for cesarean delivery.

COMPARING LABOR PROGRESSIONS

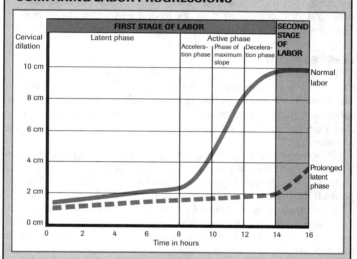

From Cohen, W.R., *Management of Labor*, 2nd ed., Aspen Publishers, Inc., 1989. Adapted with permission of the author.

abdominal cavities. In an incomplete rupture, the myometrium tears, but the peritoneal covering of the uterus remains intact.

Uterine rupture occurs more frequently after previous cesarean delivery and during prolonged labor, difficult forceps delivery, and oxytocin administration. Although signs and symptoms of uterine rupture vary widely with location and severity, they typically include abdominal pain that may decrease after rupture, vomiting, vaginal bleeding, hypovolemic shock, and fetal distress. If rupture occurs during labor, contractions may cease.

Uterine inversion is a rare, potentially life-threatening emergency in which the uterus turns inside out so that its internal surface protrudes into or beyond the vagina. Uterine inversion may occur before or after delivery of the placenta. Although the cause may not be apparent, excessive traction on the umbilical cord and attempts to deliver the placenta manually while the uterus is relaxed may be contributing factors. The patient may experience significant blood loss and shock. The clearest sign of uterine inversion is the craterlike depression that forms in the abdomen and the inverted uterus seen at the vaginal introitus.

Although uncommon, abnormalities of the uterus, cervix, and vagina may block normal labor and delivery. Improper development may produce duplications of all or part of the reproductive structures. The most common abnormality is a septate uterus.

Assessment

Nursing assessment of the patient with hypotonic or hypertonic dysfunctional labor patterns requires continuous, careful monitoring of labor progress and fetal status. To distinguish hypotonic uterine dysfunction from problems caused by CPD, the nurse-midwife or doctor may perform an amniotomy and initiate internal fetal and uterine monitoring.

When assessing contractions, keep in mind that hypertonic uterine dysfunction typically is seen during the latent phase of labor and is characterized by painful contractions of increased intensity. Though painful, the contractions do not produce normal cervical dilation.

Critical assessment criteria for possible postterm labor include accurately determining the gestational age and fetus's size. Gestational age can be determined from the patient's history, including date of last menstrual period and quickening, physical assessment, and ultrasonography. The ultrasound examination also will reveal the fetus's size.

Evidence suggests that fetal distress and meconium release and meconium aspiration syndrome occur much more frequently in postterm pregnancies than in normal pregnancies. Postterm pregnancies are also associated with larger fetal size, increasing the chance of shoulder dystocia as well. Therefore, postterm pregnancies require careful assessment of fetal well-being, including fetal monitoring according to facility policy. This may include daily fetal movement charts, non-stress tests every 2 to 3 days; and oxytocin challenge tests as indicated.

A patient with a history of precipitous labors may not progress through the stages of labor in a normal manner; monitor this patient closely.

Assessment of uterine rupture requires careful monitoring of bleeding, fetal status, the patient's vital signs, and laboratory test results.

When assessing a patient with uterine inversion, carefully monitor blood loss and vital signs to detect shock. Be prepared to assist other members of the health care team in the attempt to reverse the uterus.

Congenital and structural anomalies are assessed by the nurse-midwife or doctor. These may be diagnosed by ultrasound or during cesarean section.

Nursing diagnosis

After evaluating assessment findings, formulate appropriate nursing diagnoses. (See Appendix 1, NANDA taxonomy of nursing diagnoses.)

Planning and implementation

The fetus of a patient with a hypotonic or hypertonic uterine dysfunction may have a nursing diagnosis of *risk for fetal injury secondary to fetal hypoxia and traumatic delivery.* Continuous, careful monitoring of labor progress and fetal status is essential because fetal hypoxia may occur. Be aware of any signs of fetal distress and be prepared to intervene appropriately.

A patient with hypertonic uterine dysfunction may have a nursing diagnosis of *ineffective individual coping related to exhaustion and anxiety.* She may be given narcotic analgesia to help her sleep for several hours. Upon awakening, she may have a normal, progressive labor pattern. This intervention is used only if the membranes are intact and no evidence of fetal distress is detected because this treatment delays delivery. Provide information and support, as needed, especially if cesarean delivery becomes necessary.

A patient with hypotonic uterine dysfunction may have a nursing diagnosis of *anxiety related to abnormally prolonged labor.* Such a patient may receive an amniotomy followed by oxytocin to augment her contractions. (See "Intravenous oxytocin.") Although labor augmentation differs from labor induction with oxytocin, take similar precautions and care for the patient as if labor were being induced.

A patient with postterm labor may undergo labor induction and, if induction fails, cesarean delivery. (See "Cesarean delivery.")

For a patient with a history of a precipitous labor, carefully and constantly monitor fetal and maternal status. Prolonged periods of uterine contractions with decreased periods of uterine relaxation may lead to periods of fetal hypoxia.

If a patient experiences uterine rupture, surgical intervention must take place immediately to save the lives of the patient and the fetus. After cesarean delivery, the surgeon will repair the ruptured uterus if it can sustain a future pregnancy or remove the uterus if it cannot. If uterine inversion occurs, immediate interventions must be taken to save the patient's life, including blood transfusions and surgical reinversion of the uterus. This emergency situation requires the nurse's assistance.

Some vaginal and cervical anomalies may be repaired surgically; some may not interfere with labor and delivery. Uterine anomalies may contribute to spontaneous abortion, preterm birth, malpresentation, and uterine rupture.

Induction of labor

When medical or obstetric emergencies threaten the health of the patient or fetus, induction may be necessary. The doctor or nurse-midwife also can use labor augmentation methods to strengthen natural contractions. Occasionally, labor may be induced by choice if the patient has a term pregnancy and is free of complications.

The two most common uterine contraction induction methods are amniotomy and intravenous synthetic oxytocin hormone infusion. Another procedure involves administration of prostaglandin gel. (See *Labor induction with PGE$_2$ gel.*)

Amniotomy

To accomplish an amniotomy, a doctor or nurse-midwife artificially ruptures the amniotic membranes to augment or induce labor. Some call the procedure artificial rupture of the membranes, or AROM.

The doctor or nurse-midwife performs the procedure with the patient in the lithotomy position. During and immediately after the procedure, the obstetric team monitors the fetus to ensure its well-being and detect umbilical cord prolapse.

Amniotomy improves the efficiency of uterine contractions because the release of amniotic fluid decreases uterine volume. Amniotomy may also shorten labor when the patient's cervix is soft, dilated, anteriorly positioned, and effaced to some degree.

If amniotomy fails to induce labor, the doctor or nurse-midwife may initiate oxytocin infusion. If this fails, cesarean delivery may be required.

Intravenous oxytocin

During natural labor, the posterior lobe of the pituitary gland releases the hormone oxytocin. This hormone stimulates strong, rhythmic contractions of the uterine muscle. Estrogen production increases during pregnancy, which increases the sensitivity of the uterus to minute amounts of oxytocin. Because oxytocin stimulates such a powerful response, the doctor can induce labor by infusing minute amounts of it. The nurse must carefully administer and monitor the oxytocin via an electronic I.V. infusion pump. according to facility protocol.

Labor induction with PGE₂ gel

Prostaglandin E₂ (PGE₂) gel is used for cervical ripening and labor induction and is most effective when the patient has some cervical changes such as softening, anterior movement, or minimal dilation. The gel changes the cervix by dissolving collagen bundles and increasing the submucosal water content; then, cervical changes occur and frequently the patient goes into labor without needing oxytocin.

To administer PGE₂ gel, the doctor or nurse-midwife inserts either a 10-mg vaginal insert or uses a catheter through the cervical canal to instill 0.5 mg of the drug. The patient remains recumbent for at least 30 minutes after administration, and the obstetric team continuously monitors the fetal heart rate and uterine activity. Most patients will experience mild uterine contractions within the first hour. The patient should be observed for 30 minutes to 2 hours. If there is no uterine activity and the fetal heart rate is unchanged, the patient may be discharged. Based on the facility's protocols, a second application may be needed.

PGE₂ gel causes few side effects: hyperstimulation occurs 1% to 5% of the time; vomiting, fever, or diarrhea occurs in only about 0.2% of cases. PGE₂ administration requires cautious use in patients with glaucoma, asthma, or severe liver or kidney impairment.

Oxytocin infusion may cause excessive or tetanic uterine contractions that last longer than 70 seconds each, occur more frequently than once every 3 minutes, and increase intrauterine pressure to more than 75 mm Hg. These excessive contractions may rupture the uterus or rush labor and delivery, resulting in cervical and perineal lacerations. They may also reduce oxygen to the fetus, reducing or disrupting fetal heart rate (FHR).

Excessive contractions or reduced FHR warrants an immediate halt to oxytocin infusion. The oxytocin level will drop by half within about 3 minutes, and the tetanic contractions usually will return to a normal level.

Oxytocin has a potent antidiuretic action. An infusion of 20 mU/minute or more markedly decreases the free water clearance of the kidneys, reducing urine production. Avoid giving the patient large amounts of fluid, particularly dextrose 5% in water, during oxytocin infusion to avoid possible water intoxication.

Evaluation

For examples of appropriate evaluation statements, see page 373.

MEMBRANE AND AMNIOTIC FLUID FACTORS

Several complications may arise during labor that are linked to the membranes and amniotic fluid. They include hydramnios, oligohydramnios, and amniotic fluid embolism.

Normally, amniotic fluid volume equals approximately 1,000 ml at term. In hydramnios, volume reaches or exceeds 2,000 ml and is associated with fetal anomalies and diabetes. The most common problems are congenital anomalies of the central nervous and GI systems.

Ultrasonography and physical assessment showing significantly increased fundal height are used to diagnose this condition.

The counterpart of hydramnios, oligohydramnios refers to an abnormally small amount of amniotic fluid. Its cause is unknown, but a normal reduction in amniotic fluid after week 36 may create or aggravate the condition in postterm pregnancies. Reduced amniotic fluid is associated with maternal hypertension, fetal congenital anomalies, intrauterine growth retardation, and risk to the fetus's life. Experts are unsure about the degree to which fluid may be reduced before such adverse responses occur.

A rare obstetric disorder, anaphylactoid syndrome of pregnancy, also known as amniotic fluid embolism, has a maternal mortality rate of 60%. Profound neurologic impairment is typical in maternal survivors. The fetal mortality rate also is 70%; of the survivors, 50% have neurologic deficits. In this syndrome, amniotic fluid enters the maternal circulation and causes respiratory distress and shock. Classic symptoms include sudden onset of dyspnea, hypotension and coagulopathy possibly followed by cardiopulmonary arrest. Other significant signs include chest pain, cyanosis, tachycardia, hemorrhage, and frothy, pink-tinged sputum. Coagulopathy affects approximately 40% of patients with this syndrome and may be the cause of death in those who survive the initial hemodynamic insult.

Although it occurs primarily during labor, amniotic fluid embolism has occurred during first and second trimester abortions and even during the postpartal period. Most patients who die from this disorder do so within 30 minutes after its onset. Diagnosis is confirmed by cytologic detection of fetal squamous cells and lanugo in a blood sample aspirated through the central line used for hemodynamic monitoring.

Assessment

The patient with hydramnios may experience dyspnea during labor. The enlarged uterus also may place additional pressure on the vena cava and she may be comfortable only with the head of the bed elevated or lying on her left side. Assess the patient frequently for supine hypotensive syndrome. The fetus of a patient with ogliohydramnios may experience fetal distress from umbilical cord compression or associated fetal abnormalities and requires close monitoring during labor.

Assess vital signs closely in a patient with amniotic fluid embolism, particularly respiration and heart rate. Also monitor blood test results, particularly coagulation studies. This patient should be cared for by an intensive care unit obstetric team.

Nursing diagnosis

After evaluating assessment findings, formulate appropriate nursing diagnoses. (See Appendix 1, NANDA taxonomy of nursing diagnoses.)

Planning and implementation

The management of hydramnios depends on the severity of the patient's symptoms, which may include dyspnea and increased edema of the legs and vulva from increased uterine pressure on the venous system. The patient may experience discomfort severe enough to require hospitalization. Amniocentesis may be able to alleviate the discomfort; however, because fluid production continues, relief is temporary.

When ogliohydramnios has been diagnosed before delivery through ultrasonography, prepare the patient for possible abnormal fetal appearance, including dry, leathery skin, and urinary tract or musculoskeletal anomalies.

The treatment of a patient with amniotic fluid embolism includes maintaining oxygenation and cardiac output as well as managing any coagulation problems, recognizing the symptoms of respiratory distress and shock, and knowing emergency procedures for respiratory and cardiac arrest.

Evaluation

For examples of appropriate evaluation statements, see page 373.

UMBILICAL CORD FACTORS

Anomalies involving the umbilical cord typically are not detected until delivery. Some may threaten the fetus's life. Complications that may arise during labor include abnormal cord implantation, abnormal cord length, and cord prolapse.

Normally, the umbilical cord inserts at the center of the placenta. In a velamentous insertion, the cord vessels separate into branches before reaching the placenta and the cord inserts into the membranes rather than the placental disk. Occasionally with a velamentous insertion, fetal vessels in the membranes cross the internal os and take up a position ahead of the fetal presenting part. This potentially serious condition, known as vasa previa, may be discovered during a pelvic examination when the examiner feels vessels through the cervical os. (See *Placental and umbilical cord variations*, page 273.)

On average, an umbilical cord measures 55 cm. An excessively long cord raises the risk of knots and prolapse or a nuchal cord. A short cord may contribute to abruptio placentae or fetal distress.

Displacement of the umbilical cord to a position at or below the fetus's presenting part most commonly occurs when amniotic membranes rupture before fetal descent. The sudden gush of fluid carries the long, loose cord ahead of the fetus toward and possibly through the woman's cervix and into the vagina. Serious damage may occur when the fetus compresses the cord, interrupting blood flow from the placenta. Factors that increase the risk of cord prolapse include hydramnios, more than one fetus, AROM, a transverse or breech lie, a small fetus, a long umbilical cord, a low-lying placenta, premature delivery, and an unengaged fetal presenting part.

Umbilical cord prolapse incurs a high infant mortality rate if not detected and treated immediately. Diagnosis of cord prolapse is based on observation of the cord outside the vulva, feeling the cord during a vaginal examination, or observing fetal distress in a high-risk patient. (See *Umbilical cord prolapse*.)

Assessment

In a patient with possible cord prolapse, auscultate fetal heart tones to assess well-being. If the fetus shows any signs of distress, expect to assist with a vaginal examination.

In a patient with vasa previa, the nurse-midwife or doctor may feel the cord vessels through the cervical os. Abnormal cord length, however, cannot be assessed before delivery.

Nursing diagnosis

After evaluating assessment findings, formulate appropriate nursing diagnoses. (See Appendix 1, NANDA taxonomy of nursing diagnoses.)

Planning and implementation

In a patient with vasa previa, the examiner may feel the cord vessels through the cervical os. Because rupture of these vessels could cause the fetus to exsanguinate before emergency cesarean delivery could be performed, the patient should be kept on bed rest, and the cervical os should not be probed or manipulated. Expect a cesarean delivery.

EMERGENCY ALERT

Umbilical cord prolapse

If not corrected within 5 minutes, umbilical cord prolapse may cause fetal hypoxia, central nervous system damage, and possible death. Fortunately, rapid assessment and intervention by the health care team can help the patient and fetus survive this traumatic event. Discussed below are the signs and symptoms of cord prolapse and appropriate interventions until emergency cesarean delivery can take place.

Signs and symptoms
- Patient reports feeling the cord "slither" down after membrane rupture
- Visible or palpable umbilical cord in the birth canal or at the cervix
- Violent fetal activity
- Fetal bradycardia with variable deceleration during contractions

Nursing considerations
- Immediately summon another member of the health care team who can notify the doctor and prepare the team for a prompt delivery or emergency surgery.
- Place the patient in a Trendelenburg or knee-chest position with her hips elevated. Either position will shift the fetus's weight off the cord. The doctor, nurse-midwife, or nurse may insert two gloved fingers in the cervical opening to assist in pushing the fetus's presenting part off the cord while the operating room is prepared; the fingers should not be removed until the neonate is delivered.
- Do not attempt to press or push the cord back into the uterus. This may traumatize the cord, stop blood flow to the fetus, or start an intrauterine infection. Instead, if the cord protrudes from the vagina, lift it with gloved hands and gently wrap it in loose, sterile towels saturated with sterile saline solution.
- Expect to assist in giving the patient supplemental oxygen by face mask at 10 to 12 L/minute, initiating or increasing I.V. fluids with 5% dextrose in lactated Ringer's solution, and sending blood for type and crossmatch.
- Expect to assist in monitoring fetal heart tones with an internal fetal scalp electrode on the presenting part, if possible.
- Keep the patient informed throughout this emergency. Calmly convey the seriousness of the situation and emphasize the importance of cooperation. Reassure the patient and her family that the medical and nursing staff will do everything possible to ensure a safe and successful delivery.
- Accompany the patient to the operating room, continue to keep pressure off the cord, and monitor for signs of maternal and fetal distress.

Abnormal cord length can lead to other complications, such as cord prolapse or abruptio placentae. The nurse must know the proper nursing care for these complications.

In a patient with potential cord prolapse, a vaginal examination is performed if any signs of fetal distress exist or when the membranes rupture, especially in a patient with twins, a malpresented fetus, or an immature fetus.

Evaluation

For examples of appropriate evaluation statements, see page 373.

PLACENTAL FACTORS

Placental abnormalities may become apparent during pregnancy or they may remain undetected until labor or just after delivery. During any stage, they present a major risk to the patient and fetus. The most common placental complications include placenta previa, abruptio placentae, and failure of placental separation.

A placenta previa occurs when the placenta forms near or over the cervical os instead of taking a position higher up the uterine wall. The patient risks mild to potentially life-threatening hemorrhage, depending on the location of the placenta. Four classifications describe this abnormality:

- Complete placenta previa, in which the placenta covers the internal cervical os completely
- Partial placenta previa, in which the placenta covers the internal os partially
- Marginal placenta previa, in which an edge of the placenta meets the margin of the cervical os but does not occlude it
- Low-lying placenta, in which the placenta implants in the lower uterine segment and a placental edge lies close to the cervical os.

Placenta previa occurs in 0.5% of pregnancies. Incidence increases with previous cesarean section, induced abortion, and maternal smoking of 20 or more cigarettes a day. The main symptom of placenta previa is painless vaginal bleeding after the 20th week of pregnancy. In some patients, bleeding may not occur until labor begins. When bleeding begins before the onset of labor, it tends to be episodic, beginning without warning, stopping spontaneously, and beginning again later. The patient may experience slow, steady bleeding that could affect blood count. Typically, the uterus is soft and nontender.

Diagnosis of placenta previa is based on the patient's history, ultrasound examination, and physical assessment. Any pregnant patient who reports an episode of painless vaginal bleeding of sudden onset requires hospitalization and ultrasonography to show the location of the placenta. Laboratory studies should include a complete blood count, coagulation studies, and a type and crossmatch if bleeding is severe. To avoid potentially severe hemorrhage, the patient should not have a manual pelvic examination until results of the ultrasound examination are available. Severe hemorrhage warrants immediate emergency delivery. (See "Cesarean delivery.")

The separation of the placenta from the uterine wall before delivery of the fetus is called abruptio placentae. This condition may threaten the lives of the patient and fetus. (See *Comparing placenta previa and abruptio placentae*, page 356.)

Although the primary cause of abruptio placentae is unknown, the following conditions may contribute to it: maternal hypertension, a short umbilical cord that places traction on the placenta, external trauma, a uterine anomaly or tumor, premature rupture of membrane, cigarette smoking, and maternal cocaine use.

Whether an abruption involves a small area of the placenta or total separation, classic signs are vaginal bleeding after the 20th week of pregnancy and constant abdominal pain. Additional signs include uterine tenderness, fetal distress, frequent contractions, hypertonic uterus, preterm labor, and fetal demise. Do not rely on bleeding alone for diagnosis; it may be misleading because the presence and severity of vaginal bleeding may vary with the extent and location of placental separation. For example, vaginal bleeding will occur when a placental edge separates and blood flows between the placenta and uterine wall, escaping through the cervix. Vaginal bleeding will not occur when the center of the placenta separates but the edges remain attached. In this case, hemorrhage severe enough to cause fetal death could be concealed between the placenta and the uterine wall.

Diagnosis of abruptio placentae should be based on the patient's history, physical assessment, and ultrasound examination. Often a patient will report an episode of vaginal bleeding typically accompanied by continuous abdominal pain. In some cases, she may report uterine contractions. Fetal monitoring may show distress; ultrasound examination may reveal a retroplacental hematoma. Even if ultrasound reveals no bleeding, a tentative diagnosis of abruptio placentae should be made if the patient does not have placenta previa and preparations must be made for immediate delivery.

The placenta normally separates from the uterine wall within 10 minutes after fetal delivery. Occasionally, however, placental separation may be delayed, a condition known as retained placenta. Separation may not occur at all, a condition known as abnormal adherence that takes one of three forms: placenta acreta, placenta increta, or placenta percreta.

Comparing placenta previa and abruptio placentae

By distinguishing between similar placental abnormalities, the nurse can anticipate care measures that the health care team must take.

PLACENTA PREVIA	ABRUPTIO PLACENTAE
Description	
Development of the placenta in the lower uterine segment. Classified according to the degree that it obstructs the cervical os: low-lying, partial, marginal, and complete.	Premature separation of some or all of the normally implanted placenta from the uterine wall. Classified according to the type of hemorrhage and degree of separation.
Signs and symptoms	
Abdomen appears normal; painless bleeding; uterus soft, except during contractions; fetus palpable; fetal heart tones almost always present; fetal movement not affected.	Abdomen distended, tense, and boardlike; possible concealed hemorrhage; fetus nonpalpable; possible signs of fetal distress; if fetus has died, fetal heart tones absent, no fetal movement.
Management	
Bed rest, vaginal or cesarean delivery, Trendelenberg position to prevent shock (note: vaginal examinations are contraindicated).	Immediate cesarean or vaginal delivery to preserve the life of a live fetus or prevent further bleeding with a dead fetus.
Complications	
Hemorrhage, shock, infection, maternal or fetal death.	Hemorrhagic shock, hypofibrinogenemia, disseminated intravascular coagulation, hemorrhage into the myometrium, renal failure from acute tubular necrosis, maternal or fetal death.

When spontaneous placental separation does not occur within 30 minutes after fetal delivery, the nurse-midwife or doctor may attempt to remove the retained placenta manually. Before attempting manual removal, some physiological approaches that can be used to aid in placental separation include: nipple stimulation or putting the baby to breast to stimulate oxytocin secretion; having the mother squat and making sure the bladder is empty.

In some patients, absence of the decidua basalis allows the placenta to adhere too firmly to the uterine wall. Known as placenta accreta, this condition may occur over the entire placenta or only in a portion of it. In placenta increta, the placental villi invade the myometrium. In placenta percreta, the villi penetrate to the peritoneal covering of the uterus, sometimes causing uterine rupture.

Although the etiology of these conditions is unknown, predisposing factors may include placenta previa, previous cesarean delivery, previous curettage, and multiparity. Incidence of these abnormalities is unknown as well, but placenta accreta is the most commonly reported of the three conditions. Expect the patient to have a dilatation and curettage (D&C) to remove the placenta, and possibly a hysterectomy.

Assessment

Assessment of a patient with placenta previa includes careful monitoring of bleeding, fetal status, vital signs, and laboratory test results. Assess vaginal bleeding by monitoring the patient's perineal and bed pads. Continuous bleeding calls for I.V. fluid replacement; blood transfusions may be needed if hemorrhage occurs. Fetal monitoring may be continuous. Vital signs, level of consciousness, skin color and temperature, and pain as well as events preceding the bleeding also are necessary assessment data. Monitor the results of all laboratory tests, which will be performed more frequently if bleeding becomes more severe.

Assessment of a patient with abruptio placentae is similar to that for placenta previa. However, because fetal distress is much more likely to occur, fetal assessment must be continuous for a suspected abruption. Also, abruptio placentae can lead to disseminated intravascular coagulation (DIC); therefore, monitor the patient for signs of this condition. (See "Systemic disorders.")

The patient's history data may show previous intrauterine fetal death, placenta previa, abruptio placentae, or preeclampsia or eclampsia.

Retained placenta is assessed by measuring the time between fetal and placental delivery; an interval of 30 minutes or more indicates retained placenta. The nurse-midwife or doctor assesses for placenta accreta, increta, or percreta.

Nursing diagnosis

After evaluating assessment findings, formulate appropriate nursing diagnoses. (See Appendix 1, NANDA taxonomy of nursing diagnoses.)

Planning and implementation

Placental problems can cause unexpected complications or profuse bleeding that may alarm the patient. If placenta previa is diagnosed and the fetus is immature, the patient may be hospitalized and on prolonged bed rest. If further bleeding episodes occur, the patient may receive an intravenous line with a large-bore intra-catheter for fluid replacement and possible blood product transfusion. She may be transferred to a high-risk perinatal center for further care. The patient with placenta previa may have a nursing diagnosis of **anxiety related to uncertain maternal and perinatal outcome.** Continuously provide the patient and family with updated information to allay anxiety. Be aware of the anxiety that is experienced by the patient with placenta previa and her family. These feelings will occur not only during an episode of bleeding but until delivery because of the possibility of additional episodes of bleeding. Guidance and teaching will help the family deal with these fears and will provide an understanding of the complication and the necessary interventions.

Treatment and interventions for the patient with abruptio placentae will depend on the degree of the abruption. Nursing interventions are similar to those for a patient with placenta previa; however, fetal status must be monitored continually because fetal distress is more likely with abruptio placentae. In addition, monitor coagulation studies closely because of the risk of DIC.

If the patient with abruptio placentae requires emergency procedures, keep the family informed as they occur, and be sensitive to the family's needs during the crisis.

Prepare the patient and her family if a cesarean delivery is necessary. They may see it as a disappointment or failure, but that feeling may be balanced by the delivery of a healthy neonate.

Complete and partial previas always warrant cesarean delivery; with marginal previa or a low-lying placenta, a vaginal delivery may be possible. As pregnancy progresses and the uterine wall increases in size and rises into the pelvic cavity, the placenta frequently is moved away from the cervical os. Monitor the patient closely during labor because marginal previa may develop into a partial obstruction as the cervix dilates; prepare the patient and her family for either method of delivery.

The patient may develop a nursing diagnosis of **risk for decreased cardiac output caused by hemorrhage.** Expect immediate cesarean delivery regardless of the fetus's gestational age. However, if hemorrhage is not severe, bed rest may allow the pregnancy to continue until the fetus is viable or mature. Delivery then may be cesarean or vaginal, depending on the type of previa involved. If hemorrhage occurs, expect to monitor vital signs and fetal status and to administer fluids and blood, as prescribed.

Treatment and interventions for the patient with abruptio placentae depend on the degrees of abruption, hemorrhage, and resulting fetal distress. If abruption, hemorrhage, and fetal distress are severe, the fetus may become compromised. Emergency delivery is performed regardless of the fetus's gestational age. Support the patient and inform her about the measures that will be taken.

When blood loss is not severe and no evidence of fetal distress is found, interventions may be less urgent. If the patient is in labor with a full-term fetus, a vaginal delivery may be possible.

If a patient's placenta fails to separate spontaneously within 30 minutes after fetal delivery, the doctor may attempt to remove it manually, after administering adequate anesthesia or analgesia, by inserting one hand into the uterus and gently peeling the placenta away from the uterine wall. The patient may require D&C afterward to ensure that all fragments have been removed. She also may receive an oxytocic drug to promote uterine contractions and reduce bleeding.

The treatment of a patient with placenta accreta depends on the amount of placenta adhering to the uterine wall and subsequent hemorrhage. A small accreta may be managed by D&C; an oxytocic drug may be used to control bleeding. Total accreta, increta, or percreta require hysterectomy. Nursing care also depends on the amount of adhering placenta, the severity of blood loss, and whether hysterectomy was performed.

Cesarean delivery

Surgical incision of the abdominal and uterine walls allows cesarean delivery. There are five general reasons for cesarean delivery:

- Dystocia accounts for about 29% of all cesarean deliveries. The most common cause of dystocia is CPD, which results from a large fetus, malpresentation, a contracted pelvis, or a tumor that blocks the birth canal.
- Previous cesarean delivery is the cause in 35% of all cesarean deliveries.
- Breech presentation prompts 10% of cesarean deliveries. This indication is becoming more common, particularly in nulliparous patients. Although vaginal delivery is still the method of choice, many practitioners consider cesarean delivery safer for breech fetuses. Both are reasonable alternatives if the risk factors for each are the same.
- Fetal distress is the indication in 8% of all cases.
- Other indications account for the remaining 18% of cesarean deliveries. These include herpes simplex type 2 or condylomata acuminata lesions in the birth canal. Both are potentially dangerous if transmitted to the fetus during delivery. Condylomatous lesions also may obstruct the birth canal.

All methods of obstetric anesthesia pose some risks for the patient and fetus that must be weighed against benefits when choosing an anesthetic agent. Choice of an agent should reflect the circumstances and the patient's desires. If the patient wishes to witness the delivery, the choice typically is spinal or epidural anesthesia. In an emergency requiring immediate cesarean delivery, a rapid-induction general anesthesia may be the type of choice.

Once the patient is anesthetized, the doctor selects one of several methods to section the skin of the lower abdomen and the uterine wall. (See *Types of incisions for cesarean delivery*.)

If there is adequate time and the patient and fetus are normal, the doctor makes a transverse incision at or just below the pubic hair line.

Much less common today is the classical incision in which the doctor cuts vertically through the body of the uterus. This type of incision increases the possibility of rupture during subsequent pregnancies.

Prepare for cesarean delivery

A patient who discovers that she must undergo cesarean delivery may have a nursing diagnosis of *fear related to real or risk of threat to fetus or self.*

To prepare the patient and her family for surgery, begin by explaining all steps in the procedure and ensuring that the patient has given her written consent.

Next, take the patient to the labor and delivery area or surgical unit, according to facility policy, for physical preparation, including:

- Abdominal preparation or shaving. Facility policy may instruct the nurse to shave the entire abdomen, beginning below the nipple line and including the pubic area. Other facilities just shave the suprapubic hair line.
- Catheterization. Establish an indwelling urinary catheter with a gravity flow drainage system to prevent bladder distention during surgery.
- Laboratory tests. Obtain the tests ordered by the doctor, possibly including complete blood count, electrolytes, and type and crossmatch for blood replacement before the cesarean section, if possible.
- I.V. infusion. Begin an infusion with the prescribed solution using a 16G to 18G needle.
- Antacid administration. As prescribed, administer an antacid 15 minutes before anesthesia administration to reduce the complications associated with possible aspiration of gastric contents.
- Positioning. Assist the patient into an appropriate position on the delivery or surgical table by elevating her right hip. Manipulate the table position to prevent the gravid uterus from

Types of incisions for cesarean delivery

Skin incisions for cesarean delivery are either vertical or transverse. Uterine incisions are either vertical through the body of the uterus, vertical through the lower uterine segment, or transverse through the lower uterine segment. The type of incision used is based on a number of factors, including previous cesarean scar; fetal lie, position, and presentation; number of fetuses; structural abnormalities of the uterus or bladder; and the speed at which the delivery must take place because of fetal distress or maternal instability.

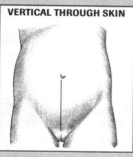

VERTICAL THROUGH SKIN

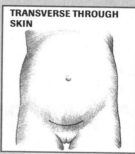

TRANSVERSE THROUGH SKIN

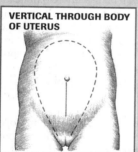

VERTICAL THROUGH BODY OF UTERUS

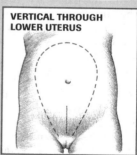

VERTICAL THROUGH LOWER UTERUS

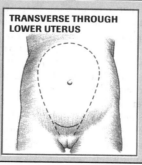

TRANSVERSE THROUGH LOWER UTERUS

compressing the inferior vena cava and to help maintain adequate placental perfusion.

- Preparation. Clean the operation site using the recommended antiseptic solution, prepare the support person if one will attend the delivery, notify the nursery staff and pediatrician, gown and glove the doctors and scrub nurses, check suction and other delivery room equipment—including a baby warmer—for proper functioning, and perform an initial sponge count.

- Assistance. During the procedure itself, assist the surgical team as needed and maintain records as required. Document the starting time of the procedure, the time of delivery, and the completion time. Immediately after delivery, assist in caring for the neonate as needed. (See Chapter 12, The second stage of labor.)

Evaluation

For examples of appropriate evaluation statements, see page 373.

PELVIC FACTORS

The relationship between the size of the pelvis and the size and presentation of the fetus is critical to normal fetal descent. Complications develop when the pelvis is too small or contracted, to allow normal fetal descent. Additional complications involving obstructed fetal descent include lacerations of the vaginal canal and surrounding soft tissues. To prevent this, the doctor or nurse-midwife may elect to do an episiotomy.

The pelvis may be contracted at the inlet, mid pelvis, or outlet, or it may be generally small. This may not be a problem with a small fetus. With a fetus of normal or above normal size, however, contracture may prevent passage.

The patient has a contracted pelvic inlet when the anteroposterior diameter measures less than 10 cm or when the diagonal conjugate measures less than 11.5 cm. The patient has a contracted midpelvis when the interspinous diameter measures less than 10 cm and a contracted outlet when the interischial tuberous diameter measures 8 cm or less. A contracted outlet rarely occurs without a contracted midpelvis.

With a normal fetopelvic relationship, uterine contractions gradually rotate the fetus's head to an anterior position that provides the most favorable adaptation between the head and the pelvis. A contracted pelvis may prevent this internal rotation, possibly placing the fetus's head in the transverse position. As with other causes of arrested fetal descent, this abnormal rotation will impair cervical dilation and may lead to a decrease in the frequency and intensity of uterine contractions. This would lead to a cesarean delivery after a diagnosis of arrest of cervical dilation is made.

During delivery, the soft tissues of the birth canal commonly sustain trauma and lacerations of the cervix, vagina, or perineum.

If the patient is bleeding heavily after expelling the placenta and her fundus is firm, suspect a cervical laceration. Small cervical lacerations occur commonly during delivery and may not need repair. Severe lacerations, possibly affecting the upper vagina, will require surgical attention. Expect the cervix to be examined after a difficult vaginal delivery.

Lacerations of the lower portion of the birth canal may be classified by severity:

- First-degree lacerations involve the fourchette, perineal skin, and vaginal mucous membranes.
- Second-degree lacerations extend to the fascia and muscles of the perineal body.
- Third-degree lacerations extend to the anal sphincter.
- Fourth-degree lacerations extend to the anal canal.

Assessment

- For a patient with structural contractures, assess labor progress, particularly cervical dilation and the frequency and intensity of uterine contractions. Because prolonged labor can endanger the fetus, monitor fetal status closely.
- Assess for abnormal bleeding in the patient with perineal lacerations.

Nursing diagnosis

After evaluating assessment findings, formulate appropriate nursing diagnoses. (See Appendix 1, NANDA taxonomy of nursing diagnoses.)

Planning and implementation

When caring for a patient in labor who has a pelvic condition that may prolong labor, be supportive and alert for impending complications. The patient with a contracted pelvis will need constant monitoring of maternal and fetal status because her labor may be arrested. Such a patient may have a nursing diagnosis of *fatigue related to prolonged labor.* Keep the patient informed of labor progress.

Lacerations of the birth canal may be prevented or minimized by episiotomy or a slow, controlled delivery.

Episiotomy may be accomplished by two methods. In the United States, the most common is a median episiotomy. Using round-tipped scissors, the doctor, or nurse-midwife cuts straight downward from the vaginal orifice toward the rectum. In the alternative method—mediolateral episiotomy—the cut angles away from the anus.

Before episiotomy takes place, the fetus's head (or buttocks in a breech presentation) should be low enough to keep the perineum stretched. Ideally, the perineum should be bulging and thinned. Waiting until this stage to perform the procedure lessens bleeding because thinner tissue contains fewer blood vessels. However, the doctor or nurse-midwife should make the incision before the muscles supporting the rectum and bladder are severely stretched.

Even with an episiotomy, delivery may extend the incision to the anal sphincter or to the anal canal. These extensions can cause pain, excessive blood loss, suture separation, fistula formation, or even permanent sphincter dysfunction. Blood loss usually is greater and repair more difficult and painful with the mediolateral episiotomy because the incision is through thicker tissue.

Patients who massage the perineum during the 6 weeks before delivery may decrease the risk of laceration and the need for episiotomy.

A patient with lacerations receives the same treatment as one who has had an episiotomy. If the lacerations are third- or fourth-degree, the patient should receive nothing by rectum, including suppositories and enemas.

The patient with a contracted pelvis may have a nursing diagnosis of *anxiety related to uncertain perinatal outcome*. The patient and her support person will need constant updating of the status of her labor. Providing support and reassurance will help them to cope with the possibility of a cesarean delivery. They also will need support and reassurance that they have not failed if a vaginal delivery is impossible.

The patient with a contracted pelvis may have a nursing diagnosis of *ineffective individual coping related to exhaustion and anxiety.* When a patient has a contracted pelvis, the fetus's presenting part may not engage in the inlet, making cesarean delivery necessary. Even if the presenting part can engage, the fetus may not descend adequately and the cervix may not dilate normally. Rupture of the membranes without adequate engagement can allow the umbilical cord to prolapse past the fetal presenting part and the pelvis. Because labor is prolonged, the patient risks exhaustion and intrauterine infection; she also may have a nursing diagnosis of *risk for fetal injury secondary to fetal hypoxia and traumatic delivery.* If the fetus passes through the contracted area, cranial molding can be excessive. Vaginal delivery may require forceps or vacuum extraction.

Forceps delivery
In this procedure, the doctor uses two curved, articulated blades to extract the fetus from the birth canal or to rotate the fetus. (See *Forceps delivery.*)

Forceps delivery

As maternal pushing efforts continue, the doctor positions and then locks the blades over the parietal bones in the fetus's skull and pulls the fetus downward and outward through the birth canal during uterine contractions. Once the fetus's head clears the perineum, the rest of the body emerges.

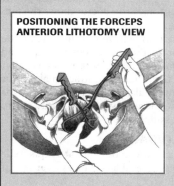

POSITIONING THE FORCEPS ANTERIOR LITHOTOMY VIEW

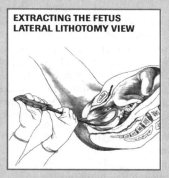

EXTRACTING THE FETUS LATERAL LITHOTOMY VIEW

Fetal station determines the type of forceps used. Outlet forceps may be appropriate when the head has reached the perineum (+2 station) and is visibly separating the labia. Forceps can help the patient push the fetus out, shortening the second stage of labor. Use of outlet forceps is relatively safe; complications usually are limited to bruising of the fetus's head and minor perineal, vaginal, or cervical trauma.

If the head is at station +2 or more and not visible at the perineum the doctor may use low forceps. Use of low forceps is still relatively safe. Use of mid-forceps is rare because it endangers the patient and fetus. Use of high forceps—when the head is unengaged and the vertex of the skull is located above the ischial spines—is not used in modern obstetrics because of the great danger to the patient and the fetus. Mid or high forceps can lead to cranial and facial nerve palsy and other morbidity. Furthermore, use of forceps does not always guarantee delivery. Today, most doctors perform a cesarean delivery rather than using mid or high forceps.

Vacuum extraction
This procedure is popular in Europe and becoming more common in the United States.

To accomplish vacuum extraction, the doctor uses a suction-cup device known as a ventouse. Ventouses are available in several diameters, including 30, 40, 50, and 60 mm. The doctor uses the largest cup size possible to minimize trauma to the fetus's scalp, especially to a suture line or fontanel.

The ventouse is attached by tubing to a suction pump. After positioning the ventouse on the fetus's scalp, air is pumped out of the space between the cup and the scalp, creating a vacuum. By pulling a chain or cord attached to the ventouse, the doctor draws the fetus through the birth canal.

Those who favor vacuum extraction believe that it decreases delivery time. They also point out that the procedure does not require additional space inside the vaginal canal; fetal head rotation can be done without impingement of maternal tissue and less intracranial pressure increases occur during traction. Contraindications to the use of the vacuum include nonvertex presentation of fetus, severe prematurity, macrosomia, and recent fetal scalp blood sampling.

Vaginal birth after cesarean (VBAC)

In VBAC, a patient who has had a cesarean delivery attempts to deliver vaginally. This approach offers several advantages over repeated cesarean deliveries:

- family experience of a normal childbirth
- reduced risk of infection and death
- less discomfort than cesarean delivery
- less recovery time than cesarean delivery
- less cost than cesarean delivery.

Patients with one prior cesarean delivery should not be discouraged from a trial of labor. As the number of cesarean deliveries increases for a patient, the rate of VBAC decreases because increased uterine scarring decreases the effectiveness of uterine contractility. One complicating issue is that the reasons for the first cesarean delivery may still be valid. Another is the risk of uterine rupture. Early studies showed that vaginal delivery after an earlier cesarean delivery performed with a low vertical uterine incision commonly led to rupture, massive maternal shock, and extrusion of the fetus into the abdomen. However, with the almost exclusive use of the low transverse uterine incision, only 0.2% to 0.5% of these scars rupture and, of those that do, about 90% involve only separation of the myometrial covering of the uterus. These ruptures cause no symptoms and little or no bleeding. No maternal or fetal deaths have been reported with such a rupture.

The American College of Obstetricians and Gynecologists (1988) established specific criteria and guidelines for the patient attempting VBAC. Criteria for VBAC include:

- previous uterine incision made in the low transverse position
- maternal desire to try vaginal delivery
- early notification of patient's wishes to the doctor
- available blood for transfusion
- an obstetric team prepared to perform cesarean delivery if necessary
- doctor available during the entire labor
- no maternal medical problems that contraindicate VBAC.

Evaluation

For examples of appropriate evaluation statements, see page 373.

SYSTEMIC DISORDERS

Complications involving hemorrhage, shock, and DIC can occur at any time during labor and delivery.

Many factors predispose the patient to hemorrhage and subsequent shock, including placenta previa, abruptio placentae, uterine rupture, and lacerations during delivery.

A pathological form of diffuse rather than localized clotting, DIC leads to massive internal and external hemorrhage as clotting factors such as fibrinogen are consumed. Intrauterine fetal death, abruptio placentae, septic shock, or amniotic fluid embolism can initiate normal clotting mechanisms. If these clotting factors are depleted, DIC may occur.

Diagnosis of DIC usually is made by laboratory studies that show a decreased fibrinogen and platelet count, increased prothrombin and partial thromboplastin times, and increased fibrinogen degradation products.

Assessment

To assess a patient who may have DIC, observe for signs of excessive or abnormal vaginal bleeding, hematuria, bleeding from the gums or nose, prolonged bleeding from injection or other trauma sites, petechiae, and ecchymoses. Determine if the patient has a history of intrauterine fetal death, abruptio placentae, or preeclampsia or eclampsia. Carefully monitor laboratory test results, particularly coagulation studies.

To assess for hemorrhage and shock, check maternal vital signs frequently for increased heart rate, decreased blood pressure, or widening pulse pressure. Assess vaginal discharge and any increase in vaginal bleeding that would indicate hemorrhage. DIC with hepatic involvement can lead to the HELLP syndrome. (See Chapter 13, The third and fourth stages of labor.)

Nursing diagnosis

After evaluating assessment findings, formulate appropriate nursing diagnoses. (See Appendix 1, NANDA taxonomy of nursing diagnoses.)

Planning and implementation

The patient with potential for hemorrhage and shock and possibly DIC is at risk, as is her fetus. She may have a nursing diagnosis of *risk for fluid volume deficit related to hemorrhage.* The patient with any bleeding condition that could possibly progress to hemorrhage, shock, and DIC should be monitored with coagulation studies. Those patients at risk for DIC have conditions that include placental abruption, fetal death with delayed delivery, amniotic fluid embolism, or traumatic delivery with hemorrhage.

Treatment of a patient with DIC must be directed to reverse defibrination. The patient may require replacement of blood components such as platelets or fresh frozen plasma. Diagnosis of DIC typically is made by laboratory studies that indicate decreased fibrinogen and platelet count; increased bleeding, prothrombin, and partial thromboplastin times; and increased levels of fibrinogen and fibrin degradation products. Vigilant monitoring of laboratory studies is essential. Prepare the patient for the possibility of blood transfusions and component replacement.

A patient who understands the seriousness of her condition may have a nursing diagnosis of *anxiety related to uncertain perinatal outcome.* Provide emotional support during emergency procedures.

Evaluation

For examples of appropriate evaluation statements, see page 373.

FETAL COMPLICATIONS

Many fetal factors can affect the progress of labor, including malpresentation, malposition, macrosomia, shoulder dystocia, and intrauterine fetal death. (See *Fetal distress.*)

When the fetal presenting part is not the head, the condition is known as a malpresentation. Examples of malpresentations include breech, shoulder, and face.

The most common malpresentation is breech, which occurs in 3% to 4% of births and more frequently in twins. Currently in the United States, 85% of breech fetuses that reach term are delivered by cesarean. However, opinions vary widely on whether cesarean delivery is necessary for such a large percentage of breech fetuses. Some doctors attempt external version to convert the breech to a vertex presentation.

EMERGENCY ALERT

Fetal distress

Fetal distress indicates that the health—and possibly the life—of the fetus is in jeopardy. For example, meconium-stained or yellow amniotic fluid signals fetal hypoxia, which can lead to anoxia, central nervous system damage, or death. The nurse can use the following lists to identify signs of fetal distress and appropriate interventions.

Signs
- Abnormal fetal heart rate (FHR) pattern, including a heart rate below 120 or above 160 beats/minute, decreased or increased variability, or periodic changes such as late decelerations or deep, wide, variable decelerations; marked bradycardia, defined as FHR of 100 beats/minute lasting for more than 10 minutes
- Increased or decreased fetal activity
- Meconium-stained or yellow amniotic fluid after membrane rupture

Nursing considerations
- Help the patient into the lateral or knee-chest position to relieve fetal pressure on the maternal vena cava, aorta, or umbilical cord, and to improve maternal and fetal circulation.
- Supply oxygen to improve oxygenation of the patient and the fetus. Administer by face mask at 8 to 10 L/minute.
- Notify the doctor, the nurse-midwife, and the surgical team.
- Initiate or increase I.V. fluids such as lactated Ringer's solution to manage hypotension or hypovolemia.
- Immediately discontinue oxytocin (if it is being administered) to improve uteroplacental perfusion.
- Remain calm and purposeful when caring for the patient. This will help prevent undue fear and anxiety that could adversely affect uteroplacental perfusion.
- Explain what is happening, and reassure the patient to help her gain control and cooperate fully. Keep her family informed and encourage their support.

Breech presentation is associated with increased incidence of preterm labor, congenital anomalies, and birth trauma. The major risk to vaginal delivery of a breech fetus is lack of adequate cervical dilation because the buttocks are smaller than the head. Therefore, after the birth of the buttocks, the cervix can entrap the head, which is larger than the buttocks.

When the head is hyperextended into a face presentation, the chin becomes the presenting part. Although vaginal delivery is possible, the neonate's face will develop temporary marked edema. Internal fetal monitoring is contraindicated because of potential damage to the face, such as skin tearing, infection, scarring, and eye injuries. When the head is midway between extension and flexion, the brow becomes the presenting part. This is a rare presentation and, because it presents the largest cephalic diameter, usually requires cesarean delivery. A transverse lie occurs when the long axis of the mother is perpendicular to that of the fetus and includes shoulder and arm presentations. Either one requires cesarean delivery .

Malposition occurs when the fetus's presenting part enters the birth canal in an abnormal position that makes delivery difficult. An example is the persistent occiput posterior position where the occiput of the fetus's head is in one of the posterior quadrants of the maternal pelvis. (See Chapter 11, The first stage of labor.) A nurse-midwife may try to have the patient rotate the head by changing her positions and rocking her hips while she stands up. Occasionally this assists the head in rotating to a more favorable position for delivery. If the occiput fails to rotate spontaneously to the anterior position, the doctor may use forceps to complete the rotation and facilitate delivery. However, forceps deliveries and rotations may put the patient and fetus at unacceptable risk.

Macrosomia is defined as a fetus that weighs more than 4,500 g. This occurs in approximately 1% of births.

A large fetus does not necessarily preclude vaginal delivery; in fact, many are delivered vaginally or with low forceps. The fetopelvic relationship must be assessed for each patient. Predisposing factors for macrosomia include maternal diabetes, multiparity, maternal age over 34, previous macrosomia, maternal height over 67″ (170 cm), and maternal weight over 154 lb (70 kg).

In shoulder dystocia, the fetus's head emerges but the anterior shoulder catches on the pubic arch, a rare condition but one that can be anticipated based on maternal evaluation. Typically in shoulder dystocia, the head emerges and is immediately pulled back tightly against the vulva. Predisposing factors include macrosomia, a prolonged second stage of labor, multiparity, prolonged pregnancy, and previous delivery of a neonate weighing more than 4,000 g. Because this condition has the potential to cause fetal trauma or death, interventions must be anticipated and immediate.

If fetal activity fails to begin or if it ceases after 20 weeks' gestation, the mother should be monitored for fetal heart tones. Absence of fetal heart tones warrants a real-time ultrasound examination to detect heart wall motion. Absence of such motion offers reliable evidence of fetal death.

In more than half the cases of fetal death, the cause can not be determined. Where the cause is known, however, it may be associated with severe maternal disease, diabetes mellitus, hypertension, abruptio placentae, erythroblastosis fetalis, and umbilical cord accidents.

The death of a fetus is a tragic loss for the couple, possibly compounded by the need to go through labor. Labor usually occurs spontaneously within 2 weeks of the fetus's death. However, an increased risk of a coagulation defect and the severe psychological stress of carrying a dead fetus may prompt the doctor to induce labor within a few days of the death. Throughout this time, coagulation studies must be carefully monitored.

Assessment

Although shoulder dystocia does not occur until delivery, the nurse may assist the nurse-midwife or doctor as described earlier. Once malposition, malpresentation, and macrosomia have been diagnosed, continue with careful monitoring of the labor for any further complications.

If a patient of 20 weeks' gestation or more reports that fetal activity has ceased, monitor fetal heart tones. If none are heard, a real-time ultrasonography is performed to check for heart wall motion. Lack of such motion is reliable evidence of intrauterine fetal death.

Nursing diagnosis

After evaluating assessment findings, formulate appropriate nursing diagnoses. (See Appendix 1, NANDA taxonomy of nursing diagnoses.)

Planning and implementation

The patient with a labor complication of fetal malpresentation may have a cesarean delivery, although some breech presentations can be delivered vaginally. An appropriate nursing diagnosis for such a patient may be *anxiety related to uncertain perinatal outcome.* For a patient with a fetal malposition, nursing interventions may assist with these problems. In some cases, version may be performed to avoid surgical intervention.

Two types of version may be performed: external, which is used to rotate the fetus from a breech or shoulder presentation to a cephalic presentation; and internal, which is used to deliver an unengaged second twin by grasping the feet.

Performed properly and gently, external version carries little risk for the patient or fetus. When external version is performed, the patient receives a drug to relax the uterus (such as ritodrine hydrochloride or terbutaline sulfate) and the doctor repositions the fetus by manipulating the patient's abdomen under sonographic observation. Rotating the fetus to a cephalic presentation increases the likelihood of successful vaginal delivery and reduces the probability of cesarean delivery. External version is more easily accomplished in multiparous patients because their abdominal walls are more relaxed than those of nulliparous patients.

Internal version may be performed to deliver a second twin when the occiput or breech is not over the pelvic inlet and external pressure fails to position a presenting part, or when uterine bleeding occurs. Expect the patient to receive an anesthetic agent. The doctor reaches one gloved hand through the vagina and cervix and into the uterus, grasps the fetus's legs, and performs a breech delivery. The doctor will attempt internal version as a last resort because it places the patient and fetus at serious risk for trauma. Failure of either internal or external version may require an emergency cesarean delivery.

A patient who knows that her fetus is in a breech position before labor begins may be able to perform version on her own. In one study, patients assumed a knee-chest position for 15 minutes, three times a day, for 7 days. In 41% of the patients studied, the fetus shifted from a breech to cephalic presentation. Another exercise involves having the patient lie in a lithotomy position with 1 or 2 pillows under her buttocks and her head on the floor. Have her lie in this position 3 to 5 times a day for 15 to 20 minutes. If she has signs of orthostatic hypotension, have her slowly roll to her left side until the symptoms subside. This exercise has also been shown to assist in rotating many breech presentations to vertex ones.

A patient experiencing any fetal complication requires sensitive, supportive nursing care. The patient experiencing a labor complicated with fetal malposition, malpresentation, and macrosomia may have a nursing diagnosis of *pain related to abnormally prolonged labor* or *risk for fetal injury secondary to fetal hypoxia and traumatic delivery.*

For a patient with shoulder dystocia, the nurse-midwife or doctor may attempt one of several maneuvers to deliver the shoulders, which may require assistance from the nurse. Downward traction may be applied to the head while an assistant applies moderate suprapubic pressure. If this fails to move the shoulder, the patient in a lithotomy position may remove her legs from the stirrups and flex them sharply against her abdomen (McRobert's maneuver) to straighten the sacrum relative to the lumbar spine and possibly free the shoulder. Fundal pressure is not to be used as it complicates the situation 77% of the time. With a shoulder dystocia, the neonatal team should be notified immediately to assist with resuscitation of the neonate as necessary.

For the patient who has experienced a stillbirth, providing nursing care is difficult. Be prepared for widely varying responses from the patient and family members. If the patient does not display grief, explore her personal feelings of anger and sadness. Prepare to refer her to counseling or support groups as needed.

A patient may have begun labor when she is told her fetus is dead, or she may have known for some time before labor begins. A nursing diagnosis of **anticipatory grieving related to death of the fetus** may apply. Be extremely sensitive to the needs of the parents and take cues from them to meet their emotional needs. Some parents may need to talk about their loss; others may not. It is essential to provide any support or opportunities for grieving that the parents may need.

Provide the same nursing care to a patient in labor with a known stillbirth as to a patient undergoing labor induction. In addition, continuously monitor her coagulation studies because of the risk of DIC.

The death of a fetus is a tragic loss for the parents that can be compounded because the patient must still go through labor. A nursing diagnosis of **powerlessness related to having to carry a dead fetus** may apply. Labor usually occurs spontaneously within 2 weeks of the fetus's death. The psychological stress of carrying a dead fetus may necessitate inducing labor within a few days of the intrauterine fetal death. Throughout this time, carefully monitor the results of coagulation studies to rule out DIC.

Give the parents an opportunity to see and hold their dead child if they wish. Wrap the child in a blanket and prepare the parents for its appearance. Give them as much time as they wish to spend with their child. Offer to provide a lock of hair, footprints, and bracelets; even if the parents decline, gather these things in case they change their minds. A Polaroid picture of the child also may be appropriate. Many parents appreciate these simple gestures, which may provide them with the only mementos of their child that they will have.

The parents may want to have their child baptized. All nurses, regardless of their religion, can perform this rite.

Evaluation

Appropriate evaluation statements for the patient and her family experiencing intrapartal complications include:

- The patient and her fetus completed labor and delivery safely with little or no additional complications.
- The patient and her support person and family received regular updates about her condition and the status of the fetus, as the situation allowed.
- The patient's coagulation studies remained within normal limits despite bleeding problems, and DIC was avoided.
- The patient remained as comfortable as possible during dysfunctional labor.
- The patient and her support person received support and encouragement from the nursing staff during complications.

NURSING CARE DURING THE POSTPARTAL PERIOD

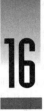

PHYSIOLOGY OF THE POSTPARTAL PERIOD

Throughout pregnancy, gradual changes occur in all body systems. The most pronounced changes are those affecting the reproductive system and the hormonal processes that regulate its function. During the postpartal period or puerperium, these changes resolve. Eventually, each body system returns to its nonpregnant state.

Although officially defined as a 6-week period, the postpartal period spans the time between delivery and the resumption of normal physiologic function. Thus its length may vary greatly, especially among lactating patients. The patient's physical capabilities and body image must adapt to postpartal changes and the restorative processes accompanying them. The nurse who understands such changes can assess the patient more proficiently and make scientifically grounded decisions, facilitating the patient's return to optimal health.

REPRODUCTIVE SYSTEM

The reproductive system recovers from pregnancy and childbirth in a unique and efficient manner. However, some structures are permanently affected.

Uterus

After delivery of the fetus and placenta, the uterus undergoes profound and dramatic changes leading to its return to a nonpregnant state. These changes, which involve both the myometrium and endometrium, take place through physiologic mechanisms not common to other organs.

Involution

A steady process, involution results from muscle contractions and autolysis, the self-disintegration or self-digestion of cells or tissue. The myometrium resumes its normal size through involution.

Immediately after delivery of the placenta, strong myometrial contractions shrink the uterus to the size of a grapefruit—roughly half its immediate predelivery size. This rapid shrinkage forces the uterine walls into close proximity, causing the center cavity to flatten.

Myometrial contractions are irregular in both timing and strength. A multiparous patient usually experiences stronger, more uncomfortable contractions than a primiparous patient—probably because the uterine muscle loses some elasticity with each pregnancy and needs to work harder to contract efficiently. Also, a lactating patient has stronger contractions than a nonlactating patient because oxytocin, while regulating milk ejection, also stimulates the uterine muscle. Oxytocin release is part of a series of events that occur with nipple stimulation such as when breastfeeding (See *How nipple stimulation affects milk production.*)

How nipple stimulation affects milk production

Nipple stimulation triggers a series of events leading to milk production, as shown in the diagram below. Continued milk production depends on the baby's suckling the breast, which stimulates the production of oxytocin by the posterior pituitary. Oxytocin causes the myoepithelial cells around the alveoli and ducts to contract, transporting the milk to the lactiferous (storage) sinuses, where it is readily available for the infant.

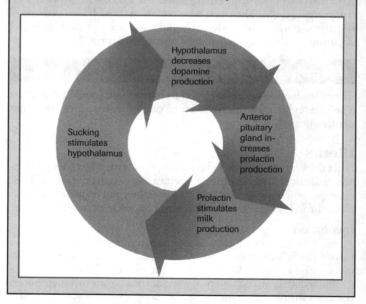

Uterine involution is rapid and steady. Just after delivery, the uterus weighs 1,000 to 1,200 g; 1 week later, it weighs 500 g. By 6 weeks post-partum, the uterus has returned to its normal nonpregnant weight of 50 to 70 g.

Uterine size decreases along with uterine weight. One hour after delivery, the fundus of the uterus is palpable at or just above the umbilicus. Each day thereafter, the uterus becomes smaller so that the fundus is palpable about one fingerbreadth lower than on the previous day. (See *Postpartal changes in fundal height*, page 378.) By 2 weeks postpartum, the uterus has returned to the pelvic cavity and no longer can be palpated as an abdominal organ. Although it never regains its nulliparous size and shape, the uterus usually resumes a nonpregnant size and contour by 6 weeks postpartum.

Through autolysis, the second mechanism leading to involution, hypertrophic uterine cells return to a nonpregnant shape and size. Autolysis is a mechanism of self-disintegration or self-digestion of cellular tissue. The number of uterine cells after delivery remains unchanged by pregnancy; the by-products of autolyzed cellular protein are absorbed and excreted by the renal system.

Endometrium

During the postpartal period, healing and regeneration restore normal endometrial structure and function. As the placenta and membranes separate from the uterine wall at delivery, the decidua basalis remains in the uterine cavity.

In the early stages of involution, myometrial contractions compress blood vessels throughout the decidua and at the placental site, leading to hemostasis. Contractions in the arteriolar walls immediately after delivery enhance hemostasis.

After the first 2 or 3 postpartal days, the decidua basalis differentiates into two distinct layers. Occlusion of decidual blood vessels leads to necrosis of the superficial layer, which is sloughed off as part of the lochial discharge. (See "Lochia.") The deeper decidual layer, or basal layer, remains attached to the uterine wall.

By 7 days postpartum, endometrial glands begin to regenerate within the basal layer. By 16 days postpartum the endometrium is completely restored, except at the placental site. Involution of the placental site and restoration of this normal tissue take longer than in the rest of the endometrium.

As the placental site heals, regenerating endometrial tissue slowly and progressively replaces the decidua basalis. At 8 weeks, it measures approximately 2 mm and still has not healed completely. Healing occurs gradually and without scarring. If healing were less efficient and the placental site became scarred, the area available for implan-

Postpartal changes in fundal height

After delivery, uterine involution progresses so rapidly that each day the level of the fundus is one fingerbreadth lower than on the previous day. Autolysis of hypertrophic uterine muscle cells also aids involution.

FUNDAL HEIGHT

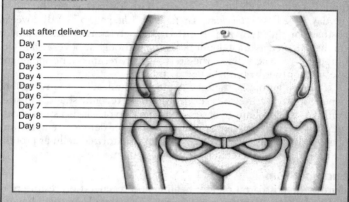

Just after delivery
Day 1
Day 2
Day 3
Day 4
Day 5
Day 6
Day 7
Day 8
Day 9

UTERINE INVOLUTION

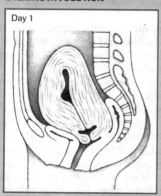

Day 1

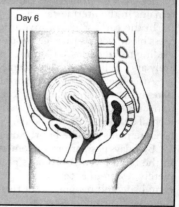

Day 6

tation of a fertilized ovum could be significantly reduced. This could contribute to reduced numbers of future pregnancies and potential for increased risk of placenta previa.

Fallopian tubes
Postpartal changes in the fallopian tubes take place mainly at the cellular level. With a gradual return to normal hormonal balance by 6 to 8 weeks postpartum, epithelial cells return to the condition seen in the early follicular phase of the menstrual cycle, with an increase in ciliated cells to help propel the ovum.

Lochia
The amount and duration of lochia—postpartal vaginal discharge—correlate with endometrial healing and regeneration. Generally, patients who have cesarean deliveries exhibit a lighter lochial flow of shorter duration than those who deliver vaginally. This probably occurs because some of the uterine debris found in lochia is removed manually during cesarean delivery. In all patients, lochial flow occurs in three gradual stages. (See *Stages of lochia.*)

Stages of lochia
Lochia progresses through three stages, each with distinctive characteristics that reflect progressive endometrial healing.

STAGE	USUAL DURATION	DESCRIPTION
Lochia rubra	1 to 4 days postpartum	Primarily contains blood and decidual tissue. May have a slightly fleshy odor.
Lochia serosa	5 to 7 days postpartum	Contains serous fluid, decidual tissue, leukocytes, and erythrocytes. Appears pink-brown. Is serous and odorless.
Lochia alba	1 to 3 weeks postpartum	Primarily contains leukocytes and decidual cells. Appears creamy white, brown, or almost colorless. May have a slightly stale odor.

Although rates of lochial discharge vary among patients, normal parameters for the amount and duration of lochia during each stage have been established. Lochia rubra, the first stage, typically lasts up to 4 postpartal days and contains a mixture of mucus, tissue debris, and blood.

As uterine bleeding subsides, lochia becomes paler and more serous, entering the second stage called lochia serosa. This pink or brownish discharge persists through 5 to 7 days postpartum. Between 7 and 14 days postpartum, sloughing at the former placental site may cause a sudden temporary increase in lochial flow or even bleeding. This self-limiting condition should last no more than 1 to 2 hours. Frequently, maternal rest will decrease this flow. The final stage of lochial discharge is lochia alba, a creamy white, brown, or colorless discharge consisting mainly of serum and white blood cells. Lochia alba usually diminishes after the third postpartal week but may persist for 6 weeks or longer. Lochia is considered abnormal if it contains clots larger than a dime or tissue fragments. Also, lochia should not have a foul or offensive odor and should not relapse to a previous stage. These changes could indicate endometritis or other infection.

Cervix

In a patient who delivered vaginally, cervical muscle tone is poor and the cervix and lower uterine segment are thin and collapsed. Examination of the external os reveals tiny lacerations and bruising. The external os contracts slowly and on the second and third days after delivery, it remains flaccid and open approximately 2 to 3 cm. By the end of the first week, the os has contracted to 1 cm and cervical tone has improved, making admission of one finger difficult. At this point, cervical edema and hemorrhage have subsided markedly and the cervical canal has begun to reform as the cervix thickens.

Although the cervix resumes its normal functional anatomy by 6 to 12 weeks postpartum, it never regains its nulliparous appearance. The external os remains widened and linear, compared to the tiny circular os of the nulliparous patient. Occasionally, the os appears fish-mouthed, particularly in cases of significant cervical trauma during delivery.

Vagina

After vaginal delivery, the vagina is smooth-walled and somewhat enlarged and edematous, with poor muscle tone. Gradually, it shrinks and the edema subsides. By the third postpartal week, rugae reappear within the vaginal walls. These rugae may remain permanently flattened to varying degrees, never returning to the nulliparous size and state (characterized by numerous mucosal infoldings). Consequently, the vaginal canal rarely resumes its nulliparous size.

The vaginal epithelium also undergoes notable postpartal changes. Vascular and well-lubricated during pregnancy because of estrogen increase, the epithelium becomes fragile and atrophic by the 3rd or 4th postpartal week. In the nonlactating patient, atrophy resolves by 6 to 10 weeks postpartum as estrogen normalizes. However, because the estrogen level remains low during lactation, the breast-feeding patient may continue to experience symptoms of vaginal atrophy. These include decreased vaginal lubrication and diminished sexual response.

External structures
The clitoris and labia may remain permanently enlarged to some extent. After vaginal delivery, the vaginal introitus remains edematous and sometimes ecchymotic. Lacerations may be apparent on the introitus and perineum, even if an episiotomy was not performed.

Without such complications as hematoma or infection, the perineum heals rapidly. Usually, the introitus and perineum resume a nonpregnant state by 6 weeks postpartum. However, the introitus may show residual gaping; typically, this change is permanent. Muscular contraction exercises, such as Kegel exercises, help the pelvic musculature regain tone.

Pelvic muscular support structures
Uterine support structures, such as the broad and round ligaments, stretch significantly during pregnancy as the uterus expands. During vaginal delivery, the support structures of the uterus, vagina, urethra, and bladder undergo trauma. Although laxity of these structures improves gradually, some pelvic relaxation may persist beyond the postpartal period, causing any of the following conditions:
- uterine prolapse
- cystocele
- rectocele
- enterocele.

Because the effects of stretching are cumulative, the likelihood of permanent relaxation of pelvic muscular support increases with each pregnancy and delivery. Kegel exercises can assist in maintaining and regaining some pelvic muscular support.

Breasts
The breast changes initiated during pregnancy—including nipple and areola enlargement, maturation of lobes and ducts, and increased vascularity—progress after delivery, particularly in the lactating patient. The size of breast cells and the number of oxytocin receptors also increase.

In the first 2 postpartal days, breast alveoli enlarge and display substantial amounts of rough endoplasmic reticulum and Golgi bodies. The reticulum and Golgi bodies play key roles in milk production. The alveoli, the basic secretory units of the breast, are the site of milk production. Surrounded by a capillary network, alveoli cluster in groups of 10 to 100 to form lobules. Each lobule is drained by a lactiferous duct. The breast contains 15 to 20 lactiferous ducts, which merge at the nipple and areola to allow emptying of the breast.

Lactation—synthesis, and secretion of breast milk—results from an interaction among several hormones. Alveolar growth and development is regulated by estrogen, progesterone, human placental lactogen (HPL), prolactin, cortisol, and insulin. Estrogen stimulates the release of prolactin and sensitizes the mammary gland to prolactin action. However, in combination with progesterone, estrogen inhibits prolactin.

The profound drop in serum estrogen and progesterone levels after delivery of the placenta removes this inhibition, allowing prolactin to stimulate initiation of milk secretion (called lactogenesis) within the alveoli.

Dopamine, a neurotransmitter originating in the hypothalamus, also inhibits prolactin (hence its alternate name, prolactin-inhibiting factor). However, nipple stimulation overcomes prolactin inhibition. When the neonate sucks on the nipple, nerve endings in the areola transmit sensory messages to the hypothalamus that reduce dopamine production; this removes prolactin inhibition. (See *How nipple stimulation affects milk production,* page 376.)

In some cases, such as when the patient chooses to bottle-feed her neonate, lactation must be suppressed. Absence of sucking and emptying of the breasts causes suppression, which usually leads to breast involution and cessation of lactation within 1 week. No longer stimulated, alveolar cells flatten and stop secreting milk; within 24 hours, cellular organelle structure begins to take on a more normal configuration, with a decrease in rough endoplasmic reticulum and Golgi bodies. Mammary blood flow decreases, leading to further involution. Over the next 3 months, connective and adipose tissue replaces glandular tissue, although the breast retains some increased glandular tissue. As involution nears completion, the breasts typically resume their nonpregnancy size. However, a mild alteration in breast shape may be permanent.

ENDOCRINE SYSTEM

Like the reproductive system, the endocrine system undergoes profound postpartal changes. Many of these changes interrelate with those of the reproductive system.

Placental hormones

With delivery of the placenta, levels of circulating placental hormones drop rapidly. The serum estrogen level plunges sharply in the first 3 hours after delivery, then more gradually until the 7th postpartal day, when it reaches its lowest level. In the nonlactating patient, estrogen begins to rise to a normal level at approximately 2 weeks postpartum. In the lactating patient, the rise is delayed, leading to such problems as vaginal mucosal atrophy. As a patient breast-feeds less frequently, her estrogen level gradually increases. Ovulation stops for some patients as they breast-feed; a lower estrogen level is a contributing factor.

Serum progesterone falls below normal luteal-phase levels by the 3rd postpartal day. After the 1st week, progesterone cannot be detected in the circulation until ovulation returns. Consequently, the first few postpartal menstrual cycles may be irregular and shorter than normal.

The two remaining placental hormones, HPL and human chorionic gonadotropin (hCG), also rapidly diminish. Circulating hCG, the hormone measured in most standard pregnancy tests, disappears within 8 to 24 hours after delivery in both lactating and nonlactating patients. The decline is so pronounced that by the end of the first postpartal week a urine pregnancy test is negative. Neither hCG nor HPL is produced until a subsequent pregnancy.

Hypothalamic-pituitary-ovarian function

Resumption of the menstrual cycle is coordinated by hormones secreted by the hypothalamus (gonadotropin-releasing hormone), pituitary gland (follicle-stimulating hormone and luteinizing hormone), and ovaries (estrogen and progesterone). Although a period of amenorrhea normally follows delivery, experts do not concur on its physiologic basis or the mechanism that reestablishes a normal cycle.

Among nonlactating patients, the average time before the return of ovulation is about 10 weeks; menstruation typically resumes by 7 to 9 weeks. Thus, for most nonlactating patients, the first postpartal menstrual period may be anovulatory.

Lactation delays the return of a normal menstrual cycle; the length of the delay depends on breast-feeding duration and frequency. For example, a patient who breast-feeds for 6 months will have longer-lasting amenorrhea than one who breast-feeds for 4 weeks. Likewise, six or more daily breast-feeding sessions decrease the chance for a normal menstrual cycle. However, poor nutritional status during lactation may delay resumption of normal hypothalamic-pituitary-ovarian function.

Return of ovulation in lactating patients also varies. For both lactating and nonlactating patients, an increased interval before the first postpartal menstrual period increases the likelihood of an ovulatory cycle. According to one extensive study, ovulation resumption is delayed with breast-feeding but lactation does not preclude early ovulation.

Reversal of other changes

The rapid decline in estrogen, progesterone, cortisol, and HPL leaves insulin relatively unopposed in the early postpartal period compared to late pregnancy. Also, for the first few postpartal days, the serum glucose level, which decreases during pregnancy, remains low. Consequently, patients with diabetes mellitus have a greatly reduced need for exogenous insulin; some require none. As hormone levels begin to stabilize, the need for exogenous insulin returns and the insulin requirement approximates the prepregnancy dosage.

RESPIRATORY SYSTEM

The postpartal period typically brings complete resolution of pregnancy-related respiratory changes and associated complaints, such as shortness of breath, chest and rib discomfort, and decreased tolerance for physical exertion.

Reversal of anatomic changes

Anatomic changes in the thoracic cavity and rib cage, caused by increasing uterine size, reverse gradually after delivery. Thus, full lung expansion returns and the rib cage regains a normal diameter. As the estrogen level declines, vascularization of the respiratory tract—increased by pregnancy—also resumes a nonpregnancy status.

Reversal of functional changes

As the serum progesterone level declines, oxygen demand decreases, and the uterus no longer impinges on the diaphragm, the following changes occur, restoring normal respiratory function.

- Tidal volume (the amount of air exchanged with each breath), minute volume (the amount of air expelled from the lungs per minute), and vital capacity (the amount of air expelled after maximum inspiration) decrease to nonpregnancy values.
- Functional residual capacity (the amount of air remaining in the lungs after normal, quiet inspiration) rises to nonpregnancy values.

CARDIOVASCULAR SYSTEM

After delivery, the cardiovascular system exhibits few subjectively no-ticeable changes as it resumes a nonpregnancy status.

Reversal of anatomic and auscultatory changes

Cardiac enlargement and displacement reverse as the uterus resumes its normal size and position. Abnormal heart sounds resulting from the anatomic and hemodynamic changes caused by pregnancy also resolve in the postpartal period.

Reversal of hemodynamic changes

Altered significantly by pregnancy, blood volume and cardiac output quickly resume a nonpregnancy status after delivery. Blood pressure and pulse undergo less dramatic changes.

Blood volume

Blood loss during delivery immediately reduces blood volume. Normal vaginal delivery leads to an average blood loss of 500 ml; cesarean de-livery, 1,000 ml or more. The increase in blood volume during preg-nancy allows the body to withstand this substantial loss. However, ex-cessive blood loss at delivery may delay functional recovery.

After delivery, extravascular fluid shifts to the circulation, lead-ing to a plasma volume increase that helps offset blood loss at deliv-ery. As postpartal diuresis occurs, this fluid is then excreted by the re-nal system—first in large amounts, then more gradually. The extra fluid is also excreted through diaphoresis, typical of the early post-partum course. Delivery of the placenta reduces the size of the ma-ternal vascular bed by 10% to 15%. Thus, a smaller blood volume is needed for tissue perfusion.

Cardiac output

Markedly increased during pregnancy, cardiac output remains high for 48 hours postpartum, then declines gradually to a nonpregnancy level. The decline is similar in lactating and nonlactating patients. Most of the decrease occurs as early as 2 weeks postpartum.

Blood pressure and pulse

Immediately after delivery, blood pressure readings should differ only slightly, if at all, from readings taken during the third trimester of preg-nancy. A decrease may indicate undiagnosed uterine hemorrhage or excessive blood loss at delivery.

An increase may signal a preeclamptic tendency, especially if accompanied by headache or visual changes. Blood pressure readings typically remain relatively stable in the first 12 weeks postpartum, then increase gradually until the 24th week when nonpregnancy readings return.

For 7 to 10 days after delivery, transient bradycardia of 50 to 70 beats/minute may occur. This finding is normal and may result from the decrease in cardiac work load that follows delivery. On the other hand, tachycardia above 100 beats/minute warrants investigation because it may reflect hypovolemia—especially in a patient with a low or decreasing red blood cell (RBC) count.

Reversal of varicose conditions

Varicosities of the legs, anus, or vulva may arise during pregnancy from diminished venous return of the legs, pressure exerted by the fetus, and straining during labor and delivery. In many patients, these conditions improve significantly or regress completely after delivery. However, signs and symptoms become more pronounced with each pregnancy. If problems persist after the postpartal period, surgical repair may be required. Mild exercise increases muscle tone which increases venous return. (See "Postpartal exercises" in Chapter 17.)

HEMATOLOGIC SYSTEM

Levels of blood constituents may vary in the postpartal period. Coagulation, enhanced during pregnancy and delivery, normalizes gradually. However, coagulatory stimulation induced by labor and delivery increases the risk of thromboembolism.

Red blood cell parameters

Immediately after delivery, the hemoglobin level and hematocrit, as well as the complete RBC count, vary from one patient to the next. Generally, for a patient who delivered vaginally without complications, these values remain near predelivery levels despite normal blood loss at delivery. This phenomenon results from hemoconcentration, which follows postpartal diuresis. In a patient who underwent cesarean delivery, increased blood loss may cause RBC parameters to fall slightly just after delivery.

In a healthy patient with adequate nutrition, all RBC parameters typically will return to nonpregnancy levels by 6 weeks postpartum. A significant or progressive decrease in these parameters in the first few postpartal days is abnormal and may indicate excessive or continued blood loss.

White blood cell count

The white blood cell (WBC) count increases, mainly in granulocytes, in the first 10 to 12 days postpartum, possibly rising as high as 25,000/mm^3. Although this change reflects a normal stress response, it may complicate diagnosis of a postpartal infection, which also increases the WBC count.

Coagulation factors

Postpartal changes in coagulation factors are gradual. Throughout pregnancy, levels of coagulation factors I (fibrinogen), VII, IX, and X rise progressively; during late pregnancy, fibrinolysis—destruction of blood clots—diminishes. These circumstances place the pregnant patient at a progressively increasing risk for thromboembolic disorders.

Delivery stimulates the coagulation system, increasing this risk even further in the early postpartal period. Studying the rate at which coagulation factors normalize after delivery, researchers found that these factors remain significantly elevated for the first 2 to 3 weeks postpartum, then fall gradually, approaching nonpregnancy levels after 6 weeks. The platelet count returns to a nonpregnancy level by 2 weeks postpartum.

However, traumatic delivery, infection, or prolonged immobility may delay the return to normal levels.

URINARY SYSTEM

Pregnancy affects both the anatomic structure of the urinary tract and the function of the urinary system. Furthermore, delivery may contribute to certain anatomic changes. Unlike most other body systems, the urinary system may show the effects of pregnancy and delivery well into and even beyond the postpartal period.

Reversal of anatomic changes

At delivery, fetal passage through the pelvis and vagina causes varying degrees of trauma to the urethra and bladder. A normal amount of trauma leads to edema and microscopic bleeding. Delivery complications, such as precipitous delivery or forceps instrumentation, may cause increased trauma, leading to laceration of the urethra or meatus. With cesarean delivery, there is the potential for surgical trauma to the bladder.

Delivery trauma accompanied by spinal or epidural anesthesia may impair bladder tone. If this occurs, the bladder may lose sensitivity, resulting in a diminished voiding urge. This contributes to postpartal urine retention.

Postpartal diuresis may cause bladder overdistention, stasis, and urine retention, possibly resulting in muscle damage, atony, and urinary tract infection. Without such complications, however, the lower urinary tract resumes normal function within 1 or 2 weeks as edema and diuresis resolve, although bladder distention may persist for 3 months.

Typically, dilation of the renal pelves, calyces, and ureters begins in the first trimester and progresses as pregnancy advances. Dilation of the renal pelves causes ureteral distention and slowing of urinary passage. Within the first 12 to 16 weeks postpartum, dilation resolves gradually, although some mild dilation may persist for years. Urinary frequency, urgency, and other symptoms caused by uterine pressure on the bladder resolve after delivery.

Reversal of functional changes
Pregnancy increases the renal plasma flow and the glomerular filtration rate (GFR). In late pregnancy, the GFR begins a gradual decline that continues into the postpartal period. Usually, the GFR returns to a nonpregnancy level by 6 weeks postpartum. Renal plasma flow also normalizes.

Urinalysis
Mild proteinuria, caused by excretion of protein by-products of uterine involution or trauma from delivery, is common after delivery but should disappear by 6 weeks postpartum. Glycosuria, another common postpartal finding, usually resolves by the end of the first week.

GASTROINTESTINAL SYSTEM
With the GI tract no longer obstructed by the expanding uterus and hormone levels declining rapidly, the GI tract quickly resumes normal function after delivery.

Appetite
After vaginal delivery, most patients are extremely hungry from lack of food intake and the exertion of labor and delivery—especially if little or no anesthesia was used. Appetite tends to subside to a normal level in 1 to 2 days, although a breast-feeding patient may maintain an increased appetite and food intake. After cesarean delivery, the patient whose appetite return is less pronounced may be started on a clear liquid diet and gradually advanced to a regular diet as GI function returns.

Bowel motility and evacuation
During pregnancy, GI motility is inhibited by the high serum progesterone level (which relaxes intestinal smooth muscle, decreasing peri-

stalsis) and by compressing the intestines with increased uterine size. With delivery resolving both factors, normal peristalsis and bowel function usually return rapidly. However, bowel motility may remain sluggish in cases of intestinal manipulation during cesarean delivery or use of anesthetic or analgesic agents.

Typically, bowel evacuation normalizes once bowel motility is restored. Nonetheless, the first bowel movement may be delayed until 2 to 3 days postpartum for reasons unrelated to intestinal function. The patient may avoid bowel evacuation, fearing it will cause pain or damage of the episiotomy. In many cases, a stool softener, laxative, or suppository may be used to reestablish normal bowel function.

Reversal of other changes

Gallbladder emptying, slowed during pregnancy, increases after delivery, reducing the risk of gallstones. The bile flow, hepatic work load, and hepatic blood flow decrease to nonpregnancy levels, and liver function studies should no longer be abnormal.

MUSCULOSKELETAL SYSTEM

Although pregnancy-related changes in the musculoskeletal system reverse after delivery, joints and muscles may show some residual effects.

Reversal of postural and joint changes

Delivery removes the mechanical strain on the musculoskeletal system and halts secretion of relaxin. Over the first 6 to 8 postpartal weeks, posture returns to normal and structural changes reverse gradually. The exact cause is unclear, but foot enlargement could be caused by the effects of relaxin on foot joints as well as weight gain and dependent edema that may persist. Thus, increased foot and shoe size tend to be a permanent reminder of pregnancy.

Reversal of muscular changes

Enlargement of breast and abdominal wall muscles during pregnancy weakens these structures. Although the damage is not permanent, many patients have trouble regaining satisfactory muscle tone in these areas.

During the third trimester, the rectus abdominus muscles may separate, causing diastasis recti abdominus. This condition sometimes can be corrected by postpartal abdominal exercises. However, it may persist indefinitely unless adequate muscle tone is restored. Poor abdominal muscle tone may contribute to back strain and low backache.

INTEGUMENTARY SYSTEM

Pregnancy-related skin changes resolve completely or partially after delivery as hormone levels decrease and the skin no longer is stretched.

Reversal of hormone–related changes

During the postpartal period, pigmentation changes caused by pregnancy—including chloasma (also called melasma, or mask of pregnancy) and linea nigra (a dark midline streak on the abdomen)—reverse gradually. However, they may never disappear completely. Pregnancy may stimulate pigmented nevi, causing them to enlarge or change color or leading to formation of new nevi. These changes tend to regress after delivery. Nevi that do not resume their prepregnancy appearance warrant further evaluation. Nipple darkening, also caused by pregnancy, reverses partially in the postpartal period. Any increased acne associated with pregnancy also resolves as hormone levels stabilize.

Pregnancy-related hirsutism also regresses. However, coarse hairs that arose during pregnancy tend to remain. Some patients complain of excessive hair loss from the head after delivery. This is a compensation for the below-normal loss during pregnancy; the postpartal loss is merely catching up with the loss that would have taken place without pregnancy. The catch-up process ends roughly 1 to 4 months postpartum.

Some vascular skin conditions observed in pregnant patients mimic those accompanying liver disease, such as spider angiomas and palmar erythema. Stemming from enhanced subcutaneous blood flow (caused by the increased serum estrogen level), these conditions disappear soon after delivery as the estrogen level falls. Changes in the mucous membranes during pregnancy—epistaxis, nasal edema with congestion, and bleeding of the gums—reverse as the estrogen level decreases. Some pregnant patients develop gingivitis, sometimes with small vascular nodules at the gum line. This condition, called epulis gravidarum, usually regresses within 1 to 2 months postpartum.

Striae or stretch marks result from increased corticosteroid levels and mechanical stretching of the skin during pregnancy. These harmless marks commonly appear over the abdomen, back, thighs, and breasts. As body size normalizes, striae shrink and fade within a year after delivery. Although they become less apparent, they never disappear completely.

Diaphoresis

In the first 2 to 3 days postpartum, many patients experience episodes of profuse diaphoresis. Associated with the postpartal fluid shift, diaphoresis is a normal mechanism that helps the renal system excrete excess fluid and waste products. It should resolve within the first postpartal week.

OTHER SYSTEMS

Metabolic, neurologic, and immunologic changes brought on by pregnancy reverse rapidly after delivery.

Metabolic system

Throughout pregnancy, the basal metabolic rate (BMR) rises until delivery, when it measures approximately 20% above normal. After delivery, the BMR decreases rapidly, approaching nonpregnancy levels by 5 to 6 days postpartum.

Neurologic system

Neurologic effects of pregnancy, which may range from minor to extremely bothersome, rarely linger after delivery.

Entrapment neuropathies

Among the most common neurologic changes caused by pregnancy, entrapment neuropathies are nerve compression disorders usually caused by fluid retention. As soft tissue becomes edematous, it exerts pressure on nerves within the tissue, causing such symptoms as numbness, tingling, and loss of function. For example, in carpal tunnel syndrome, the median nerve in the wrist is compressed. With the disappearance of edema after delivery, entrapment neuropathies usually resolve. In rare cases, surgery is required to release an entrapment.

Reversal of other changes

Other neurologic complaints during pregnancy include tension headache and syncopal or near-syncopal episodes. These conditions are associated with stress, decreased rest, poor nutritional status, increased blood glucose levels, and hormonal changes accompanying pregnancy. As delivery eliminates these factors, tension headaches and syncopal episodes diminish. With proper postpartal nutrition and rest, they disappear completely.

Immunologic system

Inhibited during pregnancy to prevent the body from rejecting the fetus as foreign matter, the immune system resumes normal function during the postpartal period. However, a patient lacking the Rh factor who delivers an Rh-positive neonate may become sensitized to the Rh antigen in neonatal RBCs and may produce Rh antibodies directed against the sensitizing antigen; this could cause problems in subsequent pregnancies. To prevent this, an Rh-negative patient must receive $Rh_o(D)$ immune globulin (RhoGAM) at 28 weeks of pregnancy and again within 72 hours after delivery.

17

NORMAL POSTPARTAL ADAPTATION

Caring for the postpartal patient offers the nurse an opportunity to promote a full and healthy recovery from delivery while helping the patient and her partner adapt to the birth of their child. As early discharge after delivery becomes increasingly common, skillful implementation of the nursing process takes on greater importance as a way for the nurse to meet the patient's physiologic, psychosocial, and teaching needs.

Assessment

Postpartal assessment begins with a review of the antenatal and intrapartal records. The nurse on the postpartal unit should make sure this information has been included in the report from the nurse who transferred the patient from the recovery unit. If the nurse is in a labor-delivery-recovery-postpartum unit, she should make sure that all information is documented on the chart. Throughout the patient's stay, the nurse must measure vital signs, determine the patient's comfort level, assess rest and sleep patterns, and evaluate the status of all body systems.

Vital signs

Obtain complete vital signs every 15 minutes for the first hour after delivery, then every hour for the next 4 hours or until vital signs are stable. Thereafter, obtain vital signs every 4 hours until 24 hours after delivery, then every 8 hours until discharge. Check the protocol of your facility to see if there are any other designated times to obtain these vital signs.

Temperature. Measure the patient's temperature orally. A slight temperature elevation from mild dehydration, caused by labor and delivery, is common during the first 24 hours after delivery. However, suspect infection if the patient has a morbid temperature, defined by the

Joint Committee on Maternal Welfare as temperature of 100.4° F (38° C) on any 2 successive postpartum days.

Pulse. The pulse may remain normal for an hour or so after delivery. During the first postpartal rest or sleep, which usually occurs 2 to 4 hours after delivery, the pulse rate typically decreases, possibly slowing to 50 beats/minute. This condition may persist for several days without ill effects and probably results from supine positioning and such normal physiologic phenomena as the postpartal increase in stroke volume and reduction in vascular bed size.

Transient tachycardia may occur during periods of excitement, incisional discomfort, or severe uterine contractions; usually, it is not a cause for concern. On the other hand, an abnormally rapid pulse may be an early sign of excessive blood loss—especially if the pulse is thready and the patient has such signs as pallor, an increased respiratory rate, and diaphoresis.

Respiratory rate. Although the respiratory rate rarely changes significantly after delivery, it may drop slightly during the first postpartal sleep or if the patient received a narcotic during labor. Like the pulse rate, the respiratory rate increases slightly during periods of excitement or discomfort. If it increases significantly, however, suspect uterine hemorrhage.

Blood pressure. Postpartal blood pressure should not differ significantly from the patient's average reading under normal circumstances. A gradual but persistent drop in blood pressure suggests excessive blood loss. A persistent elevation, especially when accompanied by edema, proteinuria, headache, blurred vision, and hyperactive reflexes, suggests pregnancy-induced hypertension (PIH), a potentially life-threatening disorder. Although most common during the antepartal period, PIH sometimes arises after delivery. To ensure prompt intervention, immediately report suspicious signs and symptoms to the doctor.

Keep in mind that certain drugs used during the intrapartal or the postpartal period may affect blood pressure. For instance, oxytocin, ergonovine, and methylergonovine may increase blood pressure.

Comfort level

Comfort is essential to the patient's postpartal recovery and adaptation to the role of new mother. However, even if she has uterine cramps, breast tenderness, or perineal discomfort, she may be too excited by the birth of her child to complain of discomfort. Stay alert for covert clues to discomfort, such as a change in vital signs, restlessness, inability to relax or sleep, facial grimaces, and a guarding posture.

Rest and sleep patterns

Fatigue is common during the first week after delivery. The tiring last few weeks of pregnancy, the exhausting work of labor and delivery, and dramatic hormonal changes contribute to postpartal fatigue. Assess the patient's rest and sleep patterns continually, keeping in mind that individual requirements for rest and sleep vary.

Reproductive system

Assess the uterus, lochia, and perineum every 15 minutes for the first hour after delivery, then hourly for at least 4 hours. Thereafter, assess every 8 hours until discharge.

Uterus. Immediately after the placenta is delivered, uterine involution should begin. A gradual process that restores the uterus to a nonpregnant state, involution involves contractions of the myometrium and self-disintegration of cells or tissue.

Assessment of the uterus helps in evaluating the progress of involution. Uterine muscle tone should be sufficient for muscles to compress vessels, thereby controlling bleeding.

To ensure accurate assessment of the uterus, ask the patient to void beforehand. Then locate the fundus, the rounded portion of the uterus above the level of the fallopian tube attachments. Just after delivery, the fundus should be located at or slightly above the midline at the level of the umbilicus. Each day thereafter, it should descend approximately 1 cm (about one fingerbreadth) toward the symphysis pubis, until about the 10th postpartal day, when it is no longer palpable as an abdominal organ. (See *Postpartal assessment techniques.*)

Next, assess the consistency of the uterus. It should feel firm. A soft, boggy uterus indicates uterine atony. This condition, which may lead to hemorrhage, most commonly results from bladder distention or excessive uterine enlargement. Multiple gestation, a macrosomic baby, and hydramnios cause overstretching of muscle fibers, which then cannot contract effectively to compress vessels. Other risk factors for uterine atony include a prolonged or accelerated labor, the use of oxytocin in labor, grand multiparity, history of postpartum hemorrhage, general anesthesia, and administration of magnesium sulfate.

If the patient has a boggy uterus, determine if it is caused by bladder distention. After delivery, the bladder may fill rapidly from postpartal diuresis, which eliminates the excess tissue fluid that accumulated during pregnancy as well as any I.V. fluids administered during labor. If bladder distention is responsible for the boggy uterus, expect the uterus to be displaced upward and to the right of the symphysis; also expect an increased lochial flow. Be sure to review the patient's labor and delivery history to check the time and amount of the last voiding or catheterization.

If the patient had a cesarean delivery, take great care when assessing the uterus. With a slow, gentle motion, press on the abdomen toward the uterus, avoiding sutures or staples. Inspect the incision site

PSYCHOMOTOR SKILLS

Postpartal assessment techniques

Through careful assessment, you can help ensure a normal postpartal recovery for the patient and prevent complications. During these assessments, provide maximum privacy and completely document each assessment. Take this time to educate the patient and answer her questions. To fully assess the patient and her condition, use the following techniques. Document all findings and make nursing diagnoses and plans based on your findings.

Assessing fundal position and bladder distention
To assess the position of the fundus place the right hand at the symphysis pubis to support the uterus while palpating the fundus with the left hand. Note the consistency of the uterus and check for vaginal bleeding at the same time. Document the fundal height in centimeters from the umbilicus and all other findings. Continue to palpate the fundus while observing the area of the bladder for any distention and check the patient's intake and output.

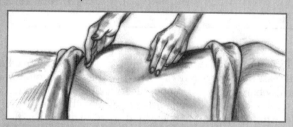

Inspecting the perineum
To evaluate for healing of an episiotomy, perineal lacerations, and the general condition of the perineum, inspect the perineum regularly, using the following technique.

Verify adequate lighting, put on disposable gloves, and position the woman appropriately. For optimal visualization with a side-lying patient, flex the top leg upward at the knee. Standing behind her, gently lift the upper buttock to expose the perineum and anus.

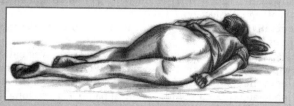

(continued)

Checking for Homans' sign

Coagulatory stimulation increases the risk of thromboembolism during the postpartal period. To assess for superficial thromboembolism, attempt to elicit Homans' sign.

Position the woman supine. With one hand supporting her knee, lift the leg and dorsiflex the foot toward the ankle. If this maneuver causes pain, suspect superficial thromboembolism.

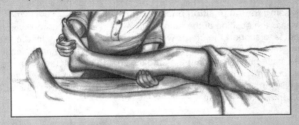

every 15 minutes for the first hour, once an hour for the next 4 hours, then at least once every 8 hours. Evaluate the site for color, warmth, edema, discharge, degree of approximation, and the condition of sutures, staples, dressing, or supportive abdominal binder.

Lochia. After the patient has delivered, lochia will begin to flow from the vagina. Normally, lochia progresses through stages marked by changes in its appearance. (See *Stages of lochia,* page 379.)

Assess the type and amount of lochia. Lochia should progress through the stages described without relapsing to an earlier stage. Evaluate the consistency of the discharge. Lochia should never contain large clots, tissue fragments, or membranes. If such material is passed, save all specimens for further evaluation. Also note the odor: normally, lochia has a fleshy, not foul, odor. A foul odor or absence of lochia may signal infection.

Generally the following classifications are used to describe the amount of lochia:

- scant: blood appears on a tissue only when the vaginal area is wiped or the stain on the perineal pad is less than 1″ long
- light: the stain on the perineal pad measures 1″ to 4″ long
- moderate: the stain on the perineal pad is 4″ to 6″ long
- heavy: the pad becomes saturated within 1 hour.

If the patient has a heavy lochial flow, begin a pad count to determine the amount of discharge more precisely. Record the number of pads used and the degree of saturation of each pad. To make lochial assessment more accurate, obtain the patient's cooperation by teaching her about the lochial stages, including how to monitor them and how to describe consistency and amount.

Expect a relatively light lochial flow in the post-cesarean patient because the uterine contents are evacuated thoroughly during this procedure. In contrast, lochial flow may be slightly heavier during and after breast-feeding sessions; the effects of oxytocin cause uterine contractions and subsequent expulsion of uterine contents. Also, lochial flow increases when the patient rises from a lying to a standing position; lochia may escape down the legs as accumulated discharge and small clots are released. Tell the patient to expect this so she will not become alarmed when it happens. To prevent her clothing from becoming stained, provide a hospital gown and disposable slippers.

Perineum. For accurate assessment of the perineum, arrange for adequate lighting and position the patient properly. The perineum can be easily visualized when the patient is lying in a lateral position with her top leg drawn up somewhat. Lifting the top buttock allows comfortable examination of the perineum.

An episiotomy or perineal laceration should appear to be healing with no exudate; the site should be clean and not excessively tender. Assess the approximation of the incision or wound and check for such abnormalities as redness, warmth, tenderness, edema, ecchymosis, discharge, and hemorrhoids. If the perineum is ecchymotic, exquisitely painful, and grossly discolored, with a collection of blood under the skin surface, suspect a hematoma and report this to the doctor.

Breasts. Breast inspection is an important part of nursing assessment during the first few days after delivery. With the patient supine and her bra removed, inspect the breasts for symmetry of size and shape. Then palpate in a circular direction as during a standard breast examination. Start by palpating the outer breast tissue, then move the fingers 1 cm toward the center of the breast and repeat. Continue with this pattern until all breast regions have been examined, noting any masses that may indicate infection or a blocked milk duct. If the breasts are tense, warm, boardlike, and painful, suspect breast engorgement, which results from transient lymphatic and venous stasis. To help determine appropriate interventions, assess the extent of engorgement. Also inspect the nipples for erectility, inflammation, tenderness, cracking, redness, and soreness.

If the patient has chosen to breast-feed her neonate, she should be able to breast-feed comfortably every 2 to 4 hours after delivery. Show the patient how to position the infant in various ways while breast-feeding, and teach her about breast care, proper latching-on, and correct removal of the infant's mouth from her breast. Colostrum, a thick, yellow liquid, is sufficient for the neonate's nutritional needs at this time. Also, the patient should be drinking an extra quart of fluids daily, increasing her food intake by 500 calories over her basic daily caloric needs, and wearing a support bra.

By the second or third postpartal day, the breast-feeding patient should begin to feel tingling and throbbing in her breasts and notice some release of mature milk when her breasts are stimulated or when she hears her neonate cry. This is called the "let-down" reflex. Mature milk is bluish in color with a thinner consistency than colostrum.

Urinary system

Assessment of urinary elimination patterns is a key component of postpartal nursing assessment. Despite rapid urine production and bladder filling after delivery, many patients have difficulty voiding. For example, the patient with severe perineal and urethral discomfort may not be able to relax the perineal muscles sufficiently to void; in the post-cesarean patient or a patient who received regional anesthesia, the bladder may lack sensitivity to pressure, impairing the urge to void.

Failure to void within 6 to 8 hours after delivery may cause excessive uterine bleeding because bladder distention prevents uterine contractions and subsequent vessel compression. When voiding finally does occur after a delay, it may be incomplete, with substantial urine remaining in the bladder. This condition, called urinary stasis, may contribute to urinary tract infection. A post-cesarean patient would have an indwelling urinary catheter in place for the immediate postpartal period but may have similar problems after its removal.

To evaluate the patient's bladder, palpate the suprapubic area. A full bladder is distended above the symphysis and can be palpated readily as a soft, movable mass. A uterus that is boggy, elevated, and deviated to one side supports the suspicion of a full bladder.

Once the patient is ambulatory and can perform satisfactory self-care, determine her urine output pattern. Note the time of each voiding and the amount voided, and ask if her bladder feels empty afterward. Also find out if she is experiencing urinary frequency, burning, or urgency.

Cardiovascular system

The hypervolemia of pregnancy protects the postpartal patient to some extent from the detrimental effects of blood loss during delivery. However, if the patient has lost more than 500 ml of blood, suspect uterine hemorrhage. Commonly, hemorrhage has a sudden onset. To ensure early detection and avert serious consequences, be sure to monitor vital signs and assess her lochia carefully. (See *Postpartal hemorrhage*.)

EMERGENCY ALERT

Postpartal hemorrhage

Postpartal hemorrhage, a leading cause of maternal mortality, demands prompt recognition and intervention to avert grave consequences. Normal blood loss at delivery is less than 500 ml. The nurse should suspect hemorrhage if the patient's estimated blood loss exceeds 500 ml. Hemorrhage is not always obvious; but may manifest as a slow but steady trickle of blood.

Postpartal hemorrhage commonly stems from uterine atony, lacerations of the cervix or vagina, or disseminated intravascular coagulation. Several weeks after delivery, the most common cause of hemorrhage is retention of placental fragments. Always be alert for postpartal hemorrhage with those patients at high risk.

If you suspect hemorrhage, notify the doctor or nurse-midwife immediately. Continually monitor the patient's vital signs, assess the condition of the uterus, evaluate the amount and character of lochia, and assess for bladder distention. Refer to the lists below to help identify signs of postpartal hemorrhage and prepare for appropriate interventions.

Signs
- Boggy (soft, pliable) uterus
- Excessively large uterus located above the umbilicus at the midline
- Excessive lochia, possibly containing large blood clots with or without tissue fragments
- Lochia that flows in a steady trickle
- Increased pulse and respiratory rate with decreased blood pressure

Nursing considerations
- Gently massage the uterus to stimulate contractions. Empty bladder as needed.
- Rapidly infuse oxytocin I.V. or administer carboprost, ergonovine, or methylergonovine by I.M. injection, as prescribed and as needed.
- Apply an ice pack to the fundus.
- Assess lochial flow to estimate the type and amount of blood loss and to detect any clots or tissue fragments. If lochia is bright red and flows in a slow trickle and the fundus is firm and located at the midline, suspect cervical or vaginal laceration as the cause of hemorrhage.
- Inspect for accumulated blood posterior to the perineum by turning the patient from side to side and checking for blood on bed sheets and the perineal pad.
- Position the patient flat on her back to facilitate circulation to vital organs.
- Make sure the blood bank has typed and cross-matched the patient for possible blood replacement. Check that the patient has no religious restrictions regarding blood replacement. If the patient's religion prohibits blood replacement, have a plasma expander ready for use if needed.
- As necessary, prepare the patient for surgery. Continuously update doctor or nurse-midwife regarding the patient's status.

Respiratory system

Assess the patient's respiratory rate, rhythm, and depth. Respiratory assessment is especially important if the patient had a prolonged labor or a complicated or surgical delivery or if she received an anesthesia that causes decreased sensation and motor activity. Because these circumstances increase the risk of respiratory complications, check for altered breathing patterns and poor gas exchange by auscultating the lungs every 4 hours for adventitious sounds, such as crackles and rhonchi. Evaluate the breathing pattern regularly until the respiratory rate normalizes and the lungs are free from adventitious sounds. Encourage the patient to breathe deeply and to cough, which helps clear the lungs. The doctor or nurse-midwife should be notified if abnormalities are heard.

Hematologic system

Usually, a complete blood count is performed 24 to 48 hours after delivery. Typically, the white blood cell (WBC) count is elevated, sometimes reaching 25,000/mm³ especially if the patient had a prolonged labor. Although the exact cause of this increase is unknown, it has been suggested that it may result from the pronounced energy expenditure and stress of labor and delivery. Consequently, an elevated WBC count is not a reliable marker of postpartal infection. However, when accompanied by other potential infection signs, it may help to confirm an infection.

Compare the postpartal hemoglobin level and hematocrit to the corresponding predelivery levels. If the postpartal hemoglobin level is more than 3 g/dl below the predelivery level, the patient is at risk for anemia; if it is 5 g/dl or more below the predelivery level, suspect heavy blood loss.

If the delivery was uncomplicated, measurement of coagulation factors usually is not necessary. Nonetheless, hypercoagulability may result if decreased plasma volume predisposes the postpartal patient to thromboembolic disease. To check for this condition, which most often affects the lower extremities as thrombophlebitis, have the patient lie supine with both legs extended. Inspect the legs for symmetry of shape and size, and palpate the thighs and calves to detect areas of warmth, edema, tenderness, redness, or hardness. Then attempt to elicit Homans' sign.

Gastrointestinal system

Assess the patient's progress toward reestablishing normal bowel function, documenting this progress daily. Bowel sounds should resume gradually on the first postpartal day. To determine the presence and quality of bowel sounds, assess the abdomen carefully in all four quadrants. Keep in mind that the post-cesarean patient may have diminished bowel sounds accompanied by abdominal distention and lack of peristalsis from immobility, surgical manipulation, and anesthesia.

Inspect the rectal area for hemorrhoids, which may cause redness, discomfort, and itching. Hemorrhoids may arise during pregnancy or from the expulsive effort of labor and delivery. Usually, they disappear in the first few postpartal weeks. Document the presence of hemorrhoids and any associated signs and symptoms. Comfort measures for this area include ice packs, xylocaine spray, witch hazel pads, sitz baths, Kegel exercises, and rectal hydrocortisone suppositories, as ordered.

Neurologic system

If the patient complains of headache, check for other signs and symptoms associated with PIH, edema, proteinuria, blurred vision, increased blood pressure, and hyperactive reflexes. Try to determine the onset, intensity, duration, and location of the headache and find out if any specific factors seem to trigger or relieve it. Keep in mind that in a patient who received some types of regional anesthesia, such as a spinal block, a postspinal headache may result from loss of cerebrospinal fluid through the dural puncture site.

During the first 4 hours after delivery, the patient who received regional anesthesia should regain full sensory and motor function. Occasionally, however, residual neurologic effects may occur. To assess for the return of sensation and movement, ask the patient to move her lower extremities and to report the level of feeling present. As sensation and motor function return, the patient may report a heightened awareness of discomfort and may need further evaluation to determine the need for pain relief. Once the cause of the headache or other discomfort is pinpointed, the nurse can administer nonpharmacologic and pharmacologic measures to reduce the patient's discomfort.

Musculoskeletal system

Assess breast and abdominal muscle tone, which commonly is diminished from overstretching and the effects of increased hormone levels during pregnancy. In some cases, the abdomen has become so stretched that the rectus abdominus muscles, which lie side-by-side, separate at the midline. This condition, called diastasis recti abdomini, rarely warrants treatment.

Many postpartal patients are concerned about poor muscle tone and eager to regain their prepregnancy figure. When conducting the assessment, provide an opening for the patient to express such concerns and recommend appropriate exercises.

Immune system

Detection of postpartal infection is a primary nursing concern. In most cases, such infection involves the reproductive system. Besides regularly assessing the patient's temperature, observe closely for subtle signs and symptoms of infection, such as chills, malaise, and pallor. Also review the patient's chart for risk factors for puerperal infection, such as prolonged labor, prolonged time since rupture of the membranes, vaginal or cervical lacerations, retention of placental fragments, and history of sexually transmitted diseases.

The patient who received regional anesthesia has an increased risk of infection because of the invasive administration route used. Regularly inspect the spinal or epidural site for redness, warmth, edema, pain, and tenderness; promptly report any of these signs to the doctor.

Also review the patient's chart to assess her Rh status and rubella status.

Psychosocial status

The postpartal nurse has a unique opportunity to assess the patient's and her partner's response to childbirth and to evaluate their interaction with the neonate. Typically, they focus initially on the neonate's sex, size, and facial similarities to their older children or to other relatives. Many facilities provide a place on the nursing record to describe parent-neonate interaction. Be sure to document this regularly.

Nursing diagnosis

After gathering assessment data, the nurse must review it carefully to identify pertinent nursing diagnoses for the patient. (See Appendix 1, NANDA taxonomy of nursing diagnoses.)

Planning and implementation

After assessing the patient and formulating nursing diagnoses, the nurse develops and implements a plan of care. When the patient arrives on the postpartal unit, identify her by checking her identification band carefully.

Provide a brief orientation to the unit, including such information as where the bathroom, telephone, and personal supplies are located and what time meals are served. Review visiting hours and rooming-in policy. If visiting hours are limited, promote compliance by explaining that such limits are imposed for the patient's and neonate's well-being. Also make sure the patient understands why visitors must comply with infection-prevention measures, such as washing hands and putting on cover gowns before handling the neonate.

Ensuring safety

Various factors may contribute to weakness and lightheadedness for the first few hours after delivery, leading to a nursing diagnosis of *risk for injury related to blood loss, fatigue, limited food intake, or med-*

ication effects. Consequently, advise the patient to call for help when getting out of bed for the first time. Also show her how to raise or lower the bed rails. To prevent injury to the neonate, caution her against falling asleep in bed with the neonate.

If the patient received regional anesthesia, she may have impaired motor or sensory function in the lower extremities. To guarantee safety, make sure all functions have returned to a satisfactory level and that her vital signs are stable before helping her out of bed.

Providing for adequate sleep and rest

For an hour or so after delivery, the patient may be too excited to sleep or rest, despite her fatigue. Within a few hours, however, she may fall into a deep, although short, sleep. This sleep is especially crucial for the patient who is recovering from a cesarean delivery or a prolonged, difficult labor and delivery. For the patient with a nursing diagnosis of *fatigue related to pregnancy, labor, and delivery,* help determine rest and sleep requirements and encourage her to limit visitors and telephone calls. The patient may choose to have the neonate room-in with her. If she is undecided about rooming-in, inform her that this arrangement does not necessarily disrupt sleep.

Promoting uterine involution and preventing hemorrhage

The uterus should have sufficient tone after delivery to contract effectively so that vessels are compressed and involution proceeds normally. If the patient has a boggy, or atonic, uterus, monitor her vital signs closely because hemorrhage can have a sudden onset. Interventions for uterine atony may vary with the underlying cause.

Facilitating voiding. If uterine atony stems from bladder distention, make every effort to keep the patient's bladder empty. Within the first 4 hours after delivery, encourage her to walk to the bathroom; if she is confined to bed, offer a bedpan. Other nursing interventions that promote spontaneous voiding include turning on the faucet in the patient's bathroom, irrigating the perineum, placing the patient's hands in water, and providing plenty of fluids.

Failure to void within 8 hours of delivery or bladder distention necessitates urinary catheterization. Fortunately, many patients regain normal urinary elimination patterns after just a single catheterization. If the patient requires catheterization, be sure to use sterile technique to minimize the risk of infection. Catheterization during the early postpartal period can cause more discomfort than usual because of the edematous, bruised condition of the bladder, urethra, urinary meatus, labia, and perineum. Conduct this procedure with extreme gentleness and privacy, offering appropriate explanations.

Massaging the uterus. When uterine atony does not stem from bladder distention, gentle massage of the uterus may be sufficient to stimulate uterine contractions, restoring firm tone. The perineum should be visualized while massaging the uterus to observe the expulsion of any lochia or clots that may have accumulated. It is important to empty the uterus of clots and blood so it can contract properly. The nurse should teach the patient how to massage her own uterus.

Administering oxytocin. If massage fails to induce contractions, expect to administer an I.V. oxytocin preparation or I.M. carboprost. (See *Drugs used during the postpartal period*.) If hemorrhage occurs despite drug therapy, expect the patient to undergo surgical exploration and evacuation of the uterus.

Relieving discomfort from uterine contractions

The severity of uterine contractions or afterpains typically varies with parity. In the primiparous patient, afterpains may not be noticeable; in the multiparous patient, they may cause severe discomfort. Because breast-feeding promotes the release of oxytocin, the breast-feeding patient typically has more severe afterpains during and after feeding sessions. For the patient with a nursing diagnosis of pain related to uterine contractions, expect to administer a mild analgesic (such as acetaminophen with codeine) or a nonsteroidal anti-inflammatory drug (such as ibuprofen). Having the patient lie prone, on her abdomen, also relieves uterine discomfort.

Reducing perineal discomfort

Perineal lacerations or an episiotomy may cause considerable pain, possibly leading to a nursing diagnosis of ***pain related to the perineal wound***. An ice pack applied to the perineum in the first few hours after delivery numbs the area and helps soothe it by constricting vessels and reducing the vascular response of inflammation.

Warmth may be applied to the perineum 12 to 24 hours after delivery. Warmth causes vasodilation, which relieves discomfort and edema and promotes the local inflammatory response by hastening the arrival of leukocytes and antibodies at the site. A warm sitz bath can provide the necessary warmth. Typically, the patient takes this treatment three or four times daily, with each bath lasting 15 to 20 minutes. The patient may continue this until the discomfort has diminished or the perineum has healed. To ensure that the patient can self-administer the bath correctly, provide complete instructions and demonstration.

A topical spray or ointment also may be applied to relieve perineal discomfort. A topical spray may be an anesthetic, which provides local pain relief, or a steroid, which reduces edema and promotes healing.

(*Text continues on page 408.*)

SELECTED MAJOR DRUGS

Drugs used during the postpartal period

These major drugs are currently used during the postpartal period.

MAJOR INDICATIONS	USUAL ADULT DOSAGES	NURSING IMPLICATIONS
codeine		
Mild to moderate postpartal pain	15 to 60 mg P.O. every 4 hours as needed (usually given with 325 to 650 mg of acetaminophen)	• Monitor respiratory and circulatory status and bowel function. • Observe the patient for drowsiness; make sure she is alert when caring for her neonate.
diphenhydramine (Benadryl)		
Nighttime sedation	50 mg P.O. at bedtime	• Observe the patient for drowsiness; make sure she is alert when caring for her neonate. • Assess the patient for nausea and dry mouth.
docusate sodium (Colace)		
Stool softener	50 to 200 mg P.O. daily or until bowel movements are normal	• Assess the patient for bowel activity, mild abdominal cramping, and diarrhea.
ergonovine maleate (Ergotrate Maleate)		
Prevention or treatment of postpartal hemorrhage from uterine atony or subinvolution	0.2 mg I.M. every 2 to 4 hours to a maximum of five doses; after the initial I.M. dose, may give 0.2 to 0.4 mg P.O. every 6 to 12 hours for 2 to 7 days	• Monitor blood pressure, pulse rate, and uterine response. This medication can increase blood pressure and pulse; it should be used prudently in selective cases. Report sudden changes in vital signs, frequent periods of uterine relaxation,

(continued)

Drugs used during the postpartal period *(continued)*

MAJOR INDICATIONS	USUAL ADULT DOSAGES	NURSING IMPLICATIONS
ergonovine maleate (Ergotrate Maleate) *(continued)*		
		• and any change in the character or amount of lochia. • If ordered for severe uterine bleeding, dilute I.V. preparation to a volume of 5 ml with normal saline solution and administer over at least 1 minute while blood pressure and uterine contractions are monitored. • Contractions begin 5 to 15 minutes after P.O. administration, 2 to 5 minutes after I.M. injection, or immediately after I.V. injection. They may continue 3 hours or more after P.O. or I.M. administration, 45 minutes after I.V. injection.
ibuprofen (Motrin)		
Mild to moderate postpartal pain	400 mg P.O. every 4 to 6 hours	• Assess the patient for signs and symptoms of GI irritation, such as nausea, vomiting, diarrhea, and gastric discomfort. • Warn the patient not to take more than 1.2 g/day without consulting her doctor.
meperidine (Demerol)		
Moderate to severe postpartal pain	50 to 100 mg P.O., I.M., or S.C. every 3 to 4 hours; or 15 to 35 mg/hour by continuous I.V. infu-	• Monitor the patient's pulse rate. • Check for signs of central nervous system (CNS) depression such as drowsiness or lethargy. Make sure the patient is alert when caring for her neonate.

SELECTED MAJOR DRUGS

Drugs used during the postpartal period *(continued)*

MAJOR INDICATIONS	USUAL ADULT DOSAGES	NURSING IMPLICATIONS
meperidine (Demerol) *(continued)*		
	sion as needed or around the clock	• Assess the patient's pain level. • To avoid toxic metabolites, give the smallest effective dosage.
methylergonovine (Methergine)		
Prevention and treatment of postpartal hemorrhage from uterine atony or subinvolution	0.2 mg I.M. every 2 to 4 hours for a maximum of 5 doses; after the initial I.M. dose, 0.2 mg P.O. every 6 to 8 hours for a maximum of 7 days	• Monitor and record blood pressure, pulse rate, and uterine response. Report any sudden change in vital signs, frequent periods of uterine relaxation, and any change in lochia. • Decrease the dosage if severe cramping occurs. • Contractions begin 5 to 15 minutes after P.O. administration, 2 to 5 minutes after I.M. injection. They continue 3 hours or more.
morphine		
Severe pain	4 to 15 mg S.C. or I.M.; may be injected by slow I.V. infusion (over 4 to 5 minutes)	• Monitor for respiratory depression and hypotension. • Check for signs of CNS depression. Make sure the patient is alert when caring for her neonate. • Drug may be injected into epidural space for prolonged pain relief. Monitor patient for delayed respiratory depression. • If the patient has pruritus after I.V. or epidural administration, expect to give antihistamines.

(continued)

SELECTED MAJOR DRUGS

Drugs used during the postpartal period (continued)

MAJOR INDICATIONS	USUAL ADULT DOSAGES	NURSING IMPLICATIONS
oxytocin (Pitocin)		
Reduction of postpartal bleeding after expulsion of the placenta	1 to 4 ml (10 to 40 units) in 1,000 ml of dextrose 5% in water or normal saline solution I.V., infused at a rate necessary to control bleeding (usually 20 to 40 milliunits/minute); or 10 units I.M.	• Administer by I.V. infusion, not I.V. bolus injection. • Record uterine contractions, heart rate, and blood pressure every 15 minutes. • Assess the amount and character of lochia and the condition of the fundus. • Check for increased pulse rate in response to pain from contractions.
simethicone (Mylicon)		
Flatulence, functional gastric bloating	40 to 125 mg after each meal and at bedtime	• Make sure the patient chews tablets thoroughly. • Assess the patient for bowel activity and abdominal distention.

Other measures to reduce perineal discomfort include using mild analgesia, witch hazel compresses, and a commercial water and disinfectant spray. Kegel exercises can also decrease pain and increase circulation, which speeds healing.

To keep the perineal region clean, show the patient how to use a perineal irrigation or squirt bottle after each voiding. The patient fills the bottle with warm water, then aims it at the perineum to rinse off any urine or lochia remaining on the surface.

Ensuring lactation success and milk production

Lactation begins as a normal response to delivery of the baby and placenta in all mothers postpartally unless effectively suppressed. For breast-feeding mothers, the two physiologic mechanisms of milk production include milk production and milk secretion or let-down. Colostrum—a thick, yellow fluid high in proteins, minerals and immunoglobulins—is initially produced and is sufficient for the neonate's needs for the first 2 to 3 days of life. The next stage of milk production involves the milk "coming in" at around 3 to 4 days postpartum. Mature milk is produced by 14 to 16 days postpartum.

Lactation is not completely understood but is an exquisite series of events that begin with the placenta's delivery, are stimulated by the neonate's suckling, and continue to produce milk by a supply and demand system. Breast milk may appear thin but is species-specific for the neonate. Breast milk has also been shown to prevent infections, thus decreasing neonatal diarrhea and GI infections.

As much as the breast-fed baby can be protected by breast milk it could also be in danger of problems due to the mother's health status and abusive behaviors. For example, the human immunodeficiency virus and various drugs (legal and illegal) can be passed from the mother to the baby in breast-milk. The nurse must be aware of this and should consult a pharmacologic specialist or guide before administering any medications to a breast-feeding mother. Furthermore, the mother should be taught about the effects of drugs on both herself and her infant. The nurse may find it necessary to refer a mother for professional counseling as indicated.

For the mother who wants to breast-feed, the nurse must teach her about supply and demand, how emotions can change her milk production, the importance of proper latching-on by the infant, and comfort measures she can use as needed. Comfort measures the patient can use include:

- Applying warm packs to her breasts or taking a warm shower to increase the let-down reflex and soothe sore areas.
- Applying a few drops of breast milk to her nipples and air-drying them between nursing sessions to decrease sore and cracked nipples.
- Properly removing the infant from the breast by gently breaking the suction to decrease tenderness.
- Wearing a supportive bra to increase her comfort.
- Alternating positions of the baby at different feedings to ensure that all areas of the breast are emptied.
- Using her hands to massage any reddened areas will help to decrease clogged milk ducts and reduce the risk of the breast infection known as mastitis.

Teach the patient to contact her health care provider if one or both breasts are extremely tender or red or if her temperature is 100.8° or greater, as these are signs of an infection.

Ensuring lactation suppression

For the mother who chooses to bottle-feed her neonate, lactation is suppressed naturally. Usually lactation ceases within 1 week.

The patient must avoid any stimulation of the breasts and nipples. She should understand that breast-feeding is a supply and demand system; once the demand decreases, the supply decreases and eventually stops. Teaching the patient that she can decrease breast stimulation by wearing a supportive bra 24 hours a day for 1 to 2 weeks, discontinuing any manual expression or massage of the breasts, and by putting ice packs on her breasts at regular intervals and no warmth to the breasts. Most importantly, give the patient ongoing reassurance that the system will work and her milk production will subside.

Promoting respiratory stability

Monitor the patient's respiratory rate and effort. For the postcesarean patient, who may have a nursing diagnosis of *ineffective breathing pattern related to immobility following cesarean delivery*, carry out measures that promote effective breathing patterns, thereby reducing the risk of pneumonia or atelectasis. For instance, have her cough and deep-breathe hourly after teaching her how to support her abdomen in order to decrease discomfort; remind her to turn every 1 to 2 hours to promote oxygenation and prevent skin breakdown. Within a few hours after delivery, teach her how to use an incentive spirometer. This device maintains lung expansion and mobilizes secretions. Also, assist her in sitting on the edge of her bed and getting out of bed as soon as possible to increase lung capacity.

Preventing hematologic complications

If the patient has a subnormal hemoglobin level and hematocrit, she has anemia. For a severely anemic patient, expect the doctor to order a blood transfusion. In less serious circumstances, provide a diet rich in iron, minerals, and vitamins and teach the patient how to prevent anemia. Generally, the patient is encouraged to continue her prenatal vitamins for at least 4 to 6 weeks until her postpartal visit.

Because the postpartal patient—especially the multiparous patient—is at risk for thrombophlebitis, stress the importance of early, moderate exercise. Unless the patient received high doses of analgesias or anesthesias during labor and delivery, she should be able to walk around within a few hours of delivery. Also, instruct in how to prevent blood stasis in the calves by wearing foot coverings that do not constrict at the knee, elevating her legs on a stool from time to time when sitting, and to avoid crossing her legs at the knee.

Promoting bowel elimination

Although bowel function usually returns to normal rapidly after delivery, various factors may hinder bowel elimination. To help avoid a nursing diagnosis of *constipation related to poor intestinal tone, diminished food intake, and immobility*, encourage early ambulation, plenty of fluids, and a well-balanced, high-fiber diet. Also advise the patient to act on any urge to defecate, taking adequate time to sit on the toilet at the time when her bowel movements normally occur. If she is reluctant to attempt a bowel movement out of fear that it will tear open her episiotomy suture line, reassure her that she will not damage the repaired wound by bearing down gently. The doctor or nurse midwife may order a stool softener to make the first postpartal bowel movement easier.

After the first few postpartal hours, the patient may be hungry and thirsty. Provide cool liquids and a light meal, regardless of the time of day, and encourage her to drink 1 or 2 quarts of fluid daily to replace fluids lost during labor and delivery.

Relieving abdominal distention and flatus accumulation

The postcesarean patient may complain of abdominal distention accompanied by flatus accumulation. Interventions for this problem include insertion of a rectal tube in the distal colon to help expel flatus or suppositories to promote bowel activity and subsequent flatus expulsion. Also, the doctor or nurse-midwife may order simethicone, which reduces flatus accumulation.

Encourage early ambulation and slow resumption of oral intake, beginning with ice chips and progressing to a liquid, then regular, diet. Advise the patient to avoid carbonated beverages and gas-forming foods such as cabbage, asparagus, and brussels sprouts.

Relieving hemorrhoidal discomfort

If the patient has hemorrhoids, assure her that the acute discomfort should last only 2 to 3 days. In the meantime, apply soothing witch hazel compresses, ice packs, or an anesthetic or steroid-based cream, or administer anti-hemorrhoidal suppositories. Other measures that help relieve hemorrhoidal discomfort include mild analgesics, sitz baths, sitting on a foam ring, and a side-lying position. Sometimes the hemorrhoid discomfort can be reduced by pushing the inflamed tissues back into the rectum with a finger cot or a gloved, lubricated finger; if appropriate, teach the patient how to do this herself. Teach her how to perform Kegel exercises to reduce hemorrhoids as well.

Avoiding neurologic complications

The patient who received spinal anesthesia may develop postspinal headache. If so, position her flat; or, if she is permitted to lie on her side, make sure her head is elevated no more than 30 degrees. Make sure she remains supine for 8 to 10 hours after anesthesia administration or as long as identified in the facility's anesthesia protocols. Monitor her response to positioning; if she reports that the headache has worsened, lower the head of the bed. Because fluid replacement helps prevent postspinal headache, monitor fluid intake in a patient at risk for this problem.

When headache results from PIH, interventions may include bed rest and administration of magnesium sulfate or sedatives. Monitor her blood pressure as well.

Correcting musculoskeletal deficits

Beginning immediately after delivery, suggest mild exercises to improve muscle tone, such as arm, head, and shoulder raises or deep abdominal breathing with contraction of the abdominal muscles. Within a few days of delivery, the patient may begin abdominal exercises, alternately contracting and relaxing the abdominal muscles to reduce the diastisus recti. As a general rule, lochial flow increases with stress, overexertion, and fatigue. Advise her to reduce or stop exercising if lochial flow increases or if she becomes uncomfortable or fatigued.

Ensuring adequate immunologic status

If the patient has signs and symptoms of postpartal infection, expect to administer antibiotics and to carry out measures to minimize or reverse any precipitating factors, such as anemia.

To prevent isoimmunization, all Rh-negative pregnant women now receive Rh immune globulin (RhoGAM) during or near the 28th week of pregnancy. Cord blood is sampled after delivery to determine the neonate's Rh status. If the neonate is Rh-positive, make sure the mother receives an additional RhoGAM injection within 72 hours of delivery, even if she received a prenatal injection.

If the mother's antenatal rubella titer test is less than 1:10, she lacks immunity. She should be immunized before discharge. If she will receive the live vaccine (Meruvax II), warn her to avoid becoming pregnant for 3 months after immunization. Caution is advised if the mother is breast-feeding and needs this immunization. At this time, there is no adequate data on the vaccine's effect on the neonate. A few rare neonatal rubella cases have implicated this vaccine as the cause. It has been found that the active virus is secreted in breast milk and can cause the neonate to contract rubella.

Promoting psychosocial adaptation

Postpartal hospitalization provides the patient and her partner with an opportunity to adjust to their new role as parents and to review and receive information and feedback about the childbirth experience. The nurse should encourage the patient to express her feelings about the experience. (See *Assessing psychosocial adaptation*, page 414.) The patient's progression through the stages of maternal adaptation should be noted, including evaluation of her emotional status and any signs of postpartal depression. If the patient does not have a partner, identify a support person with whom she can share her feelings. If appropriate, suggest that the patient's partner participate in a fathers' support group to help him learn child-care skills and coping strategies and to provide a forum in which he can express his feelings

Provide the patient with positive feedback about her behavior during labor and delivery and her ongoing acquisition of parenting skills. If she has a negative perspective about the childbirth experience based on a misperception, provide a brief explanation to clarify the situation and promote positive feelings.

Adolescent patients pose a special challenge. To promote psychosocial adaptation, the nurse must understand adolescent behavior—especially the drive for independence, which plays a major role in adolescent judgment and decision making. A nonjudgmental approach is essential to developing a positive relationship with this adolescent, and may necessitate self-exploration of the nurse's own feelings and attitudes toward adolescent sexuality, pregnancy, and motherhood.

Promoting positive parent-neonate interaction

Positive interaction between the parents and neonate promotes healthy bonding. Such interaction depends on the ability of both parties to send, receive, and interpret messages correctly.

Optimal conditions for interaction. The best time for interaction is when both the parent and neonate are rested, focused, and attentive; preferably, the neonate should be in a quiet, alert state. The first period of reactivity may be such a time.

Health also is important. Prematurity or illness may restrict the neonate's ability to interact. Likewise, if the mother is fatigued or suffering postpartal discomfort or complications, her desire, energy, and attention for interacting may be limited. Under these conditions, bonding may take longer to achieve. Furthermore, it is important for the mother to understand that a neonate has optimal focusing of his or her eyes at 18 to 20 inches from the subject. If the baby is closer than that, it may attempt to pull away, giving the appearance of disinterest in interacting with that person.

Assessing psychosocial adaptation

Depending on the patient's and family's circumstances, the nurse may ask questions similar to those below to determine how the mother feels about her neonate and how she perceives her family's responses to the birth of the neonate. Rationales are given to explain the purpose of each question.

How do you feel about being a parent to this infant?
Rationale: This question gives the mother a chance to express her concerns about parenting. The answer may reveal problems in bonding or in adaptation to the parental role. The remaining questions may help pinpoint some of her concerns.

How do you feel about your infant's behavior?
Rationale: If the mother perceives the behavior as troublesome or abnormal, mother-infant interaction may be in jeopardy and the neonate may be at risk for abuse.

Does your infant look the way you expected?
Rationale: If the mother perceives the neonate as unattractive or as having the "wrong" features, interaction may be compromised.

How do you feel about having a boy (or girl)?
Rationale: If the mother was anticipating a child of the opposite sex, she will need to grieve over the loss of the fantasy child before she can bond with the real child.

Is the infant's father pleased with the infant?
Rationale: The mother who receives and perceives support from the neonate's father has a better chance for a healthy adaptation to the parenting role.

Does the infant's father plan on helping you at home?
Rationale: The father who participates in child care or household tasks shows positive adaptation to his new role and tasks. This may promote the mother's adaptation.

How do you feel about having someone help you at home?
Rationale: Rejection of help or other indications of possessiveness toward the neonate may signify a problem in adaptation.

How do your other children feel about this infant?
Rationale: This question gives the mother a chance to express any concerns she may have about the neonate's siblings. If the siblings are having problems adjusting to a new brother or sister, the mother may need help coping.

What have the baby's grandparents said about this infant?
Rationale: Failure of the grandparents to accept the neonate or to offer emotional support to the mother may make it difficult for her to adapt to the parental role.

Neonatal attentiveness and temperament. By altering the degree of attentiveness to stimuli, the neonate can affect the interaction with the parent. A neonate who is attentive and responsive rewards the parent's interactive efforts; this encourages the parent to continue such interaction. Thus, the more attentive and responsive the neonate, the more frequently the parent will interact.

Temperament also plays a part. A neonate who smiles frequently, eats well, is easy to console, and remains alert for long periods is more pleasant to interact with than one who is irritable and difficult to console. Parents should be counseled about both types of temperaments and given suggestions about how to deal with each.

Communication cues, reciprocity, and synchrony. The neonate presents predictable, behaviorally organized communication cues that reflect neonatal needs and normally elicit a response from the parent or other caregiver. Prematurity, illness, temperament, and other factors can affect a neonate's ability to send communication cues.

Parental sensitivity to neonatal cues is essential to the developing parent-child relationship. As part of this relationship, parents also exhibit communication cues that elicit a response from the neonate. Parents typically vary in their ability to interpret neonatal cues and respond appropriately.

Communication cues can be verbal or nonverbal. Verbal cues used by neonates include crying and cooing. Nonverbal cues include reaching movements, facial expressions, staring, and gaze aversion due to boredom or overstimulation. By refusing to focus on the person offering stimulation, the neonate signals that he or she does not want additional stimulation at that time.

The process by which the neonate gives cues and the parent interprets and responds to these cues is known as reciprocity. Through reciprocity, which may take several weeks to develop, the interaction is maintained and the parent-neonate relationship develops.

Appropriate action and reaction to cues by parents and neonate is called synchrony. A synchronous, reciprocal interaction is mutually rewarding and is ideally established within the first few weeks of delivery.

Verbal communication and entrainment. At first, parent-neonate communication takes on unique qualities. Mothers often speak to their neonates as they held them in the en face position. To soothe a neonate, parents frequently speak softly and slowly; to gain the neonate's attention, they use fast, high-pitched speech. Parents also use such games as "peek-a-boo" to communicate with their neonate verbally.

Healthy neonates move in rhythm with adult speech. This phenomenon, known as entrainment, is essential to parent-infant bonding, rewarding the parent and encouraging further communication. Entrainment continues as the child learns speech.

Nonverbal interaction. To interact nonverbally, parents may imitate the neonate's facial expressions. This helps the neonate develop communication skills by demonstrating that the parent responds to nonverbal interaction and that nonverbal behaviors have a meaning between people.

Initial touching between mother and neonate often progresses in a typical pattern. First, the mother touches the neonate with her fingertips only; then, she progresses to whole-hand touching, and finally embraces the neonate with her arms. Primiparous and multiparous women demonstrate the same progression, although the latter progress to the embrace more rapidly.

One study found that fathers use the same touching pattern; in a later study, they found that medical students also used this pattern, even though they were unrelated to the neonates with whom they were interacting. These findings suggest that such touching is a human behavior pattern not restricted to parents.

Nursing care. Observe the patient and neonate together and assess their interaction. If possible, observe them during a feeding session; this is when the mother and neonate are most likely to interact. To ensure accuracy, assess interaction on at least two occasions; if the mother is fatigued or in discomfort during one assessment, her behavior may give a false impression.

Note the amount of eye contact between the mother and neonate. Does she pay more attention to the observer or the neonate? Also note whether she holds the neonate close or at a distance, and assess the quality of her touch. Does she stroke, kiss, and fondle the neonate, or is her touch rough, quick, and unaffectionate? Does she talk to, smile at, or sing to the neonate when changing the diaper? These behaviors show that the mother acknowledges the neonate's presence and seeks a response.

Listen to the mother talk to her neonate. Does she speak directly in a soothing or playful way? If her tone is continually demanding or rejecting, try to identify the cause.

Find out if the mother worries about the neonate when the two are apart and if she believes the neonate knows her voice and notices her presence. Also pay close attention to her comments about the neonate. Does she express pleasure and satisfaction with the way her child is feeding? How does she talk about the neonate's characteristics? Note whether she uses "claiming" expressions such as "He's got his daddy's eyes." The patient who claims her child has reconciled the real child with the "fantasy" child and has placed the child within the family context; this shows that interaction has begun. Other indications of claiming include referring to the neonate as "my baby" or "our baby" and calling the neonate by name rather than "it."

Also listen for attribution of negative personality traits to the neonate for example, such statements as, "This baby is so stubborn; she just won't breast-feed." Lack of interaction also may be signaled by such comments as, "He's mad at me today" or, "She doesn't like me." In some cases, the mother may state that the neonate prefers to be held by someone other than herself. Expression of continued disappointment with the neonate's gender or physical appearance also warns of a relationship at risk.

Promoting psychosocial adaptation in special-needs patients
Special-needs patients include adolescent and older mothers and those with sensory, mental, or physical disabilities. Teaching should be adjusted appropriately for each particular patient and her level of understanding.

Expect the adolescent to have a greater need for teaching about neonatal and infant care. Ask how she plans to care for her child after discharge. If her arrangements seem inadequate, refer her to the appropriate resources.

The first-time mother over age 30 may feel anxious about her caregiving skills and her changing role. Particularly if she gave up a career to have a child, she may have a nursing diagnosis of **parental role conflict related to the birth of a new family member.** Urge this patient to express her feelings about becoming a mother; if appropriate, refer her for counseling.

A patient with a disability may need individualized nursing care to ease the transition to parenthood. (See *Helping the disabled patient adapt to parenthood*, pages 418 and 419.) However, she may have adequate services and support systems already in place. The nurse must evaluate each case individually and involve the entire health care team as indicated.

Implementing patient teaching
The trend toward early discharge has made postpartal teaching increasingly important. Maternal teaching may be carried out by the postpartal nurse or a nurse who provides follow-up care at home after early discharge.

Teaching should focus on self-care and neonatal care. The former include such topics as postpartal danger signs, rest, nutrition, and exercises. (See *Self-care after discharge*, pages 420 and 421.)

Especially for the patient with a nursing diagnosis of **knowledge deficit related to self-care or parenting skills,** consider using both

Helping the disabled patient adapt to parenthood

Most disabled patients can develop a full, rewarding parenting role. Nursing care for these patients and their families necessitates extra creativity, empathy, and emotional support, with emphasis on communication and individualized interventions.

The nurse will often need to change the plan of care to fit the patient's specific situation. Extra time is needed to assess the level of intervention needed for the patient, and to ensure that she sufficiently understands all the nurse has taught.

Vision-impaired patient
Although a vision-impaired patient cannot make eye contact with her neonate, she can use other senses to develop a bond. Give her the opportunity to touch, hear, and smell the neonate. Be sure to provide a thorough orientation to the surroundings, because the health care facility is an unfamiliar environment.

To help the mother feel comfortable and confident when performing physical caregiving tasks, describe the motions involved. For example, when teaching her how to wrap the neonate in a blanket, describe the process step by step. Have her feel the position of the blanket and neonate at each stage, then guide her as she performs the actions, giving her ample time to become familiar with each step through touch.

Hearing-impaired patient
When working with a hearing-impaired patient, first determine if she can read lips or use sign language. The nurse who does not know sign language should seek help from a knowledgeable resource person. In some cases, a magic slate or tablet and pen can be used to communicate. Be aware that federal law stipulates that facilities receiving federal funds must provide alternative ways of communicating with hearing-impaired patients.

Although the mother cannot hear her neonate, she may be able to feel sound vibrations. If she can vocalize, encourage her to do so with the neonate. Also consider recommending that she obtain a device that converts sound waves into a flashing light signal; this device can be placed on the nursery door at home to alert the mother when the child is crying.

Mentally impaired patient
A multidisciplinary team approach incorporating family and community support is required to address the needs of this mother and her child. Unless severely impaired, the mentally impaired mother can learn caregiving skills. If her social, communication, daily living, and independent living skills have not been assessed, refer her to the appropriate professional for evaluation.

Helping the disabled patient adapt to parenthood *(continued)*

If the patient functions well enough to care for her neonate, implement a thorough plan for teaching child care tasks, taking into account her best learning method. Keep the teaching environment free from distractions, and ask the patient to give return demonstrations of skills taught. Use an appropriate teaching pace, and repeat teaching points as necessary.

Be sure to identify support resources and incorporate them into discharge planning. If the patient lacks adequate support, help her make contact with a local support group, such as a parenting group. Refer her to a community health nurse or visiting nurse for follow-up assessment of her daily living skills.

Physically disabled patient

Before making multiple referrals, assess what facilities and support people the patient has available to her to make her role as a caregiver easier. Many parents with physical disabilities are quite creative when performing caregiving tasks. Base interventions on the patient's particular strengths and weaknesses. For example, a patient with psychomotor dysfunction may require referral to an occupational therapist, adaptation of the home environment, and an assistant caregiver until a comfortable and safe caregiving routine has been established.

individual and group teaching. Keep in mind that creative teaching strategies make learning more enjoyable. Always summarize important points in writing, perhaps listing them in a pamphlet that the patient can take home to review.

Individual teaching allows the nurse to interact with the patient on a one-to-one basis and may allow the patient to be more open with information and questions. Group teaching offers the advantage to the nurse of being able to teach more patients at once, thereby decreasing the need for the same information to be taught multiple times. A group also encourages patients to share their experiences and knowledge with other mothers, which can be an invaluable way to learn. Different patients have different learning styles and needs; it is up to the nurse to work with mothers to determine what is best for individual situations.

Postpartal examination. Make sure the patient knows that she must visit the nurse-midwife or doctor 4 to 6 weeks after delivery for the postpartal examination. Provide a written reminder to reinforce this information. Also review danger signs the patient should watch for after discharge. (See *Self-care after discharge*, pages 420 and 421.) Most facilities have printed postpartal instructions and danger signs for each

Self-care after discharge

As you recover from delivery and welcome a new child into your life, you may experience dramatic physical and emotional changes. The guidelines below will help ensure your well-being during this challenging period and help you understand what to look for and when to contact your doctor or nurse-midwife. Remember that these are just guidelines, and if you are unsure about something regarding your physical or emotional status, you should contact your health care provider.

Postpartal warning signs
If you have any of the following problems after discharge, notify your doctor or nurse-midwife promptly:
• heavy vaginal bleeding or passage of clots or tissue fragments; foul-smelling vaginal discharge
• a fever of 100.2° F or higher for 24 hours or longer with or without chills
• a red, warm, painful area in either breast
• excessive breast tenderness not relieved by a support bra, pain pills, or warm or cool compresses
• pain on urination or voiding of only small amounts of urine
• a warm, red, tender area on either leg, especially the calf, possibly accompanied by pain on walking or with flexion of the feet
• a feeling of extreme sadness, depression, or inability to get out of bed in the morning.

Hygiene, rest, and nutrition
During your recovery, take the following measures to maintain adequate hygiene, rest, and nutrition:
• When using a sanitary belt and perineal pad, change the pad every 4 hours. To prevent contamination from fecal organisms, apply and remove the pad from front to back. Do not use tampons until after your 6-week postpartum checkup.
• Before emptying your bladder or moving your bowels, remove the perineal pad. Afterward, use a perineal squirt or spray bottle to cleanse the perineum. Wipe or pat the area gently with toilet tissue, again moving from front to back; then, apply a fresh pad.
• After urinating or moving your bowels, wipe from front to back, then wash your hands thoroughly to prevent fecal contamination of the vagina, perineum, and urethra.
• Take a shower or bath daily.

HOME CARE

Self-care after discharge *(continued)*

- Engage in sexual intercourse if it is comfortable. Discuss contraception with your health provider to avoid unwanted pregnancy.
- Rest frequently during the day, especially if you must awaken during the night to care for your infant.
- Consume a nourishing diet—at least 2,200 calories daily or 2,500 calories if you are breast-feeding. Include foods from all four food groups. If you have trouble moving your bowels, add high-fiber foods (such as fresh fruits and vegetables, bran, and prunes) to your diet.

patient to take home with her. Make sure that these are in her preferred language and that she is able to read and understand them. Advise her to call the nurse-midwife or doctor if any danger signs arise.

Breast care. Regardless of the infant feeding method the mother is using, teach her to inspect her breasts daily, using a circular palpation pattern. This also is a good time to stress the importance of the monthly breast self-examination.

With the bottle-feeding mother, who must suppress lactation, inform her that she may notice an occasional release of milk and may experience some breast fullness and discomfort until milk production ceases. Instruct her to drink adequate, but not excessive, amounts of fluids. For severe breast discomfort, recommend a mild analgesic.

Rest and sleep requirements. Advise the patient to anticipate increased sleep and rest requirements after discharge. Also counsel her to have realistic expectations of herself, her neonate, and her family. Some patients assume that they will be able to resume their usual schedule immediately, preparing all meals or returning to full-time work at home or at the office. Such expectations may prevent satisfactory adjustment to the new role. Consequently, recommend that the patient limit her activities to caring for herself and the neonate for the first week after discharge, then increase other activities gradually over the following weeks.

If the patient has limited support and must be self-sufficient after discharge, help her set priorities and reasonable goals so that she can get adequate rest. Also urge her to ask a friend or relative to help during the first week or two at home if possible. Such a person could assist with laundry, shopping, cooking, and care of older children.

Resumption of sexual activity. If the patient does not ask when she can resume sexual intercourse, provide an opening, for instance, by saying, "Many patients are not sure when they can safely resume sexual intercourse and have questions about birth control." Inform her that she should consult her nurse-midwife or doctor. If her postpartal recovery is satisfactory, the nurse-midwife or doctor probably will inform her that she may resume sexual intercourse. However, advise her that intercourse must be gentle at first because the vaginal and perineal areas may remain tender. Also, she may need to use a lubricant because postpartal hormonal changes may cause vaginal dryness.

Caution her that she can become pregnant during the postpartal period—whether or not she is breast-feeding. Identify her need for family planning information by determining how she and her partner would feel about another pregnancy occurring so soon after this one. Based on her teaching needs, review family planning methods and refer her for appropriate follow-up resources.

Postpartal exercises. Provide the patient with teaching materials on exercises. Show her how to do the exercises that she can do at this time. Explain to her the need to gradually increase her exercise. Also inform her that after the postpartal examination, the nurse-midwife or doctor may approve more vigorous exercise, such as paced walking, swimming, and low-impact aerobics. If appropriate, recommend a community exercise program supervised by an experienced teacher.

For the patient with especially poor abdominal tone, institute a teaching plan focusing on improving body tone before discharge or refer her to a postpartal exercise program.

Community resources. Despite the advantages of early discharge—lower health care facility costs, reduced exposure to pathogens, and enhanced parent-infant bonding—the practice has some drawbacks. Home visits to patients who were discharged early have uncovered breast-feeding problems, transitory depression, fatigue, neonatal icterus, and poor parent-infant bonding. To help prevent or minimize such problems, inform the patient about community resources that can help her and her partner make a more satisfactory adjustment to parenthood. In many regions, community health nurses make home visits to provide guidance, support, and counseling as well as assess the health of the mother and neonate. The nurse also may offer information and support through follow-up telephone calls.

Preparing the patient for discharge

When the patient is ready for discharge, make sure she has sufficient supplies, such as perineal pads, a 24-hour supply of infant formula if necessary, and satisfactory clothing for the neonate. If the family is having financial problems, refer them to a social worker, who may be able to provide some of these items.

If the family plans to go home by automobile, make sure an infant car seat or restraint is available; in most states, such a seat is required by law. Some states and facilities offer a program whereby the patient can borrow or rent (at a nominal fee) a car seat as long as she needs it for her infant. Inform the parents that studies show that an adult's lap is not a safe place for the neonate to ride. In fact, a neonate held on the lap may suffer fatal injury in an accident.

Evaluation

The following examples illustrate appropriate evaluation statements for the postpartal patient:

- The patient maintained vital signs within a normal range.
- The patient's uterus remained firm and the fundus descended 1 cm toward the symphysis each day.
- The patient had a normal lochial flow with no large clots, tissue fragments, or membranes or foul odor.
- The patient demonstrated adequate healing of the episiotomy with no exudate.
- The patient ambulated within 2 hours of vaginal delivery.
- The patient showed positive interaction with the neonate.
- The patient knows how to care for her perineum.
- The patient can determine whether her lochial flow is normal.
- The patient can state danger signs to stay alert for after discharge.
- The patient can state when to return to her nurse-midwife or doctor for the postpartal examination.
- The patient had early contact with the neonate and showed positive bonding behaviors, such as fondling, kissing, and cuddling.
- The patient expressed an understanding of the best times to interact with the neonate.
- The patient has responded appropriately to neonatal communication cues.
- The patient showed increasing proficiency and confidence in caregiving skills.

18 POSTPARTAL COMPLICATIONS

The immediate postpartal period is a time of significant physiologic and psychological stress. Fatigue caused by labor, blood loss during delivery, and other conditions brought on by childbirth can cause complications—some of them critical—in the postpartal patient. Prevention of such complications is a major focus of nursing care. Once a complication occurs, of course, the nurse must work to promote the patient's recovery and ensure that the problem does not jeopardize the developing mother-neonate relationship.

PUERPERAL INFECTION

Puerperal infection—an infection of the genital tract occurring during the postpartal period—was once a leading cause of childbearing-associated morbidity and mortality throughout the world. However, recent studies show a 4% to 8% incidence of maternal mortality from infection in the U.S.

Labor and delivery reduce resistance to infection from bacteria normally found in or on the body. Puerperal infections generally result from such bacteria as beta-hemolytic streptococci, staphylococci, and coliform and various other organisms. It is imperative that the nurse understand the possibility of death from these infections. The nurse must also know that prevention, including good hand-washing techniques and patient teaching, can significantly reduce the incidence of puerperal infections. Sterile technique should also be used as indicated. Furthermore the nurse must be acquainted with the signs and symptoms of these infections in order to notify the doctor or nurse-midwife early in the process so that action may be taken in a timely manner. (See *Risk factors for puerperal infection*.)

The duration of labor, rupture of membranes, number of vaginal exams, and amount of intrauterine manipulations are all directly proportional to the incidence of infection. Thus, the health care team

Risk factors for puerperal infection

The nurse should stay alert for signs and symptoms of infection in a postpartal patient with any of the risk factors below.

Prenatal risk factors
- Anemia
- History of venous thrombosis
- Lack of prenatal care
- Poor nutrition
- History of untreated vaginal or cervical infection or sexually transmitted disease

Intrapartal risk factors
- Cesarean delivery
- Chorioamnionitis
- Episiotomy; perineal or vaginal lacerations
- Forceps delivery
- Prolonged rupture of membranes
- Numerous vaginal examinations during labor, especially with ruptured membranes
- Intrauterine fetal monitoring
- Improper perineal care or breaks in aseptic technique

Postpartal risk factors
- Inadequate infection control
- Postpartal hemorrhage
- Retained placental fragments
- Inadequate hand-washing technique

must be vigilant about good hand-washing and aseptic technique when in contact with a patient in the labor, delivery, and postpartal periods.

Types of puerperal infection

A puerperal infection develops at one site (or lesion) or its extension. With a local lesion, the infection remains within the original infection site. The vagina, the cervix, a hematoma, an episiotomy, and any laceration of the vulva, vagina, or perineum are potential entry points for pathogenic organisms. An incision also may be the source of infection; the mortality rate from puerperal infection is much higher after cesarean than after vaginal delivery. Many studies have demonstrated that socioeconomic status and the use or nonuse of antibiotics have significant effects on the numbers of maternal deaths from puerperal infections.

Extension of the original lesion occurs when a localized infection spreads to other areas via the blood or lymphatic vessels, leading to such infections as salpingitis, parametritis, peritonitis, or thrombophlebitis.

Localized wound infections

A localized infection may arise from a repaired external or internal wound. With infection of an external wound, such as an episiotomy, the apposing wound edges become edematous and separate; the wound then exudes purulent and possibly sanguineous discharge. An internal wound, such as a vaginal laceration, may become infected directly or by extension from the perineum. In this case, the vaginal mucosa becomes edematous and red; necrosis and sloughing follow. Cervical infection, which typically develops from a cervical laceration, may serve as the origin for a more distant infection.

Endometritis

After placental delivery, the placental attachment site is less than 2 mm thick, contains many small openings, and is infiltrated with blood, making it highly vulnerable to bacterial penetration. The remaining decidua also is susceptible to bacteria. Endometritis, the resulting infection, may involve the entire mucosa and sometimes impedes uterine involution.

Salpingitis

Commonly caused by gonorrheal organisms, this infection develops from bacterial spread into the lumen of the fallopian tubes. It usually manifests during the second week postpartum.

Parametritis

This infection, also called pelvic cellulitis, involves the retroperitoneal fibroareolar pelvic connective tissue; severe cases may involve connective tissue of all pelvic structures. Transmission may occur via lymphatic vessels from an infected cervical laceration or from a uterine incision or laceration. In some cases, however, parametritis represents ascent of an infection that began in a cervical laceration.

Peritonitis

This infection of the peritoneum develops in the same manner as parametritis. Generalized peritonitis poses a grave threat; bowel loops may become bound together by purulent exudate and abscesses may develop in various pelvic sites causing decreased peristaltic activity and potential bowel blockage.

Thrombophlebitis

This venous inflammation occurs when a puerperal infection spreads through veins. In thrombophlebitis, a thrombus or clot forms and attaches to the vessel wall. The condition is known as pelvic thrombophlebitis when it involves the uterine and ovarian veins, and it is called femoral thrombophlebitis when it involves the femoral, popliteal, or saphenous veins. (See "Vascular complications" for more information on thrombophlebitis.)

Bacteremic (septic) shock

Parametritis, peritonitis, or thrombophlebitis may lead to systemic infection of the bloodstream, resulting in bacteremic shock, most frequently stemming from gram-negative organisms. In this condition, vascular resistance decreases, causing a severe blood pressure decline and the threat of imminent death.

In toxic shock syndrome (TSS), a form of bacteremic shock, *Staphylococcus aureus* enters the bloodstream through microulcerations, or small abrasions, in the vaginal or cervical mucosa. Because vaginal and cervical lacerations are common during vaginal delivery, the postpartal patient is at increased risk for developing TSS.

Assessment

Review the patient's history for risk factors. Because puerperal infection is associated with temperature elevation, obtain vital signs regularly. Suspect an infection if the patient has a morbid temperature, defined by the Joint Committee on Maternal Welfare as one that exceeds 100.4° F (38° C) on any 2 days after delivery, excluding the first 24 hours, to be taken orally at least 4 times daily. However, be aware that a low-grade fever is common during the first 24 hours after delivery; it is often due to dehydration.

Be sure to note any complaints of chills, malaise, or generalized pain or discomfort because these are common signs and symptoms of infection. Assess uterine tone and fundal height, and evaluate lochial discharge, noting the amount, color, consistency, and odor. Also obtain information about the patient's sleep and rest patterns and hydration and nutritional status.

Laboratory analysis should be documented. If infection is present, analysis typically reveals an elevated white blood cell count and an increased erythrocyte sedimentation rate. Blood and vaginal cultures may be analyzed to isolate the causative organism; however, isolation typically proves difficult because a blood or vaginal culture may become contaminated.

Localized wound infection

Inspect for localized areas of edema, erythema, and tenderness; purulent drainage; gaping of wound edges; and dysuria. Stay alert for complaints of pain in a specific area. Lochial evaluation can be important;

in a localized episiotomy infection, for instance, lochia may have a foul odor and appear yellow. Note the color, amount, consistency, and odor of the lochia.

Endometritis

Check for a fever (which may range from low-grade to 103° F [39.4° C]), malaise, lethargy, anorexia, chills, a rapid pulse, lower abdominal pain or uterine tenderness, and severe afterpains. Lochia may range from normal to foul-smelling, scant or profuse, and bloody to serosanguineous and brown.

Salpingitis

Signs and symptoms of salpingitis include fever with chills, elevated erythrocyte sedimentation rate, and the simultaneous presence of lower abdominal pain with or without rebound tenderness, cervical motion tenderness, and adnexal tenderness. The presence of vaginal discharge is not generally considered in diagnosing salpingitis.

Parametritis

Besides the signs and symptoms seen in endometritis, this condition may cause a prolonged, sustained fever and tenderness on one or both sides of the abdomen.

Peritonitis

The clinical picture presented by peritonitis also resembles that of endometritis. Other possible findings include vomiting, diarrhea, anxiety, tachycardia, shallow respirations, and bowel distention. Also check for abdominal guarding, rigidity, and rebound tenderness.

Thrombophlebitis

Assess for tenderness, warmth, and redness in a portion of the vein. Try to elicit Homans' sign. Assess for low-grade fever, and a slight increase in the pulse. (See "Vascular complications.")

Bacteremic shock

In the patient who has a suspected or diagnosed infection, stay alert for signs of fever, confusion, nausea, chills, vomiting, and hyperventilation. In early shock, arterial blood gas (ABG) measurements typically reflect respiratory alkalosis. Later, the patient becomes apprehensive, restless, irritable, thirsty, flushed, tachycardiac, tachypneic, hypothermic, and anuric. ABG findings may show a progression to metabolic acidosis with hypoxemia.

Besides ABG analysis, the doctor will order various studies to verify the diagnosis and guide intervention—hematologic tests, leukocyte analysis, creatinine and blood urea nitrogen tests, central venous pressure, pulmonary artery and wedge pressures, and hemodynamic values.

Nursing diagnosis

After gathering all of the assessment data, the nurse must review it carefully to identify pertinent nursing diagnoses for the patient. (See Appendix 1, NANDA taxonomy of nursing diagnoses.)

Planning and implementation

For the patient with a nursing diagnosis of *risk for infection related to broken skin or traumatized tissue,* prevention is the best intervention. Careful aseptic technique, especially thorough hand washing, is crucial. Any change in the patient's status should be reported and documented.

To prevent cross-contamination among patients, make sure the patient has her own sanitary supplies and that nondisposable items are cleaned after each use. Monitor the patient for changes in vital signs. Instruct her on good hand-washing technique. Also teach the patient techniques that help prevent the spread of infection. To prevent contamination of the vagina with rectal bacteria, instruct her to use a front-to-back motion when applying perineal pads and when cleansing the vulvar and perineal area. Note the percentage of perineal pad saturation and time required for saturation. Also note the appearance of the affected area, if applicable.

For the patient with a diagnosed infection, expect to administer antimicrobial and antipyretic therapy. The doctor or nurse-midwife will choose an antibiotic based on the location and severity of the infection, the causative organism, and the patient's physiologic status. They usually take an aggressive treatment approach, choosing a broad-spectrum antibiotic. Many patients require a combination of oral and I.V. antibiotics.

The doctor also may order analgesics to help relieve general malaise, headache, and backache. For a localized wound infection, the doctor may incise the infected area or remove sutures to promote drainage.

Independent nursing actions for the patient with a puerperal infection focus on alleviating signs and symptoms and helping to meet the patient's psychosocial needs. Thus, be prepared to carry out comfort measures, ensure adequate rest, and provide a relaxed, quiet environment to counter malaise. To promote healing, provide sitz baths as prescribed. Teach the patient how to clean and change the dressing over the infected area and how to remove and apply perineal pads properly. Also, make sure the patient's fluid intake is 2 qt (2 L) per day.

Allow the mother and neonate to spend as much time together as possible. If the patient has a nursing diagnosis of *knowledge deficit related to the etiology and treatment of the postpartal complication,* teach her and her family about her condition and treatment, and provide emotional support and encouragement. Encourage them to express their feelings to help them work through anxiety and discouragement.

Evaluation

During this step of the nursing process, the nurse assesses the effectiveness of the plan of care by evaluating subjective and objective criteria. Evaluation findings consist of actions performed or outcomes achieved for each goal. The following examples illustrate appropriate evaluation statements for the patient with a postpartal complication:

- The patient's verbal and nonverbal behavior reflected an increased comfort level.
- The patient's vital signs improved or remained within normal limits.
- The patient exhibited adequate wound healing.
- The patient was able to interact with her neonate.
- The patient demonstrated how to perform perineal hygiene and uses good hand-washing techniques.

For the patient with a puerperal infection, these additional evaluation statements may be appropriate:

- The patient's temperature is normal and drainage is no longer purulent.
- The patient expressed an understanding of infection control measures.

POSTPARTAL HEMORRHAGE

Postpartal hemorrhage occurs when a patient loses more than 500 ml of blood during or after the third stage of labor. Blood loss commonly is underestimated at the time of delivery because precise measurement is difficult; actual loss usually is twice that of estimated loss.

Postpartal hemorrhage may occur early or late. Early postpartal hemorrhage arises within 24 hours after delivery. Late (or delayed) hemorrhage develops 2 days to 6 weeks postpartum.

Potential sequelae of postpartal hemorrhage include transfusion reactions, hepatitis, and renal failure from prolonged hypotension. Rarely, patients who recover from severe postpartal hemorrhage suffer anterior pituitary gland necrosis or Sheehan's syndrome.

Causes

Any condition that results in trauma during childbirth can lead to postpartal hemorrhage. The most common causes are uterine atony; lacerations of the vagina, cervix, perineum, or labia; and retained placental fragments.

Uterine atony

This condition may stem from uterine over-enlargement caused by hydramnios, multiple gestation, or delivery of a very large neonate. As the uterus enlarges, its muscle fibers become overstretched and cannot contract effectively to compress vessels; thus the uterus continues to bleed, setting the stage for hemorrhage.

Other causes of uterine atony include a prolonged or accelerated labor, general anesthesia, or administration of magnesium sulfate. Also, a patient with a history of postpartal hemorrhage has an increased risk for uterine atony.

Lacerations

Laceration of the vagina, cervix, perineum, or labia provides a potential hemorrhage site. A cervical laceration is particularly likely to hemorrhage because of increased cervical vascularity during pregnancy and immediately after delivery. Perineal and vaginal lacerations also may contribute to postpartal blood loss. However, these wounds are more likely to cause long-term damage by weakening the perineal muscles, which may necessitate later surgery.

Retained placental fragments

Retained placental fragments, the major cause of late postpartal hemorrhage, sometimes adhere to the uterus and cause hemorrhage by impeding uterine contractility. In cases with a retained placenta, the entire placenta remains in the uterus at least 30 minutes after the second stage of labor.

Other causes

Postpartal hemorrhage also may result from various other conditions.

Hematoma. This collection of extravasated blood forms when blood escapes into the connective tissue beneath the skin of the external genitalia (vulvar hematoma) or beneath the vaginal mucosa (vaginal hematoma).

Episiotomy dehiscence. An episiotomy may dehisce in response to such factors as pressure caused by a vaginal hematoma. Also, a patient who is obese or who has diabetes mellitus is more susceptible to episiotomy dehiscence because these conditions impair healing.

Uterine inversion. Hemorrhage immediately follows this condition, in which the uterus is turned inside out.

Uterine subinvolution. Uterine atony, retained placental fragments, or postpartal endometritis may cause this condition, in which the uterus fails to return to a nonpregnant size and condition after delivery.

Assessment

This condition can progress to shock, so be sure to assess the patient carefully and thoroughly. Because hemorrhage usually can be predicted, review the patient's history for such predisposing conditions as a prolonged labor or prenatal anemia. (See *Predisposing factors for postpartal hemorrhage.*) If possible, quantify blood loss, keeping in mind that a loss exceeding 500 ml is ominous.

Early postpartal hemorrhage may manifest either as a large gush or as a slow, steady trickle of blood from the vagina. Even a seemingly innocuous trickle may lead to significant blood loss, which becomes increasingly life-threatening.

Late postpartal hemorrhage usually has a sudden onset; shock may ensue rapidly. When this occurs, immediate intervention is crucial to prevent cardiac arrest and death. Because late postpartal hemorrhage typically occurs after discharge and without warning, it can be especially dangerous to the unsuspecting woman.

Predisposing factors for postpartal hemorrhage

To anticipate the possibility of postpartal hemorrhage, the nurse should review the patient's chart for the following predisposing factors:
- cesarean delivery
- forceps or mid-forceps rotation at delivery
- hematoma
- history of postpartal hemorrhage and uterine atony
- intrauterine manipulation
- lacerations of the birth canal
- manual removal of the placenta
- multiparity
- overdistention of the uterus (as with a large neonate, multiple gestation, polyhydramnios)
- oxytocin augmentation or induction
- pregnancy-induced hypertension
- magnesium sulfate use during labor
- premature placental separation
- prenatal anemia
- prolonged labor
- rapid labor or precipitous delivery
- retained placental fragments
- uterine inversion
- uterine subinvolution.

To detect trends that may reveal deteriorating status in a patient with significant blood loss, measure vital signs regularly and assess skin turgor and color. A serious hemorrhage may cause the skin to turn pale and clammy. It also may trigger chills, visual disturbances, and a rapid, thready pulse. However, keep in mind that pulse and blood pressure may not change significantly until the patient loses more than 10% of her blood volume. At this point, compensatory mechanisms triggered by hemorrhage fail and shock ensues; signs and symptoms then vary according to the stage of shock.

Determining the cause of hemorrhage

In a patient with excessive vaginal bleeding, try to determine the cause to help guide intervention. For instance, assess uterine tone; a firmly contracted fundus rules out uterine atony and suggests an unrepaired cervical laceration as the cause of bleeding. (See *Postpartal hemorrhage*, page 399.)

If the patient has severe perineal pain with sensitive ecchymosis, suspect vulvar hematoma as the cause of hemorrhage. A vaginal hematoma, on the other hand, manifests as severe rectal pain and pressure and inability to void. Be aware that a vaginal hematoma is more difficult to visualize than a vulvar hematoma.

To assess for episiotomy dehiscence, another possible cause of hemorrhage, carefully inspect the area surrounding the episiotomy sutures and assess general perineal healing at least three times daily. Pain, a gaping suture line, and a reddened, edematous episiotomy suggest dehiscence.

Signs and symptoms of uterine subinvolution include a large, noncontracted uterus positioned above the umbilicus, prolonged lochial discharge, backache, and a heavy sensation in the pelvis.

Nursing diagnosis

See Appendix 1, NANDA taxonomy of nursing diagnoses.

Planning and implementation

Early identification and prompt, aggressive intervention are necessary to avert grave consequences of hemorrhage. As with puerperal infection, prevention is the best defense.

Prevention strategies. Prevention of hemorrhage hinges on averting or treating underlying causes. To detect retained placental fragments, the nurse-midwife or doctor will inspect the delivered placenta for completeness; missing pieces warrant uterine exploration.

After placental separation, the doctor or nurse-midwife may order an oxytocic drug to prevent uterine atony. When administering an oxytocic drug, monitor vital signs and uterine contractions every

15 minutes. Gently massage the uterus to help stimulate uterine contractions. If oxytocic therapy and uterine massage fail to stimulate contractions, expect surgical exploration and evacuation of the uterus.

To prevent hemorrhage from a deep cervical laceration, immediate suturing is necessary. However, perfect repair is difficult, and suturing sometimes causes further complications such as cervical eversion and exposure of the endocervical glands.

Blood loss from a hematoma commonly is underestimated, so be prepared for the possibility of hemorrhage in the patient with a vulvar or vaginal hematoma. Small hematomas, however, usually reabsorb naturally. To prevent serious blood loss from a hematoma, the doctor may incise and evacuate, or drain, the hematoma. Because incision and evacuation may cause infection, be sure to practice aseptic technique and teach the patient how to perform perineal hygiene, especially if she has a nursing diagnosis of **knowledge deficit related to aseptic technique and perineal hygiene.** Expect antibiotic therapy to be ordered. The doctor will incise and drain the area to prevent serious hemorrhage from episiotomy dehiscence. If dehiscence results from an infection, the doctor will order antibiotic therapy. Aseptic technique, frequent perineal pad changes, and careful hygiene are critical in the treatment of dehiscence.

If the patient has suffered uterine inversion, immediate manual replacement—and perhaps blood or surgical replacement—are needed to save her life.

To avert hemorrhage from uterine subinvolution, the doctor may prescribe oxytocic agents to stimulate uterine contraction or increase uterine tone. Curettage may be performed to remove retained placental tissue. Because breast-feeding stimulates uterine contractions, encourage the patient to begin or continue breast-feeding if she has chosen this feeding method.

General interventions. When caring for the patient with postpartal hemorrhage, be sure to conduct frequent, careful observations to detect status changes early. Closely monitor the following:

- vital signs, including central venous pressure (CVP) measurements
- fundal status, the amount and frequency of uterine massage administered, and any blood clots expressed
- number and weight of perineal pads used, the percentage of pad saturation, and the time required to saturate the pad
- amount, color, consistency, and odor of lochia
- fluid intake and urine output of at least 30 ml/hour, monitoring frequently according to facility protocol.

Check the patient's level of consciousness frequently and report any changes to the doctor or nurse-midwife. Be sure to maintain fluid replacement carefully because the patient will have a nursing diagnosis of **fluid volume deficit related to active postpartal hemorrhage.** When

administering oxytocic therapy, check I.V. lines for patency, and document the effectiveness of therapy. Also document CVP recordings and perform CVP maintenance as necessary. As prescribed, type and cross-match blood in anticipation of transfusion or surgery. Because this patient has a nursing diagnosis of *altered peripheral tissue perfusion related to hypovolemia,* be prepared to carry out the following measures:
- Increase the existing I.V. infusion rate or start an I.V. drip to boost circulating blood volume, as prescribed.
- Assist with insertion of a CVP catheter as needed.
- Administer an I.V. oxytocic agent as prescribed and evaluate effectiveness of oxytocic therapy.
- Give supplemental oxygen at 6 L/minute, as prescribed.
- Insert a urinary catheter, as prescribed.
- Lower the head of the bed (generally to Trendelenburg's position) and place the patient in a supine position.
- Monitor the patient's vital signs, urine output, blood loss, and general condition.
- Massage the fundus gently but firmly.
- Draw blood for a complete blood count; type and crossmatch the patient's blood for possible transfusion, as prescribed.
- Monitor vital signs every 5 to 15 minutes.
- Provide simple, appropriate explanations to the patient to allay her anxiety.
- Keep a count of perineal pads applied, and document the percentage of saturation and saturation time.

Evaluation

The nurse assesses the effectiveness of the care through ongoing evaluation of subjective and objective criteria. For the patient with postpartal hemorrhage, these evaluation statements may be appropriate:
- The patient's uterine tone improved.
- The patient's lochial flow decreased to within normal limits.
- The patient's vital signs are within normal limits.

BIRTH CANAL INJURIES

Many patients suffer lacerations of the vagina and cervix during childbirth. Also, labor and delivery normally cause changes in the position of pelvic structures.

Types of birth canal injuries

Birth canal injuries include vaginal and perineal lacerations, cervical lacerations, levator ani injuries, pelvic joint injuries, pelvic relaxation, and fistula.

Vaginal and perineal lacerations

Lacerations of the anterior vagina near the urethra are relatively common intrapartal events. Typically, these injuries are accompanied by perineal lacerations; a deep perineal laceration may involve the anal sphincter and extend through the vaginal walls. Lacerations of the middle and upper thirds of the vagina, less common than anterior lacerations, usually result from forceps delivery and may lead to copious blood loss.

Cervical lacerations

Cervical lacerations up to 2 cm long are common during childbirth. Normally, they heal uneventfully within 6 to 12 weeks and cause no further problems; however, the external os remains elongated permanently.

Deep cervical lacerations, an occasional result of precipitous labor, may lead to serious hemorrhage because of increased vascularity of the cervix and fragility of surrounding tissues. The tear may involve one or both sides of the cervix, possibly reaching up to or beyond the vaginal junction.

Levator ani injuries

The levator ani is one of a pair of muscles that lies across the pubic arch and pelvic diaphragm, supporting the perineal floor. Injury to this muscle results from overdistention of the birth canal; this, in turn, may cause muscle fibers to separate or decrease in tone. As a result, the pelvis becomes relaxed; urinary incontinence may develop if the pubococcygeal muscle is involved.

Pelvic joint injury

Pelvic immobility and subsequent joint injury may occur if the patient's legs are positioned improperly during delivery or if she remains in stirrups for a prolonged period.

Pelvic relaxation

Exaggeration of the normal relaxation of pelvic support structures during childbirth may cause displacement of the uterus and other pelvic structures. Uterine prolapse occurs in varying degrees. In mild prolapse, the cervix descends below its normal position in the vaginal canal; in moderate prolapse, the cervix reaches the introitus; in severe prolapse, the entire uterus protrudes from the vagina.

Enterocele (prolapse of the intestine into the posterior vaginal wall), cystocele (prolapse of the bladder into the anterior vaginal wall), and urethrocele (prolapse of the urethra into the anterior vaginal wall) sometimes accompany uterine prolapse. The combination of marked cystocele and uterine prolapse may cause obstruction of the lower ureter, with resulting hydronephrosis and renal dysfunction.

Fistula

A fistula, or abnormal passage, may follow a traumatic delivery and be vesicovaginal or rectovaginal. A vesicovaginal fistula is an opening between the vagina and the urinary tract; urine passes involuntarily into and discharges from the vagina. A rectovaginal fistula is an opening between the rectum and vagina; flatus and stool may be involuntarily discharged through the vagina. This type of fistula usually forms after unsuccessful repair of an episiotomy or laceration. Although a portion of the anal sphincter heals after repair, the area above the sphincter may break down.

Assessment

Injury to the birth canal may cause a wide range of signs and symptoms. These problems must be detected promptly to prevent further complications. Review the patient's history, especially the intrapartal records, for risk factors, including:

- prolonged labor with protracted descent
- delivery of a large neonate
- abnormal fetal presentation
- cesarean, forceps, version, or vacuum extraction delivery
- previous history of cesarean delivery, traumatic delivery, uterine surgery, or postpartal hemorrhage
- uterine retroversion or anomaly.

Other key factors to assess for include the amount and color of vaginal bleeding, level of consciousness, subjective expressions of well-being, vital sign measurements and patterns, and fundal height and tone. Stay alert for signs of impending shock.

Vaginal and perineal lacerations

An extensive perineal laceration usually is apparent; this wound may bleed and interfere with normal voiding. A vaginal laceration may bleed and is visible on pelvic examination. The Redness, Edema, Ecchymosis, Discharge, Approximation (REEDA) scale may be used to assess the condition of the perineum. This scale, which provides a means for objective assessment, evaluates the five components of healing, as its name suggests. The total score may range from 1 to 15; the higher the total, the worse the condition of the perineum. Daily documentation allows tracking of the healing.

Cervical lacerations

Signs and symptoms of a deep cervical laceration include bright red (arterial) vaginal bleeding with a firmly contracted uterus. The cervix appears lacerated, edematous, bruised, and ulcerated.

Levator ani injuries

When the patient resumes sexual intercourse, she may report a reduction in pleasure. Urinary incontinence may occur if the pubococcygeal muscle also was involved. If the injury caused weakening of the perineal floor, intercourse may be painful, a condition known as dyspareunia.

Pelvic joint injuries

The most common of all pelvic joint injuries is the separation of the symphysis pubis, although it occurs infrequently. The patient will report hearing a "popping" sound during delivery and severe tenderness of the suprapubic area afterward. She may complain of being unable to have her baby lie on her abdomen because of the pain. Supportive care and teaching regarding the course of recovery are vital nursing roles with this injury.

Pelvic relaxation

Uterine prolapse is visible on vaginal examination. To help determine the degree of prolapse, the examiner may ask the patient to bear down during the examination. Also, the patient may report a sensation of a lump in the vagina during prolonged standing or straining. If the cervix is irritated or eroded from its descent, vaginal discharge may occur. With cystocele and urethrocele, the patient may retain urine, which may lead to frequency and urgency on urination and other signs and symptoms of urinary tract infection.

Pelvic relaxation may cause stress incontinence. Diagnosis of stress incontinence can be made on pelvic examination by manually restoring and maintaining the normal posterior ureterovesical angle to check for deformity reflected by an increased angle.

Fistula

Definitive diagnosis of a fistula is made by the doctor or nurse-midwife during a pelvic examination. The patient may complain of urinary or fecal incontinence or urine and fecal discharge from her vagina, leading to the possible diagnosis of fistula. Referrals should be made accordingly.

Nursing diagnosis

See Appendix 1, NANDA taxonomy of nursing diagnoses.

Planning and implementation

Any birth canal injury may cause fatigue and stress. Therefore, group nursing procedures together to promote sleep and rest. Evaluate fundal height and uterine tone. Also, help the patient participate in her recovery to the extent that she can. To help avoid a nursing diagnosis of *sexual dysfunction related to altered body structure secondary to a birth canal injury,* teach her how to perform Kegel exercises to strengthen pelvic floor muscles.

Depending on their size and location, some perineal and vaginal lacerations heal on their own. For the patient with a nursing diagnosis of *pain related to birth canal injury,* provide pain relief measures and teach her how to manage pain by using sitz baths, topical or oral medications, and distraction. Evaluate the perineal area and note the status of the injury, as well as the patient's complaints.

If the patient has difficulty voiding, insert an indwelling catheter, as prescribed, until healing begins.

An extensive perineal or vaginal laceration that bleeds profusely requires suturing, as does a deep cervical laceration. Because of their location, labial lacerations are difficult to repair and cause much discomfort during healing.

For a levator ani injury, medical and nursing management vary depending on the severity of the injury as well as the emotional impact on the patient and family. In some cases, surgery is necessary; in others, the injury heals spontaneously.

For uterine prolapse, the doctor manually repositions the uterus in the pelvis and may insert a pessary to elevate it and support the ligaments. Usually, the doctor inserts the pessary initially; then the patient removes it before going to bed and reinserts it each morning. Teach the patient how to insert the pessary correctly; teach her to wash it with a mild antiseptic solution and to rinse it thoroughly before each insertion, using clean hands.

For a vesicovaginal fistula, the doctor will attempt surgical repair. After surgery, the bladder must be drained for 10 days via an indwelling catheter. If surgical repair is not possible, the doctor will order continuous bladder drainage because spontaneous closure of the fistula sometimes occurs. For a rectovaginal fistula, management involves surgical repair and antibiotic therapy. Because this patient may have a nursing diagnosis of *body image disturbance related to birth canal injury,* be sure to provide emotional support. Passage of urine or stool through a fistula can make this injury particularly stressful for the patient. Monitor bowel status including the presence or absence of bowel sounds and bowel movements. Be sure to note patient teaching and nursing interventions including the comfort measures used and their effectiveness.

Evaluation

The nurse assesses the effectiveness of the care through ongoing evaluation of subjective and objective criteria. For the patient with a birth canal injury, these evaluation statements may be appropriate:

- The patient demonstrated knowledge of pelvic floor exercises.
- The patient expressed her feelings regarding this complication of birth.

VASCULAR COMPLICATIONS

The postpartal period is marked by a series of complex physiologic adjustments. During this time, the patient continues to be at risk for vascular complications. Prevention or early detection is vital to minimize difficulties during this period.

Types of vascular complications

Vascular complications of the postpartal period include pregnancy-induced hypertension (PIH) and venous thrombosis.

Pregnancy-induced hypertension

PIH refers to hypertensive disorders that develop between the 20th week of pregnancy and the end of the first postpartal week. Preeclampsia refers to hypertension with albuminuria or edema. Eclampsia occurs in a patient who has seizures in addition to preeclampsia, possibly with coma; untreated, eclampsia usually is fatal.

Although the cause of PIH is unknown, inadequate prenatal care may be a contributing factor. Other possible predisposing factors include primigravidity, multiple gestation, preexisting diabetes mellitus or hypertension, and hydramnios. (See *Pathophysiology of pregnancy-induced hypertension,* pages 133 and 134.)

Venous thrombosis

Venous thrombosis is relatively rare. Because early ambulation has become the norm, the frequency of venous thrombosis has decreased dramatically. Predisposing conditions include increased levels of certain blood-clotting factors; greater platelet number and adhesiveness; release of thromboplastin substances from deciduous tissues, placenta, and fetal membranes; and increased fibrinolysis inhibition. Hydramnios, preeclampsia, cesarean delivery, and immobility are additional risk factors.

When venous thrombosis occurs in response to inflammation of the vein wall, it is known as thrombophlebitis. When no inflammation is present, it is called phlebothrombosis. In thrombophlebitis, the thrombus is attached firmly to the vein wall; it is less likely to break away and form a life-threatening pulmonary embolus than in phlebothrombosis, in which the thrombus is attached more loosely.

Typically, thrombophlebitis lasts 4 to 6 weeks, with symptoms subsiding gradually. In severe cases, potentially fatal abscesses develop. Thrombophlebitis is most common in a superficial vein but may develop in a deep leg vein. Typically, superficial thrombophlebitis manifests on the third or fourth postpartal day.

Assessment

Evaluate the patient for evidence of PIH and venous thrombosis.

Pregnancy-induced hypertension

Usually, signs and symptoms of PIH subside rapidly after delivery. However, in the high-risk patient, monitor blood pressure closely during the first 24 hours postpartum. As a rule of thumb, suspect PIH if systolic pressure rises at least 30 mm Hg and diastolic pressure increases at least 15 mm Hg above the baseline value. A persistent diastolic blood pressure of 90 mm Hg is abnormal. Be aware that an increase in blood pressure may signify an impending seizure. With mild preeclampsia, expect generalized edema and proteinuria in addition to hypertension. With severe preeclampsia, blood pressure increases more sharply and the patient typically complains of a severe, persistent headache and visual disturbances. She also may have epigastric pain, hyperreflexia, vomiting, apprehensiveness, photophobia, and sensitivity to noise.

Inspect the patient's hands and feet for edema. Weigh the patient daily to assess fluid retention. Be sure to assess fluid intake and urine output; the latter may drop below 30 ml/hour. Generally, an indwelling catheter is placed for the first 24 hours in the severely preeclamptic patient to accurately measure urine output.

Promptly report urine output below 30 ml/hour, proteinuria, and other suggestive findings to the doctor. In the preeclamptic patient, blood volume may decrease with an accompanying increase in hemoglobin, due to the fluid shift of intravascular fluid to interstitial spaces. Thus, an accurate hemoglobin measurement is important. The doctor usually orders clotting studies to rule out disseminated intravascular coagulation.

Venous thrombosis

Check the patient's history for the following risk factors:

- obesity
- age over 40
- parity greater than three
- previous history of venous thrombosis
- anemia
- heart disease
- venous stasis from prolonged inactivity, such as after anesthesia and surgery.

With superficial thrombophlebitis, the affected vessel feels hard and thready or cordlike and is extremely sensitive to pressure. The surrounding area may be erythematous and feel warm; the entire limb may be pale, cold, and swollen. The patient may have a low-grade fever.

In a woman with suspected deep vein thrombosis (DVT) or one who is at risk for DVT, perform a general assessment, including temperature measurement. Stay alert for complaints of cramping or aching pain in a specific region, especially if that region appears stiff, swollen, and red. Attempt to elicit Homans' sign. However, be aware that a negative Homans' sign does not rule out DVT. Other manifestations of DVT include malaise, edema of the ankle and leg with taut, shiny skin over the edematous area, fever, and chills. Measure leg, calf, and thigh circumferences to document any edema.

When the popliteal vein is involved, expect pain in the popliteal and lateral tibial areas. With anterior and posterior tibial vein involvement, the entire lower leg and foot are painful. Inguinal pain suggests femoral vein involvement; lower abdominal pain, iliofemoral vein involvement.

Pulmonary embolism, a potential complication of venous thrombosis, may manifest as sudden onset of dyspnea accompanied by diaphoresis, pallor, confusion, and a blood pressure decrease. The patient may complain of chest pain accompanied by anxiety, tachycardia, and weakness. If these signs and symptoms occur, notify the doctor immediately. Prompt initiation of therapy improves the chance for recovery.

Nursing diagnosis
See Appendix 1, NANDA taxonomy of nursing diagnoses.

Planning and implementation
Skilled nursing intervention for the postpartal patient with PIH or venous thrombosis can help avert a negative outcome of these complications.

Pregnancy-induced hypertension
Nursing management for preeclampsia and eclampsia focuses on preventing seizures and monitoring signs and symptoms of these disorders. The ultimate goal is to stabilize the patient's status by intervening appropriately, providing optimal environmental conditions, and promoting psychosocial adjustment.

Nursing interventions. If the patient was diagnosed as preeclamptic during pregnancy, the doctor may order I.V. magnesium sulfate postpartally to increase the seizure threshold, provide sedation, and dilate blood vessels. A narcotic also may be prescribed. Immediately report any change in the patient's condition. Weigh the patient daily and monitor fluid intake and output. Note the presence of urinary protein, headache, visual disturbances, or epigastric pain. Also note any signs and the degree of edema, the status of deep tendon reflexes, and the patient's level of consciousness.

Usually, the preeclamptic patient will not receive oxytocic agents postpartally because of their hypertensive qualities; therefore, be sure to massage the uterus frequently to promote uterine contractions. Also encourage frequent voiding to keep the bladder empty and thus help avoid uterine atony.

The eclamptic patient has a nursing diagnosis of *risk for injury related to seizure secondary to eclampsia.* To help ensure the patient's safety in case of a seizure, make sure bed rails are padded, an airway is at the bedside, and emergency equipment is readily available. During a seizure, do not attempt to force open the patient's mouth. Strong muscle contractions prevent the jaws from opening without injury; also, the patient may bite off a portion of any object in her mouth and aspirate it during the seizure. After the seizure is over, move the tongue aside with a tongue depressor and insert an oral airway.

Environmental management. Maintaining an optimal environment is crucial for the patient with PIH. Minimize external stimulation by keeping the room dark and removing the telephone and television; the ring of a telephone or a flickering image on the TV screen may cause a seizure. Keep visitors to a minimum and visits short. Once the patient shows signs of improvement, external stimuli can be reintroduced gradually.

When providing care, be thorough and efficient so as to disturb the patient as little as possible. For instance, group together vital sign checks, hanging of I.V. solutions, dressing changes, pain assessments, and other routine nursing procedures. As soon as the patient's condition improves, extend the time between vital sign checks.

Psychosocial management. The patient who is not critically ill probably will express concern about her own and the neonate's physical safety, leading to a nursing diagnosis of *anxiety related to perceived health status.* Assure her that her condition is not permanent and will reverse. If the neonate is in the neonatal intensive care unit (NICU), encourage her to keep in touch with the NICU staff by telephone. Urge family members to visit the nursery so that they can tell the mother about the neonate. If possible, place a photograph of the neonate at the mother's bedside.

On the other hand, if the patient is too ill or too sedated to inquire about the neonate or even to remember the delivery, suggest that the nurse who attended during labor and delivery talk to her to help her understand the circumstances. The nurse must be available to actively listen to the patient and her family as they voice their concerns and anxieties.

Venous thrombosis

Preventing and detecting pulmonary embolism are the highest priorities when caring for the postpartal patient with venous thrombosis who has a nursing diagnosis of *risk for injury related to dislodgement of a blood clot.* Monitor the patient for dyspnea, a low-grade fever, tachycardia, chest pain, a productive cough, pleural friction rub, and signs of circulatory collapse. As prescribed, administer an anticoagulant, and monitor for therapeutic efficacy and adverse effects of the drug. Observe closely for signs of bleeding, and teach the patient about the drug's purpose, adverse effects, and interactions with any other medications she is receiving. For thrombophlebitis, also expect to administer antibiotics.

Be sure to note assessment findings, interventions, and patient teaching. Do not massage or rub the affected extremity and caution the patient never to do this, especially if she has phlebothrombosis. Because the thrombus is loosely attached to the vessel wall, rubbing can dislodge it, increasing the risk of embolism. Management of the patient with superficial thrombophlebitis typically involves local heat application, elevation of the affected limb, bed rest, analgesics, and use of elastic stockings to help prevent blood from pooling in the legs. If these interventions are ineffective, the doctor may prescribe an anticoagulant. For DVT, treatment typically includes I.V. heparin therapy, bed rest, analgesics, elevation of the affected limb, and elastic stockings.

Once symptoms subside, the patient can resume ambulation gradually. Instruct her to wear elastic support stockings and to perform prescribed leg exercises. Caution her not to stand or sit for long periods and to avoid crossing her legs because this reduces circulation. Make sure she knows how to identify signs and symptoms of thrombus formation, and advise her to call the doctor when they occur. Also teach her how to manage symptoms and relieve pain. For instance, applying warm, moist soaks increases circulation to the affected area and taking analgesics provides pain relief. Throughout her stay in the health care facility, encourage her to visit with the neonate frequently to promote bonding. The nurse should actively listen to the patient and her family regarding their concerns.

Evaluation

The nurse assesses the effectiveness of the plan of care through ongoing evaluation of subjective and objective criteria.

For the patient with PIH, these evaluation statements may be appropriate:

• The patient's blood pressure declined to within normal limits.
• The patient remained free from seizures.
• The patient maintained normal reflexes (2+).
• The patient's edema decreased.
• The patient maintained a urine output greater than 30 ml/hour.

For the patient with venous thrombosis, these evaluation statements may be appropriate:
- The patient's condition remained stable, with no signs of pulmonary embolism.
- The patient walked increasing distances without pain.
- The patient's leg circumference decreased.
- The patient expressed an understanding of the purpose, dosage, and adverse effects of anticoagulant medication and the necessity for continued medical supervision.

OTHER POSTPARTAL COMPLICATIONS

Other complications of the postpartal period include mastitis, urinary tract disorders, diabetes mellitus, substance abuse, and postpartal psychosis.

Causes

These postpartal complications have a variety of causes, depending upon the disorder.

Mastitis

This inflammation of the breast, which occurs in 2% to 3% of breast-feeding women, involves the tissue around the nipple and sometimes the periglandular connective tissue as well. The most common cause is infection by *Staphylococcus aureus* bacteria; other causative organisms include beta-hemolytic streptococci, *Haemophilus influenzae*, *H. parainfluenzae*, *Escherichia coli*, and *Klebsiella pneumoniae*. The pathogenic organism generally, but not always, enters through a crack or abrasion in the nipple. Frequent breast-feeding and position changes of the infant while nursing help prevent mastitis. (See "Ensuring lactation success and milk production" on page 408.)

Urinary tract disorders

Because of normal postpartal diuresis, urine production increases markedly—up to 500 ml to 1,000 ml—in the first 48 hours after delivery. This increase in urine production heightens the risk of urinary tract infection associated with bladder distention and increased exposure to catheterization.

Cystitis. This inflammatory condition of the bladder and ureters may result from retention of stagnant urine in the bladder, catheterization, or bladder trauma during delivery. Usually, the infecting organisms ascend from the urethra to the bladder and can spread to the kidneys.

Pyelonephritis. This diffuse pyogenic inflammation of the pelvis and parenchyma of the kidney occurs when a bladder infection spreads to the ureters and kidneys; it begins in the interstitium and rapidly extends to the tubules, glomeruli, and blood vessels.

Urinary incontinence. Urinary incontinence may result from bladder distention with overflow or from relaxation of the pelvic floor muscles.

Diabetes mellitus

Diabetes mellitus refers to a group of endocrine disorders characterized by impaired carbohydrate metabolism secondary to insufficient insulin secretion or resistance to insulin by target tissue. Because pregnancy alters carbohydrate metabolism and increases the need for insulin, the blood glucose level may be difficult to control during pregnancy. Thus, a pregnant patient with previously stable diabetes may suffer postpartal complications.

In the early postpartal period, the diabetic patient may need little or no exogenous insulin because the rapid postpartal decline in placental hormones and cortisol reduces opposition to insulin. However, as hormone levels begin to stabilize, the need for exogenous insulin increases. Throughout the postpartal period, the insulin dosage must be readjusted to achieve diabetic control in patients with insulin-dependent and noninsulin-dependent diabetes. Patients diagnosed with gestational diabetes usually resume a normal glucose status postpartally.

Substance abuse

In some patients, substance abuse is not detected until the postpartal period, when the neonate shows neurobehavioral abnormalities or other effects of maternal substance abuse. The reason is twofold: Many pregnant substance abusers do not seek prenatal care and, even if signs of substance abuse manifest earlier, the patient may deny her problem because of fear of possible legal and social ramifications.

Postpartal psychiatric disorder

Childbirth can sometimes precipitate a major depressive episode. In many cases, the patient with a major depressive episode must be admitted to a psychiatric hospital for treatment.

Assessment

Assess the patient for evidence of mastitis, urinary tract disorders, diabetes mellitus, substance abuse, and postpartal psychiatric disorder.

Mastitis

Signs and symptoms of mastitis typically do not arise until 2 to 3 weeks after delivery. A portion of the breast is firm, tender, reddened, and warm; axillary lymph nodes may become enlarged. The patient reports chills, malaise, headache, nausea, and aching joints. Typically, the body temperature measures 102° to 104° F (38.8° to 40° C). A culture of breast milk or the neonate's throat will identify the causative organism; elevated leukocyte and bacterial counts indicate infectious mastitis.

Urinary tract disorders

With cystitis, expect urinary urgency and frequency, dysuria, discomfort over the bladder area, hematuria, and a low-grade fever. With pyelonephritis, expect urinary urgency, dysuria, nocturia, cloudy urine, chills, and flank pain accompanied by a temperature of 102° F or higher.

Bladder distention causes a boggy (soft) uterus that is displaced upward and to the right. Bladder distention with overflow is characterized by frequent voiding of small amounts (less than 75 ml per voiding).

Diabetes mellitus

If the patient's history indicates that she has diabetes, be aware that she is at increased risk for developing other postpartal complications, including infection, hemorrhage, hypoglycemia, and hyperglycemia. Also, because of cardiovascular degeneration, the risk of preeclampsia is up to four times greater in diabetic patients than in the general population.

Infection in the diabetic patient typically involves the urinary tract; the vagina is also vulnerable because of altered pH and glycosuria, conditions conducive to bacterial growth. If the patient had a cesarean delivery, monitor her closely for infection at the incision site and the indwelling catheter site. If she delivered vaginally, assess episiotomy healing and evaluate lochia for signs of infection such as foul odor or a yellow or greenish color.

Also assess for signs of hemorrhage; its risk in the diabetic patient stems from her predisposition to hydramnios and fetal macrosomia causing uterine overdistention, which can lead to uterine atony and subsequent postpartal hemorrhage. Hyperglycemia or hypoglycemia may develop as plunging levels of placental hormones alter postpartal glucose metabolism. Psychological stressors, such as strong postpartal emotions and the physical work of labor, contribute to glucose alterations. To detect hyperglycemia, which can lead to diabetic ketoacidosis, assess for thirst, hunger, weight loss, fruity breath, and polyuria. Also check for indications of hypoglycemia—tremulousness, cold sweats, piloerection, hypothermia, and headache. Confusion, hallucinations, bizarre behavior and, ultimately, seizures and coma may occur in late hypoglycemia.

Substance abuse

Because postpartal hospital stays are shorter than ever, remain alert for and report possible signs of substance abuse. These signs fall into three categories: physical, psychosocial, and obstetric.

Physical signs of substance abuse include chronic nasal congestion, dilated pupils, anorexia nervosa, tachycardia, irregular pulse,
needle tracks, and marks on the skin. Physical signs in the neonate
also may suggest substance abuse.

Psychosocial signs of substance abuse include memory loss, frequent mood swings, hostile or violent behavior, low self-esteem, and
a drastic change in financial or social status.

Suggestive obstetric findings include a previous preterm delivery,
history of abruptio placentae, hypertension, precipitous delivery, and
previous delivery of a low-birth-weight neonate.

The substance-dependent patient may develop cardiovascular and
central nervous system complications. Cocaine and certain other vasoconstrictive drugs may cause a transient increase in blood pressure,
which may be mistaken for preeclampsia.

Abusing multiple substances is common and may complicate assessment, hindering anticipation of maternal and neonatal needs. To
help detect any drugs ingested in the previous few hours or days, the
doctor or nurse-midwife may order toxicologic urine and blood screening. When assessing a patient suspected of abusing drugs, try to establish a rapport and convey a caring, nonjudgmental attitude. If she admits to abusing substances, attempt to elicit the following information:

- extent and type of substance abused
- any substance abused by the patient's partner
- previous or current participation in a substance-abuse treatment
program
- degree of a commitment to stop substance abuse.

Postpartal psychiatric disorder

This disorder usually begins within 4 weeks postpartum and presents
with mood lability and delusions generally about the neonate. The occurrence is 1 in 500 to 1,000 and the incidence is increased in patients
with previous mood disorders or a family history of bipolar disorders.
Therefore, a review of the patient's history and her family's history may
help anticipate a problem. In both psychotic and nonpsychotic postpartal depression, signs and symptoms include suicidal ideation, lack of
concentration, psychomotor agitation, and obsessional thoughts regarding violence to the neonate.

Signs and symptoms of postpartal major depressive episode—the
most serious postpartal psychiatric disorder—include depressed mood,
markedly diminished interest or pleasure in activities, significant
weight loss or gain, anxiety, panic attacks, insomnia, psychomotor agitation, fatigue, and crying long past the typical 3 to 7 days postpartum. At least five of these symptoms must be present and at least one
of them must be either depressed mood or loss of interest.

Nursing diagnosis

See Appendix 1, NANDA taxonomy of nursing diagnoses.

Planning and implementation

Nursing care for these widely varying complications depends on the specific disorder. For example, in cases where the patient abuses substances or has postpartal psychosis, a multidisciplinary management approach is particularly important. If the patient suffers from other disorders, such as mastitis, urinary tract disorder, or diabetes mellitus, keys to her recovery include the nurse and the nurse's assessment, planning, and implementation of care.

Mastitis

Because this infection usually manifests after discharge, teach the patient how to prevent and detect mastitis when preparing her for discharge. The first line of defense against mastitis is prevention of cracked nipples. Advise her not to use soap or alcohol to clean the nipples because these substances have a drying effect. Instead, instruct her to use plain water, allow the nipples to air-dry, then apply a breast cream that does not contain lanolin. To avoid undue tension on the tissues, instruct her to remove the neonate from her breast carefully at the end of a feeding session. Mastitis also may result from milk duct blockage and subsequent milk stasis; advise the patient to breast-feed frequently (holding the neonate to her breast in various positions to completely empty each breast) and to call the doctor or nurse-midwife if her breasts become severely engorged.

Treatment for mastitis includes a full course of organism-specific antibiotic, bed rest for at least 48 hours, close monitoring, and patient teaching. (See *Self-care for mastitis*, page 450.)

An untreated breast infection may result in an abscess, necessitating surgery. Even after surgery, however, the patient usually can continue breast-feeding with no ill effects. However, teach or remind her how to place the neonate's mouth carefully on the nipple. If postoperative breast-feeding is contraindicated, advise her to pump her breasts for several days until breast-feeding can be resumed. This may avert a nursing diagnosis of *ineffective breast-feeding related to an interrupted breast-feeding schedule* or *inability to initiate breast-feeding*.

Urinary tract disorders

Expect to administer antimicrobial therapy, provide comfort measures, and apply topical antiseptics. Catheterization may be necessary to prevent urine from accumulating in the bladder. Ensure a fluid intake of more than 3,000 ml/day, and record fluid intake and output. As prescribed, collect urine specimens for culturing.

HOME CARE

Self-care for mastitis

To help ensure a complete recovery from mastitis, follow the guidelines below.
- Breast-feed your infant at least every 2 or 3 hours.
- Immediately before each feeding, apply a warm, wet washcloth to the affected area. Repeat this as often as desired.
- Begin breast-feeding with the affected breast and continue with this breast until it feels completely soft.
- To allow your breast to empty completely, do not wear a brassiere or other restrictive clothing when breast-feeding.
- Breast-feed in different positions during each feeding session to promote full drainage of all milk ducts.
- Gently massage the affected area while you breast-feed. Apply a few drops of breast milk to your nipples and allow them to air-dry after each feeding. Do not use a petroleum jelly product because it causes the skin to dry out.
- Express by hand or pump any milk your infant does not remove from your breast.
- Increase your daily fluid intake by several glasses. Complete the entire course of antibiotics, even if you begin to feel better before the medication is finished.
- Rest as much as possible, and ask your family and friends for help with other children and household chores.
- Contact the doctor or nurse-midwife if your infant develops diarrhea or if you do not feel better after 48 hours of antibiotics and breast-feeding. This may mean that your mastitis medication should be changed.

This teaching aid may be reproduced by office copier for distribution to patients.
© 1998, Springhouse Corporation.

Diabetes mellitus

Caring for the postpartal diabetic patient can be challenging because her blood glucose level may fluctuate widely, causing rapid changes in her exogenous insulin requirement. A multidisciplinary medical management team focuses on returning the patient gradually to her prepregnancy insulin dosage, which may take 48 hours to 1 month postpartum. The postpartal insulin dosage typically is half—or even less—of the prepregnancy dosage.

Nursing care centers on monitoring serial blood glucose measurements and observing for signs of hypoglycemia and hyperglycemia, preventing or controlling complications of diabetes, and teaching the patient about her insulin needs. Monitor for signs or symptoms of preeclampsia, infection, or hemorrhage. Also, ensure proper nutrition and promote mother-infant bonding.

Monitoring blood glucose. Monitor the patient's blood glucose level every 4 hours or more frequently, as needed. Some facilities order a fasting glucose and a 2-hour postprandial test. Instruct her to call for help immediately if she notices signs or symptoms of hypoglycemia or hyperglycemia. If hyperglycemia occurs, monitor urine for ketones every 4 hours. Note any insulin administered.

Preventing or controlling complications. This patient has a nursing diagnosis of **risk for infection related to broken skin, traumatized tissue, and altered blood glucose level.** To help detect infection, monitor the patient's temperature at least every 4 hours for the first 24 hours postpartum, and notify the doctor or nurse-midwife if it reaches 100.4° F (38° C) or more. To prevent hemorrhage, assess uterine tone and fundal height; evaluate lochia amount, color, and odor; check perineal pad saturation; and monitor bladder status. Good perineal hygiene and frequent hand washing are imperative infection control practices.

Maternal teaching. Make sure the patient understands the expected postpartal changes in her dietary and insulin requirements, especially if she has a nursing diagnosis of **knowledge deficit related to dietary and insulin requirements**. Teaching should also include review of a blood glucose monitoring schedule, signs and symptoms to report to a doctor, discussion of exercise, and the need for regular follow-up medical care. Emphasize that she should remain flexible and patient because it may be difficult to achieve postpartal diabetes control, which may cause frustration and anger. Also, stress that she should not consider herself "cured" of diabetes if she is able to go a day or two without insulin and eat a regular diet during the postpartal period. Offer active listening so the patient can voice her concerns and frustrations.

Because insulin does not enter breast milk, the patient can breast-feed if she wishes. However, caution her that the additional 300 to 500 calories/day required to maintain breast-feeding will necessitate insulin adjustments, as may altered postpartal sleeping and eating patterns. Also inform her that the glucose content of breast milk rises along with the maternal blood glucose level.

If the patient had gestational diabetes, advise her to have a follow-up oral glucose tolerance test 6 to 8 weeks postpartum. Inform her that she has an increased risk of developing diabetes mellitus later in life, and advise her to seek prenatal care early if she becomes pregnant again.

Substance abuse

The substance-abusing postpartal patient requires a multidisciplinary treatment approach. Besides the nurse and doctor, a social worker, child protection worker, and community health worker may be involved in her care. Treatment depends on her willingness to admit her problem and comply with a drug treatment program.

The patient may be difficult to care for—irritable, manipulative, angry, defensive, and fearful. If necessary, set limits on acceptable behavior. However, remain nonjudgmental and avoid exacerbating any guilt the patient may feel about her substance abuse, especially if her neonate is congenitally malformed or suffering other effects of maternal substance abuse.

Substance abuse may complicate accurate pain assessment and relief. To be effective, any analgesic administered must be equianalgesic to that of the substances the patient is accustomed to taking. Document the patient's response to prescribed analgesia. Creative nonpharmacologic pain relief methods—such as distraction, music therapy, and biofeedback—may prove challenging. However, having the patient rate her pain on a scale of one to ten may aid efforts to evaluate the effectiveness of pain medication. Also, when possible, group together nursing procedures to decrease stimulation and increase rest for the patient. Be aware, too, that care is more likely to be effective when provided consistently by a familiar staff. Note any signs or symptoms of drug withdrawal or continued drug use during hospitalization.

Keep in mind that a substance-dependent patient will not recover from her addiction during her short postpartal stay. Treatment takes time, and its success depends greatly on the patient's commitment and the treatment approach. The patient who received methadone before delivery should remain on the drug during the postpartal period. To establish trust and prevent drug withdrawal, make sure she receives the correct methadone dosage at the right time.

Note any expressions of the patient's willingness to be treated for substance abuse. For information about community substance abuse treatment programs, call the national drug treatment referral hotline (1-800-662-HELP), or urge the patient to call this number. Provide the patient with the telephone number of a crisis intervention or parent support hotline and arrange for follow-up medical care for both the mother and neonate. This is especially important if she has a nursing diagnosis of *ineffective individual coping related to a deficit in problem-solving skills* or *altered health maintenance related to decreased capacity for deliberative and thoughtful judgment.* Evaluate the mother's interaction with the neonate, the absence or presence of signs of mother-infant bonding, and the extent of her interactions with her partner and the health care team.

Breast-feeding concerns. If the patient expresses a desire to breast-feed, explain to her that the substance or substances she has been using may appear in her breast milk. If she seems likely to continue her substance abuse after discharge, explain the dangers to the neonate of breast-feeding under these conditions.

Legal and ethical considerations. The increasing problem of maternal substance abuse has sparked debate on such issues as the rights of substance-abusing patients and their neonates and the responsibilities of all parties involved in their care.

Most states allow a substance-abusing mother to be discharged from the health care facility with her neonate unless she has previously abused a child or if health care professionals have sufficient reason to believe the neonate is at high risk for neglect or abuse. Early consultation with a social worker can initiate child welfare visits if the neonate is determined to be at high risk for abuse or neglect. A history of substance abuse usually is sufficient documentation to initiate such visits. Assess for other support systems the patient may have.

Postpartal psychiatric disorder

Supportive therapy, such as psychiatric consultation, should begin as early as possible. Some patients require hospitalization and psychotropic drugs or electroconvulsant therapy. The nurse must remember that once a patient has an episode of postpartal depression, there is a 30% to 50% risk of recurrence. Nursing interventions, referrals, and contact with other health practitioners such as a psychiatrist should be made accordingly. Document any treatment plans.

Allow the patient to express her feelings freely and respond in a supportive, empathetic manner. To give her a sense of control, encourage her to participate in her care and the neonate's care as much as possible. Recognize and reinforce all positive parenting behaviors. Evaluate the patient's verbal and nonverbal behavior toward the neonate. Also provide information and teaching, as needed, to the patient's support personnel.

Postpartal mood swings may manifest as maternity blues, as more severe alteration in mood swings, or as a major depressive episode. If the patient's behavior warrants a nursing diagnosis of ***risk for violence: self-directed or directed at others related to postpartal psychiatric disorder,*** notify the doctor at once and, if necessary, initiate appropriate emergency procedures, as specified by facility policy. Make sure the patient remains under observation at all times.

Evaluation

During this step of the nursing process, the nurse assesses the effectiveness of care through ongoing evaluation of subjective and objective criteria. Evaluation findings should be stated in terms of actions performed or outcomes achieved for each goal.

For the patient with diabetes, these evaluation statements may be appropriate:
- The patient's blood glucose level remained within normal limits.
- The patient showed no signs or symptoms of hypoglycemia or hyperglycemia.
- The patient remained free from infection.
- The patient expressed an understanding of the effects of nutrition, rest, and breast-feeding on her insulin requirements.

For the substance-abusing patient, these evaluation statements may be appropriate:
- The patient acknowledges that she has been abusing substances.
- The patient expressed readiness to enter an appropriate treatment program.

For the patient with mastitis, these evaluation statements may be appropriate:
- The patient expressed an understanding of self-care for mastitis.
- The patient's temperature returned to normal.

For the patient with urinary tract disorders, these statements may be appropriate:
- The patient states that she understands the need for increased fluid intake and for completing her entire antibiotic regimen.
- The patient demonstrates good perineal hygiene habits.

For the patient with postpartal psychiatric disorder, these evaluation statements may be appropriate:
- The patient expresses relief at her diagnosis and hospitalization.
- The patient expresses understanding of her need for psychiatric consultation.

19

MATERNAL CARE AT HOME

Increasingly, patients are leaving the health care facility within 2 to 24 hours of delivery with no further contact with a health-care professional for 3 to 6 weeks. This scenario is not always the decision of the doctor or nurse-midwife; it is one made by the insurance companies and health maintenance organizations. Some states are beginning to regulate third-party payers, mandating that they pay for longer hospital stays.

These changes in health care significantly affect the patient, her family, and the health care team. Therefore, it is imperative to prepare the patient and family prenatally and postpartally for her discharge to home. Further, it is of utmost importance for the nurse to be the primary contact for these patients; nursing interventions that are implemented are key to good follow-up care. Thus, nurses now offer continued support for childbearing families in the home.

The challenge for the home care nurse is to ensure continuity of care and maintain a high quality of care while taking advantage of the benefits of the home setting. By allowing a broader perspective for understanding the postpartal family, nursing care in the home enhances family-centered care. Because patients are more relaxed in their own surroundings than in an institutional setting, mutual trust is easier to establish. At home, the nurse can incorporate the realities of the patient's home situation into all aspects of care, making that care holistic and more relevant. For the patient, home care means that daily routines and schedules are dictated not by health care facility policy but by the family's normal activities and requirements. The patient is free to decide on her own visiting hours as well. An added benefit is that nosocomial infections are not acquired in the home.

NURSING STRATEGIES

The key to the success of home health care is close cooperation between health professionals within the health care facility and those providing care at home. The home care nurse should obtain a copy of the discharge plan and review it carefully before the first home visit.

Although most assessment methods and interventions used in the home are similar to those used in the health care facility, home care calls for thorough planning coupled with a flexible, innovative approach. Also, because the nurse is a guest in the patient's home, establishing rapport and showing a regard for family customs and routines take on paramount importance.

Planning ahead

Unavoidable disruptions and distractions add an element of uncertainty to the home visit. Telephone calls and unplanned visits by relatives and friends may cause interruptions; noise made by children, televisions, and stereos may break the concentration needed in a teaching session. However, careful timing of visits can minimize this problem.

Setting specific appointment times and verifying them the day before helps minimize interruptions. Determine whether the patient requested the visit herself or was referred by a third party. If she was referred, find out if she understands the reason for the referral; a patient who does not know why the nurse is there may refuse to share information freely or even to become involved in the process.

Establishing rapport

To provide family-centered care, establish a rapport based on mutual trust. Unlike the health care facility, the home is the family's territory. The family's unwritten rules, not health care facility policy, dictate acceptable behavior. Recognize and respect family beliefs, customs, and routines. In a home where domestic violence is present, it may be difficult for the patient to have a trusting relationship with the nurse. It is imperative that the nurse evaluate and carefully assess each of these situations. Keep in mind that some people are uncomfortable when a stranger comes into the home. To put the patient at ease, begin the first visit by making introductions, then clarify the purpose of the visit and describe the services the nurse can provide.

Maintain a friendly but professional manner and convey a caring attitude; also offer an accurate, complete description of the purpose and nature of home nursing visits.

The informality of a home visit can lead to role confusion. To avoid this problem, keep in mind that the nursing role, unlike friendship, is goal directed; the nurse and patient continually evaluate progress toward goal achievement.

Be sure to consider how the patient's cultural background may be affecting her postpartal recovery and her general lifestyle. Explore the patient's culturally related beliefs about childbirth, postpartal recovery, and child rearing. Keep in mind that for some cultures, routine Western postpartal practices—early ambulation, exercise, showering, and warm sitz baths—may seem incomprehensible or even dangerous. In many cultures and religions there are significant differences and expectations. The nurse will have a much smoother home visit with the patient if this information is gathered before the actual visit. This allows the nurse to research the cultural differences before arriving at the woman's home.

Assessment

For the postpartal patient at home, a complete assessment includes a history, physical examination, psychosocial assessment, evaluation of mother-neonate interaction, and home assessment. However, not all patients may wish to be examined or to answer questions about their personal relationships; thus, the nurse must be sensitive to the patient's right to refuse. (See *Home assessment of the postpartal patient*, page 458.) Assessment in the home has important advantages. If the patient was discharged early, thorough assessment is particularly important to detect postpartal complications. Also, assessment in the home yields in-depth data about the patient's role in her family, her family, lifestyle, beliefs, values, customs, and interests—information available only indirectly in an institutional setting.

If other family members are home during the assessment, the nurse can observe family interactions.

To avoid infringing on the patient's or family's privacy or personal space, use sensitivity, tact, and creativity. Let the patient choose the best time and location for personal discussions and potentially embarrassing assessment procedures, and obtain her verbal permission before beginning the assessment. If other members of the household are within hearing range, maintain confidentiality by conducting the assessment in another part of the home or tactfully asking others to move to another room for a few minutes.

History

The nurse who has had no previous contact with the patient should review the antepartal and intrapartal records carefully.

When reviewing the immediate past pregnancy and delivery, note:
- whether it was a planned or unplanned pregnancy
- the extent of the patient's prenatal care and any problems
- hazardous exposures during pregnancy
- hospital admissions or problems during pregnancy
- labor and delivery course and outcome.

Home assessment of the postpartal patient

Once the patient has delivered her neonate and is discharged from the hospital, the nurse's role changes to meet the needs of the mother and her new infant. As always, the nurse must establish a trusting relationship with the patient and her family and objectively evaluate the entire home situation.

Before the visit, the nurse should review the delivery records and know what her facility requires and recommends. Thereafter, the nurse can customize the standard assessment as appropriate for the patient's situation. Below are the standard areas that need to be evaluated for all postpartal patients.

- Patient's overall mental status: postpartal blues versus postpartal depression, domestic violence indicators, and patient complaints and concerns
- Vital signs: temperature, heart rate, respirations, and blood pressure
- Breasts: lactating or nonlactating, nipple status, engorgement, latching-on success
- Abdomen: status of incision from cesarean delivery, if pertinent
- Fundus: consistency and location, diastasis recti muscle status
- Lochia: type, amount, and odor
- Perineum: intact, tender, edematous, or ecchymotic
- Extremities: edema, deep tendon reflexes, clonus, varicosities
- Self-care: as described by patient
- Baby: alertness, eating patterns, sleep habits, and vital signs
- Patient's follow-up appointments, teaching, and questions
- Other assessments as appropriate to the patient's case

Assess the patient's breast-feeding experience, if relevant, and ask about family planning and contraceptive use. Also question her about her sleeping and eating patterns and comfort level.

Physical examination

To assess the patient's postpartal recovery and help detect or prevent complications, conduct a brief physical examination that focuses on evaluating postpartal recovery. During the examination, teach the patient about postpartal physiologic changes and show her how to assess her progress toward recovery.

Obtain vital signs to rule out infection, hemorrhage, pregnancy-induced hypertension, or other postpartal complications. Conduct a review of body systems to check for expected reversal of the changes that took place during pregnancy. Assess uterine involution (by the 10th day postpartum, it should no longer be palpable as an abdominal organ). Determine whether lochia is progressing through the normal stages and examine the perineum to determine if an episiotomy or laceration is healing properly. Check the breasts for engorgement, lactation stage, and nipple condition.

Psychosocial status

Ideally, obtain a psychosocial history, emphasizing such topics as psychological problems after previous deliveries, the patient's social support systems, and any recent or current family stress. Also assess the patient's economic status, review her work history, and ask about her child care plans. Evaluate for domestic violence indicators. (See Chapter 6, High-risk antepartal patients.) Most postpartal patients express satisfaction and positive feelings; some, though, have ambivalent feelings, which may indicate conflicts that could compromise postpartal adaptation. Assess for other potential signs of poor adaptation, such as disinterest in the neonate, adults, or adult activities; lack of social participation; and social isolation

The postpartal patient may experience mood swings and emotional lability. To check for these problems, ask the patient to describe her moods and feelings; be alert to extremes, such as elation and depression.

Maternity blues, a transient mood alteration, is characterized by sadness, crying episodes, fatigue, and low self-esteem. Usually arising within the first 10 days postpartum, this condition is self-limiting and is experienced by 50% to 80% of postpartal patients.

A more severe alteration in mood swings occurs in approximately 20% of postpartal patients and manifests as tearfulness, despondency, feelings of guilt and inadequacy, and inability to cope with neonatal care. Generalized fatigue and complaints of ill health also are common. Signs and symptoms typically arise within the first 4 weeks of delivery and may last from a few weeks to years.

Major depressive episode, a severe form of depression, occurs in approximately 0.1% of postpartal patients and in many cases requires hospitalization. A patient with a major depressive episode will have at least five of the following symptoms: depressed mood, markedly diminished interest or pleasure in activities, significant weight loss or weight gain, insomnia or hypersomnia, psychomotor agitation, fatigue or loss of energy, feelings of worthlessness, diminished ability to think, and recurrent thoughts of death. At least one of the symptoms of this psychiatric disorder is depressed mood or loss of interest or pleasure. (See *Assessing your patient's psychosocial status*, page 460.)

Mother–infant interaction

In the home, the nurse can observe mother-infant interaction over time and within the natural setting, taking into account the effects of other family members and the home surroundings. An optimal time

HOME CARE

Assessing your patient's psychosocial status

To assess your patient's adaptation to her new role as a mother, begin by asking her open-ended questions that allow her to explore her feelings. Clarify or reword questions if necessary; if the patient won't answer a particular question, go on to the next one. Conduct the assessment in a private area, away from the patient's family members, to make it easier for her to answer your questions. Below are examples of questions to use while evaluating your patient's psychosocial status.

Handling daily responsibilities
- How well are you managing day-to-day activities?
- How is your appetite?
- How do you feel about the amount you are sleeping?
- How effectively do you feel you are managing your responsibilities?

Considering the impact of childbirth
- How do you feel about your childbirth experience?
- How well do you think you dealt with that experience?
- What aspects of the experience are particularly important to you? Why?

Interacting with the infant
- What feelings do you have about being a mother?
- How well do you think you interact with your infant?
- What are you thinking and feeling when you are with your infant?
- Do you have any concerns about your infant's health and safety? How do you handle these concerns?

Resuming social activities
- Have you resumed socializing with other adults?
- Which social interactions have you enjoyed most? Which have you enjoyed least?
- How has your relationship with your infant's father changed?

Evaluating self-esteem
- How well do you feel you are adjusting to your new role as a mother?
- How would you describe your mood these days?
- What are your thoughts about your future?

to observe is during a feeding session, when the mother and infant are most likely to interact closely. The nurse must also be skilled in newborn assessment and care. Sometimes the nurse does a complete follow-up visit of the infant as well as the mother. Teaching the mother how to perform tasks of daily living for herself and her infant and then observing as the patient performs these tasks is an excellent way to evaluate and change nursing interventions as needed.

Home environment
Determine if the home is conducive to safe, adequate care of the mother and neonate and whether it promotes positive psychosocial adaptation. For example, check for safety hazards and availability of basic necessities such as water, electricity, and heat, and determine whether the patient can obtain privacy in the home.

Nursing diagnosis
After gathering all of the assessment data, the nurse must review it carefully to identify pertinent nursing diagnoses for the patient. (See Appendix 1, NANDA taxonomy of nursing diagnoses.)

Planning and implementation
After assessing the patient and formulating nursing diagnoses, the nurse develops and implements a plan of care. Nursing goals for the postpartal patient receiving care at home include promoting postpartal recovery, helping the patient adapt to the maternal role, promoting parenting skills, enhancing the couple's relationship, and helping siblings adapt to the birth of a new family member. Depending on the number of visits the nurse will make, meeting all of these goals may be a challenge. As appropriate, refer the patient to community resources, such as self-help groups or parenting classes.

Promoting postpartal recovery
If assessment reveals postpartal complications or delayed postpartal recovery, intervene as appropriate, referring the patient to a doctor or nurse-midwife as necessary. For example, after inspecting the episiotomy site, the nurse may determine that the patient has a nursing diagnosis of *pain related to the perineal wound.* In this case, recommend a sitz bath three or four times daily, with each bath lasting 15 to 20 minutes. If the patient does not know how to administer this treatment, provide teaching.

Helping the patient adapt to the maternal role
To help avoid a nursing diagnosis of *ineffective individual coping related to adaptation to the maternal role,* use interventions that help

the patient regain control of her life if she has not been able to do so independently.

Offer praise and reassurance for her efforts to fulfill her responsibilities. If she feels overwhelmed by the tasks of her new role as a parent, help her break down large tasks into smaller, more manageable parts. Keep in mind that a new mother needs some mothering herself, so encourage her to nurture and pamper herself, paying attention to her own needs as well as to those of the neonate.

If the patient has a nursing diagnosis of *risk for altered parenting related to postpartal mood swings*, refer her for counseling or therapy. Also, because sleep deprivation may contribute to postpartal mood swings, help her plan ways to get adequate rest. (See *Nursing interventions for postpartal mood swings.*)

For the patient with a nursing diagnosis of *social isolation related to the neonate's constant care demands*, help her develop contacts within the community and refer her to appropriate community resources, such as counseling services, self-help groups, and babysitting services.

Promoting parenting skills

The roles of parents in our society are ever-changing and there are many demands on parents. Further, more mothers are working outside the home and one-parent families are increasing. However, our society fails to adequately prepare adults for the demands of parenting. As a result, the patient or couple may have a nursing diagnosis of *knowledge deficit related to parenting and neonatal care*.

To increase their competence and confidence in caring for the neonate, help the parents by reinforcing discharge teaching of neonatal care-giving skills and providing information about infant growth and development. As appropriate, recommend fourth trimester classes, which offer anticipatory guidance and provide a forum for parents to share their concerns. Also teach the parents about their neonate's capacities and behavioral traits.

Most new parents also benefit from discussing their concerns with other parents such as a parent support group. Besides offering first-hand knowledge and advice from experienced parents, a parent support group helps new parents feel that they are not alone in their concerns and that their child is not the first to behave in unexpected ways.

Enhancing the couple's relationship

The birth of a neonate leads to wide-ranging changes in family dynamics and interrelationships. The nurse who makes home visits can help the family adapt to these changes.

Ask the couple what they each enjoy most about their new role as parents, what they find most difficult about being parents, and how

Nursing interventions for postpartal mood swings

There are four areas of concern for the patient with postpartal mood swings, sometimes described as postpartal blues—the overwhelming nature of neonatal care, the meaning of motherhood, self-concept, and the relationship with her partner. The chart below shows nursing interventions to help the patient deal with each concern. If the patient exhibits signs of postpartal depression, as described in Chapter 18, refer her to her doctor or nurse-midwife immediately.

PATIENT CONCERN	INTERVENTION
Overwhelming nature of neonatal care The time involved in caring for a neonate may seem overwhelming to the new mother. Her concept of herself as a mother may hinge on her ability to feed the neonate and cope with the neonate's crying; when feeding does not go well or the neonate is fretful, she feels she has failed.	• Mobilize the patient's support system. • "Mother" the patient. • Explore child care options. • Refer the patient to a support group. • Teach the patient various approaches to coping with a crying neonate. • Solicit the partner's support. • Advise the patient to sleep when the neonate sleeps. • Instruct the patient to break down large tasks into small, manageable parts. • Give positive reinforcement for a job well done.
Meaning of motherhood For the patient with postpartal mood swings, the romanticized view of motherhood that she may have developed during pregnancy is replaced by feelings of confinement, isolation, and lack of time to herself. She feels overwhelmed by the responsibilities of being a mother 24 hours a day and may feel guilty about neglecting her partner and other children.	• Help the patient grieve over the loss of her fantasies about motherhood. • Encourage the patient to express her anger. • Help the patient make social contacts so that she can share her concerns with other mothers. • Help the patient find time to spend with her other children.

(continued)

Nursing interventions for postpartal mood swings (continued)

PATIENT CONCERN	INTERVENTION
Self-concept After delivery, a patient's self-concept may dramatically change. Disappointment related to the childbirth experience—for instance, an unexpected cesarean delivery—may lead to feelings of failure and guilt. Weight gain and poor muscle tone may cause the patient to feel overweight and unattractive. In some patient, role conflicts lead to resentment and depression. For instance, the patient may resent the neonate for interrupting her career; or, if she is compelled by economic circumstances or peer pressure to return to her job, she may feel guilty about leaving the child with someone else.	• Review the events of childbirth with the patient and help her accept, understand, and integrate the experience. • Provide diet counseling. • Teach the patient how to perform postpartal exercises, such as leg rolls, abdominal breathing, and arm raises, to help her regain her prepregnancy figure and thereby enhance her self-esteem. • Encourage the patient to find time for herself.
Relationship with her partner The birth of a new family member triggers many changes in the couple's relationship. The neonate's constant care demands may restrict the couple's freedom, impose on their privacy, alter their sexual relationship, and result in general lifestyle changes. Also, the patient may have role expectations that her partner cannot—or will not—fulfill.	• Reinforce the strengths of the relationship. • Provide counseling about resumption of sexual intercourse and family planning. • Explore the division of household labor and suggest changes, if necessary. • Encourage the partners to communicate openly.

they expected the neonate's birth to affect their roles and relationships. Also ask how their relationship has changed and how they would like it to be. Point out that changes in a relationship affect both partners; the neonate's father may feel driven to work harder out of a sense of increased responsibility, whereas his partner may want him to help with child care. Each may feel that the other has the easier job. Discussing the division of household labor, as described earlier, may help clarify or resolve inequities in household responsibilities.

The birth of a child usually alters the couple's sexual relationship. Frequency of and desire for sex declines during the postpartal period. However, be aware that the couple may be embarrassed to ask questions about sex. Consequently, approach the topic gently by asking them to describe the changes that have taken place in their relationship, then asking, "And what about sex?" Urge them to share their feelings about sex with each other, emphasizing that many postpartal couples have concerns about sex.

Some patients are reluctant to resume sex out of fear of discomfort, leading to a nursing diagnosis of *altered sexuality patterns related to a painful episiotomy or fear of conception.* If this is the case, point out that intercourse usually can resume once the perineum has healed, bleeding has stopped, and the partners feel ready. However, caution the patient that the first intercourse after childbirth may be somewhat painful because of perineal tenderness or vaginal dryness induced by hormonal changes. Recommend the use of lubricating jelly and positions that do not put pressure on the episiotomy or laceration sites, especially for the first postpartal intercourse. Make sure the patient understands that petroleum jelly is not a lubricant and can cause drying; therefore, it should not be used for vaginal lubrication. If the patient is afraid to resume sex out of fear of conception, provide teaching about family planning. Keep in mind that because oral contraceptives are contraindicated during breast-feeding, the breast-feeding patient who used this contraceptive method before pregnancy may have special teaching needs in the early postpartal weeks. The couple must also understand that they can become pregnant again before the patient has her first period and that there are alternative ways to share intimacy besides sexual intercourse. Education and active listening by the nurse are extremely important at this time.

Helping siblings adapt

Siblings may react to the birth of a neonate with jealousy, anger, and other negative behaviors, which may lead to a nursing diagnosis of *altered family processes related to the birth of a neonate.* The parents must understand that generally there will be some degree of regression in each sibling. Help the parents deal with this problem by advising them to spend time alone with each sibling and to let siblings participate in neonatal care. This intervention will vary based on the individual's age and that person's belief in how the neonate will change the family dynamics.

Evaluation

For postpartal home visits, the nurse makes two types of evaluations. Formative, or ongoing, evaluation takes place at the end of each visit as the nurse reviews mutually set goals and determines whether the patient met the goals. Later, when the nurse and patient decide to discontinue home visits, the nurse conducts summative evaluation.

The following examples illustrate appropriate evaluation statements for the patient receiving nursing care at home:

- The patient's postpartal recovery is progressing normally without complications.
- The patient and her partner show competence and confidence in neonatal care-giving skills.
- The patient shows a positive adaptation to the maternal role.
- Other family members demonstrate a healthy adjustment to the birth of the neonate.

APPENDICES

NANDA TAXONOMY OF NURSING DIAGNOSES

A taxonomy for classifying nursing diagnoses has evolved over several years. The current list is grouped around nine human response patterns endorsed by the North American Nursing Diagnosis Association.

Pattern 1. Exchanging (Mutual giving and receiving)

1.1.2.1	Altered nutrition: More than body requirements
1.1.2.2	Altered nutrition: Less than body requirements
1.1.2.3	Altered nutrition: Risk for more than body requirements
1.2.1.1	Risk for infection
1.2.2.1	Risk for altered body temperature
1.2.2.2	Hypothermia
1.2.2.3	Hyperthermia
1.2.2.4	Ineffective thermoregulation
1.2.3.1	Dysreflexia
1.3.1.1	Constipation
1.3.1.1.1	Perceived constipation
1.3.1.1.2	Colonic constipation
1.3.1.2	Diarrhea
1.3.1.3	Bowel incontinence
1.3.2	Altered urinary elimination
1.3.2.1.1	Stress incontinence
1.3.2.1.2	Reflex incontinence
1.3.2.1.3	Urge incontinence
1.3.2.1.4	Functional incontinence
1.3.2.1.5	Total incontinence
1.3.2.2	Urinary retention
1.4.1.1	Altered (specify type) tissue perfusion (renal, cerebral, cardiopulmonary, gastrointestinal, peripheral)
1.4.1.2.1	Fluid volume excess
1.4.1.2.2.1	Fluid volume deficit
1.4.1.2.2.2	Risk for fluid volume deficit
1.4.2.1	Decreased cardiac output

1.5.1.1	Impaired gas exchange
1.5.1.2	Ineffective airway clearance
1.5.1.3	Ineffective breathing pattern
1.5.1.3.1	Inability to sustain spontaneous ventilation
1.5.1.3.2	Dysfunctional ventilatory weaning response (DVWR)
1.6.1	Risk for injury
1.6.1.1	Risk for suffocation
1.6.1.2	Risk for poisoning
1.6.1.3	Risk for trauma
1.6.1.4	Risk for aspiration
1.6.1.5	Risk for disuse syndrome
1.6.2	Altered protection
1.6.2.1	Impaired tissue integrity
1.6.2.1.1	Altered oral mucous membrane
1.6.2.1.2.1	Impaired skin integrity
1.6.2.1.2.2	Risk for impaired skin integrity
1.7.1	Decreased adaptive capacity: Intracranial
1.8	Energy field disturbance

Pattern 2. Communicating (Sending messages)

2.1.1.1	Impaired verbal communication

Pattern 3. Relating (Establishing bonds)

3.1.1	Impaired social interaction
3.1.2	Social isolation
3.1.3	Risk for loneliness
3.2.1	Altered role performance
3.2.1.1.1	Altered parenting
3.2.1.1.2	Risk for altered parenting
3.2.1.1.2.1	Risk for altered parent, infant, or child attachment
3.2.1.2.1	Sexual dysfunction
3.2.2	Altered family processes
3.2.2.1	Caregiver role strain
3.2.2.2	Risk for caregiver role strain
3.2.2.3.1	Altered family process: Alcoholism
3.2.3.1	Parental role conflict
3.3	Altered sexuality patterns

Pattern 4. Valuing (Assigning relative worth)

4.1.1	Spiritual distress (distress of the human spirit)
4.2	Potential for spiritual well-being

Pattern 5. Choosing (Selecting alternatives)

5.1.1.1	Ineffective individual coping
5.1.1.1.1	Impaired adjustment
5.1.1.1.2	Defensive coping

5.1.1.1.3	Ineffective denial
5.1.2.1.1	Ineffective family coping: Disabling
5.1.2.1.2	Ineffective family coping: Compromised
5.1.2.2	Family coping: Potential for growth
5.1.3.1	Potential for enhanced community coping
5.1.3.2	Ineffective community coping
5.2.1	Ineffective management of therapeutic regimen (individuals)
5.2.1.1	Noncompliance (specify)
5.2.2	Ineffective management of therapeutic regimen: Families
5.2.3	Ineffective management of therapeutic regimen: Community
5.2.4	Effective management of therapeutic regimen: Individual
5.3.1.1	Decisional conflict (specify)
5.4	Health-seeking behaviors (specify)

Pattern 6. Moving (Involving activity)

6.1.1.1	Impaired physical mobility
6.1.1.1.1	Risk for peripheral neurovascular dysfunction
6.1.1.1.2	Risk for perioperative positioning injury
6.1.1.2	Activity intolerance
6.1.1.2.1	Fatigue
6.1.1.3	Risk for activity intolerance
6.2.1	Sleep pattern disturbance
6.3.1.1	Diversional activity deficit
6.4.1.1	Impaired home maintenance management
6.4.2	Altered health maintenance
6.5.1	Feeding self-care deficit
6.5.1.1	Impaired swallowing
6.5.1.2	Ineffective breast-feeding
6.5.1.2.1	Interrupted breast-feeding
6.5.1.3	Effective breast-feeding
6.5.1.4	Ineffective infant feeding pattern
6.5.2	Bathing or hygiene self-care deficit
6.5.3	Dressing or grooming self-care deficit
6.5.4	Toileting self-care deficit
6.6	Altered growth and development
6.7	Relocation stress syndrome
6.8.1	Risk for disorganized infant behavior
6.8.2	Disorganized infant behavior
6.8.3	Potential for enhanced organized infant behavior

Pattern 7. Perceiving (Receiving information)

7.1.1	Body image disturbance
7.1.2	Self-esteem disturbance
7.1.2.1	Chronic low self-esteem
7.1.2.2	Situational low self-esteem
7.1.3	Personal identity disturbance
7.2	Sensory or perceptual alterations (specify visual, auditory, kinesthetic, gustatory, tactile, olfactory)
7.2.1.1	Unilateral neglect
7.3.1	Hopelessness
7.3.2	Powerlessness

Pattern 8. Knowing (Associating meaning with information)

8.1.1	Knowledge deficit (specify)
8.2.1	Impaired environmental interpretation syndrome
8.2.2	Acute confusion
8.2.3	Chronic confusion
8.3	Altered thought processes
8.3.1	Impaired memory

Pattern 9. Feeling (Being subjectively aware of information)

9.1.1	Pain
9.1.1.1	Chronic pain
9.2.1.1	Dysfunctional grieving
9.2.1.2	Anticipatory grieving
9.2.2	Risk for violence: Self-directed or directed at others
9.2.2.1	Risk for self-mutilation
9.2.3	Post-trauma response
9.2.3.1	Rape-trauma syndrome
9.2.3.1.1	Rape-trauma syndrome: Compound reaction
9.2.3.1.2	Rape-trauma syndrome: Silent reaction
9.3.1	Anxiety
9.3.2	Fear

North American Nursing Diagnosis Association. *NANDA Nursing Diagnoses: Definitions and Classification 1997-1998*. Philadelphia: NANDA, 1997.

2

AWHONN STANDARDS FOR THE NURSING CARE OF WOMEN AND NEWBORNS

The Association of Women's Health, Obstetric, and Neonatal Nurses (AWHONN) has issued eight universal standards encompassing the field of nursing care of women and newborns. The first three are the universal standards of nursing practice, health education and counseling, and policies, procedures, and protocols. The remaining five are generic standards that relate to all aspects of nursing. They include professional responsibility and accountability, utilization of nursing personnel, ethics, research, and quality assurance.

Standard I: Nursing practice
Comprehensive nursing care for women and newborns focuses on helping individuals, families, and communities achieve their optimum health potential. This is best achieved within the framework of the nursing process.

Standard II: Health education and counseling
Health education for the individual, family, and community is an integral part of comprehensive nursing care. Such education encourages participation in, and shared responsibility for, health promotion, maintenance, and restoration.

Standard III: Policies, procedures, and protocols
Written policies, procedures, and protocols clarify the scope of nursing practice and delineate the qualifications of personnel authorized to provide care to women and newborns within the health care setting.

Standard IV: Professional responsibility and accountability
Comprehensive nursing care for women and newborns is provided by nurses who are clinically competent and accountable for professional actions and legal responsibilities inherent in the nursing role.

Standard V: Utilization of nursing personnel

Nursing care for women and newborns is conducted in practice settings that have qualified nursing staff in sufficient numbers to meet patient care needs.

Standard VI: Ethics

Ethical principles guide the process of decision making for nurses caring for women and newborns at all times and especially when personal or professional values conflict with those of the patient, family, colleagues, or practice setting.

Standard VII: Research

Nurses caring for women and newborns utilize research findings, conduct nursing research, and evaluate nursing practice to improve the outcomes of patient care.

Standard VIII: Quality assurance

Quality and appropriateness of patient care are evaluated through a planned assessment program using specific, identified clinical indicators.

Source: NAACOG. (1991). *NAACOG Standards for the Nursing Care of Women and Newborns,* 4th ed. Washington, D.C.

3

NUTRITIONAL GUIDELINES AND WEIGHT TABLE

The U.S. government's nutritional guidelines and weight table reflects the use of a health-based definition for desirable weight, a focus on the total diet, and a focus on specific foods in the diet. Modifications in the dietary guidelines address the intake of calories, fat, cholesterol, sodium, complex carbohydrates, and fiber. Excess intake of the first four and insufficient intake of the last two have been linked with obesity, heart disease, high blood pressure, stroke, diabetes, and some forms of carcinomas. Summaries of the specific recommendations follow.

Eat a variety of foods

Because no single food can supply all nutrients in the amounts needed, a nutritious diet must contain a variety of foods. More than 40 nutrients are required to maintain health, including vitamins, minerals, amino acids, certain fatty acids, and sources of calories. To ensure variety, select foods daily from the five major food groups:

- vegetables
- fruits
- breads, cereals, rice, and pasta
- milk, yogurt, and cheese
- meats, poultry, fish, dried beans and peas, eggs, and nuts.

Many pregnant women, women of childbearing age, teenage girls, and young children need an iron supplement. Also, some pregnant or breast-feeding women may need supplements to meet their increased requirements for other nutrients.

Maintain healthful weight

Excess or inadequate weight increases the risk of developing health problems. Excess weight has been linked with hypertension, heart disease, stroke, diabetes mellitus, certain carcinomas, and other problems. Inadequate weight is associated with osteoporosis in women and an increased risk of early death in both sexes.

A healthful weight depends on how much of the weight is fat, where the fat is located, and whether the person has weight-related problems or a family history of such problems. Healthful weight cannot be determined exactly; researchers are trying to develop more precise ways to describe it. However, the following guidelines can help the nurse judge whether a patient's weight is healthy.

- A weight within the range in the table for the patient's age and height. The table allows higher weights for people ages 35 and older compared to younger adults because research suggests that slightly increased weight among older people is not associated with health risks. The weight ranges given here are likely to change based on ongoing research. Also, the table shows weights in ranges because people of the same height with equal amounts of body fat may differ in amount of muscle and bone. The higher weights in each range are suggested for people with more muscle and bone. Weights above the range are unhealthful for most people; weights below the range may be healthful for some small-boned people but have been linked to health problems.
- Body shape. For adults, health depends on body shape as well as height. Research suggests that excess abdominal fat poses a greater health risk than excess fat in the hips and thighs.

To assess body shape, find the waist-to-hip ratio. First, measure around the waist near the navel as the patient stands relaxed. Then measure around the hips, over the buttocks where they are largest. Divide the waist measurement by the hip measurement to find the ratio. A ratio above 1 suggests a greater risk for several diseases.

Choose a diet low in unsaturated fat, saturated fat, and cholesterol

Most health experts recommend that Americans eat less fat both unsaturated and saturated fat and cholesterol. Populations with high-fat diets have more obesity and certain types of carcinomas; high amounts of saturated fat and cholesterol increase the risk of cardiac disease. Also, with a low-fat diet, the variety of foods needed for nutrients can be consumed without exceeding caloric needs because fat contains more than twice the calories of an equal amount of carbohydrates or protein. A diet low in saturated fat and cholesterol can help maintain a desirable blood cholesterol level. (A blood cholesterol level above 200 mg/dl increases the risk of heart disease.)

For adults, dietary fat should account for 30% or less of the total calories needed for healthy weight; saturated fat should provide less than 10% of calories. Because animal products are the source of all dietary cholesterol, eating less fat from animal sources will help lower both saturated fats and cholesterol.

Choose a diet with plenty of vegetables, fruits, and grain products

Americans and other populations with diets low in dietary fiber and complex carbohydrates (such as starch) and high in fat tend to have more heart disease, obesity, and some carcinomas. To help ensure a varied diet, increase dietary fiber and carbohydrate intake, and decrease dietary fat intake, adults should eat at least three servings of vegetables, two servings of fruits, and six servings of grain products daily. Preferably, most dietary fiber should come from foods rather than supplements.

Use sugar in moderation

Sugar and most foods containing large amounts of sugar are high in calories and low in essential nutrients. Therefore, most healthy people should eat these foods in moderation; people with low caloric needs should eat them sparingly. Sugar also contributes to tooth decay.

Use salt and sodium in moderation

Most Americans consume more salt and sodium than they need. In populations with diets low in sodium, hypertension is less common than in the United States. Restriction of dietary salt and sodium may help reduce the risk of hypertension and usually helps decrease blood pressure in people with hypertension.

Drink alcoholic beverages in moderation, if at all

Alcoholic beverages provide calories but little or no nutrients; they are linked to many health problems and accidents and can be addictive. Therefore, they should be consumed in moderation, if at all. The following individuals should not consume any alcoholic beverages:

- pregnant women or women trying to conceive
- people who plan to drive or engage in other activities requiring attention or skill
- people taking medications
- people who cannot limit their alcohol intake.

Weight table

The following table reflects ongoing research, which presently suggests that people can carry somewhat more weight as they age without added health risk. Because people of the same height may differ in muscle and bone makeup, weights are shown across a range for each height.

HEIGHT*	WEIGHT IN POUNDS†	
	Ages 19 to 34	Ages 35 and over
5'0"	97-128	108-138
5'1"	101-132	111-143
5'2"	104-137	115-148
5'3"	107-141	119-152
5'4"	111-146	122-157
5'5"	114-150	126-162
5'6"	118-155	130-167
5'7"	121-160	134-172
5'8"	125-164	138-178
5'9"	129-169	142-183
5'10"	132-174	146-188
5'11"	136-179	151-194
6'0"	140-184	155-199
6'1"	144-189	159-205
6'2"	148-195	164-210
6'3"	152-200	168-216
6'4"	156-205	173-222
6'5"	160-211	177-228
6'6"	164-216	182-234

*without shoes
†without clothes

Source: U.S. Department of Agriculture, U.S. Department of Health and Human Services (1990). *Nutrition and Your Health: Dietary Guidelines for Americans,* 3rd ed. Washington, DC.

4 UNIVERSAL PRECAUTIONS

Universal precautions should be observed in maternity care. The nurse must assume that all human blood and body fluids are infectious for human immunodeficiency virus, hepatitis B virus, and other blood-borne pathogens and are potentially hazardous. Below are examples of universal precautions.

General precautions

- Wash hands with plain soap and water after touching any contaminated items, after removing gloves, or between patients.
- Wear gloves when touching body fluids or contaminated items, changing gloves frequently, and disposing of gloves properly after removal.
- Wear a mask and eye protection to protect eyes, nose, and mouth.
- Wear a gown to protect skin and clothing from contamination.

Patient-care equipment

- Discard all single-use items.
- Ensure that all reusable items are properly cleaned.

Environmental control

- Follow agency procedure for cleaning and disinfecting supplies.
- Wear gloves when disposing of contaminated linen.

Occupational health and bloodborne pathogens

- Never recap needles.
- Use puncture-resistant container for sharps.

REFERENCES

General references
Carpenito, L., *Nursing Diagnosis: Application to Clinical Practice*, 7th ed. Philadelphia: Lippincott-Raven, Publishers, 1997.

DeCherney, A.H., and Pernoll, M.L. *Current Obstetric and Gynecologic Diagnosis and Treatment*, 9th ed. East Norwalk, Conn.: Appleton & Lange, 1997.

Guidelines for Perinatal Care, 4th ed. Washington, D.C.: American Academy of Pediatrics and American College of Obstetricians and Gynecologists, 1997.

Guyton, A. *Textbook of Medical Physiology*, 9th ed. Philadelphia: W.B. Saunders Co., 1995.

NANDA Nursing Diagnoses: Definitions and Classification 1997-1998. Philadelphia: North American Nursing Diagnosis Association, 1997.

Scott, J.R., ed. *Danforth's Handbook of Obstetrics and Gynecology*. Philadelphia: Lippincott-Raven, Publishers, 1996.

Sparks, S., and Taylor, C. *Nursing Diagnosis Reference Manual*, 4th ed. Springhouse, Pa.: Springhouse Corp., 1998.

Unit I: Overview of maternity care
Cunningham, F., et al. *Williams Obstetrics*, 20th ed. East Norwalk, Conn.: Appleton & Lange, 1997.

Kenner, C.A., and MacLaren, A. *Essentials of Maternal and Neonatal Nursing*. Springhouse, Pa.: Springhouse Corp., 1993.

NANDA Nursing Diagnoses: Definitions and Classification 1997-1998. Philadelphia: North American Nursing Diagnosis Association, 1997.

Speroff, L., and Glass, R. Clinical Gynecology, Endocrinology, and Infertility, 2nd ed. Baltimore: Williams & Wilkins, 1994.

Suddarth, D.S. Lippincott Manual of Nursing Practice, 7th ed. Philadelphia: Lippincott-Raven, Publishers, 1996.

UNIT II: Nursing care during the antepartal period

"AIDS and Human Immunodeficiency Virus Infection in the United States: 1996 Update," Centers for Disease Control and Prevention Morbidity and Mortality Weekly Report 38(S4):1-38, 1996.

Barron, W.M., et al., eds. Medical Disorders During Pregnancy, 2nd ed. St. Louis: Mosby–Year Book, Inc., 1995.

Battaglia, F., and Meschia, G. An Introduction to Fetal Physiology. Orlando, Fla.: Academic Press, 1986.

Beischer, N.A., and MacKay, E.V. Obstetrics and the Newborn, 3rd ed. Philadelphia: W.B. Saunders Co., 1997.

Creasy, R.K. "Preterm Labor and Delivery," in Maternal-Fetal Medicine: Principles and Practice, 3rd ed. Edited by Creasy, R.K. and Resnick, R. Philadelphia: W.B. Saunders Co., 1994.

Davis, L. "Daily Fetal Movement Counting: A Valuable Assessment Tool," Journal of Nurse-Midwifery 32(1):11-19, 1987.

Foley, M., and Strong, T. Obstetric Intensive Care: A Practice Manual. Philadelphia: W.B. Saunders Co., 1997.

Hetteberg, C., et al. "Substance Abuse in Perinatal Care," in Nursing Care of Clients with Substance Abuse. Edited by Sullivan, E.J. St. Louis: Mosby–Year Book, Inc., 1995.

Joesoef, M.R., et al. "Intravaginal Clindamycin Treatment for Vaginosis: Effects on Preterm Delivery and Low Birth Weight," American Journal of Obstetrics and Gynecology 1733:1527, 1995.

Kimberlin, D.F., et al. "The Effect of Maternal $MgSO_4$ Treatment on Neonatal Morbidity in <1,000 Gram Neonates," American Journal of Obstetrics and Gynecology 175:382, 1996.

McIntosh, G.C., et al. "Paternal Age and Risk of Birth Defects in Offspring," *Epidemiology* 6:282-87, 1995.

Niswander, K.R. *Manual of Obstetrics*, 5th ed. Philadelphia: Lippincott-Raven, Publishers, 1996.

Papatsonis, D.N.M., et al. "Tocolytic Efficacy of Nifedipine Versus Ritodrine: Results of a Randomized Trial," *American Journal of Obstetrics and Gynecology* 174:306, 1996.

Poole, G.V., et al. "Trauma in Pregnancy: The Role of Interpersonal Violence," *American Journal of Obstetrics and Gynecology* 1174:1873, 1996.

Remington, J.S., and Klein, J.O., eds. *Infectious Diseases of the Fetus and Newborn Infant*, 4th ed. Philadelphia: W.B. Saunders Co., 1995.

Standards for Isolation Precautions: Infectious Disease. Atlanta: Centers for Disease Control and Prevention, 1996.

Sweet, R.S., and Gibbs, R.L. *Infectious Diseases of the Female Genital Tract*, 3rd ed. Baltimore: Williams & Wilkins, 1996.

Varney, H. *Varney's Midwifery*, 3rd ed. Sudbury, Mass.: Bartlett & Jones, 1997.

Watt-Morse, M.L., et al. "Magnesium Sulfate Is a Poor Inhibitor of Oxitocin-Induced Contractility in Pregnant Sheep," *Journal of Maternal/Fetal Medicine* 4:139, 1995.

Worthington-Roberts, B.S., and Rodwell Williams, S. *Nutrition in Pregnancy and Lactation*, 6th ed. Dubuque, Iowa: Brown & Benchmark Publishers, 1997.

UNIT III: Nursing care during the intrapartal period

Apgar, V. "The Newborn (Apgar) Scoring System: Reflections and Advice," *Pediatric Clinics of North America* 13(3):645-50, 1966.

Bobrowski, R.A., and Bottoms, S.F. "Underappreciated Risks of the Elderly Multipara," *American Journal of Obstetrics and Gynecology* 172:1764, 1995.

"Cultural References," Technical Bulletin No. 207, American College of Obstetricians and Gynecologists, July 1995.

Friedman, E. *Labor: Clinical Evaluation and Management,* 2nd ed. East Norwalk, Conn.: Appleton-Century-Crofts, 1978.

Friedman, E. "The Graphic Analysis of Labor," *American Journal of Obstetrics and Gynecology* 68:1568-75, 1954.

Hannah, M.E., et al. "Induction of Labor Compared to Expectant Management for Prelabor Rupture of Membranes at Term," *New England Journal of Medicine* 334:1005-10, 1996.

Hellman, L.H., and Prystowski, H. "The Duration of the Second Stage of Labor," *American Journal of Obstetrics and Gynecology,* 61: 1223-33, 1952.

Johnson, S., and Rosenfeld, J.A. "The Effect of Epidural Anesthesia on the Length of Labor," *The Journal of Family Practice* 40(3):244-47, 1995.

Lubarsky, S.L., et al. "Obstetric Characteristics Among Nulliparas Under Age 15," *Obstetrics and Gynecology* 84:365, 1994.

"Nursing Responsibilities in Implementing Intrapartum Fetal Heart Rate Monitoring," Statement by Association of Women's Health, Obstetric, and Neonatal Nurses, Washington, D.C., 1997.

"Practice Patterns: Monitoring, Interpretation and Management," Technical Bulletin No. 1, American College of Obstetricians and Gynecologists, August 1995.

"State-Specific Pregnancy and Birth Rates Among Teenagers: United States, 1991-1992," *Centers for Disease Control and Prevention Morbidity and Mortality Weekly Report* 44:677, 1995.

"Trends in Sexual Risk Behavior Among High School Students, United States, 1990-1993," *Centers for Disease Control and Prevention Morbidity and Mortality Weekly Report* 44:121, 1995.

UNIT IV: Nursing care during the postpartal period

Brazelton, T.B. *Neonatal Behavioural Assessment Scale*, 3rd ed. Cambridge: Cambridge University Press, 1995.

Briggs, G.B., et al. *Drugs in Pregnancy & Lactation*, 4th ed. Baltimore: Williams & Wilkins, 1998.

DSM-IV Diagnostic and Statistical Manual of Mental Disorders, 4th ed. Washington, D.C.: American Psychiatric Association, 1994.

Scanlan, K.A., ed. *Managed Care*. Washington, D.C.: American College of Nurse-Midwives, 1996.

Sweet, R.L., and Gibbs, R.S. *Infectious Diseases of the Female Reproductive Tract*, 3rd ed. Baltimore: Williams & Wilkins, 1995.

Worthington-Roberts, B.S., and Rodwell Williams, S. *Nutrition in Pregnancy and Lactation*, 6th ed. Dubuque, Iowa: Brown & Benchmark Publishers, 1997.

INDEX

---

i refers to an illustration; t refers to a table.

---

i refers to an illustration; t refers to a table.

i refers to an illustration; t refers to a table.

---

i refers to an illustration; t refers to a table.

---

i refers to an illustration; t refers to a table.

i refers to an illustration; t refers to a table.

i refers to an illustration; t refers to a table.